Praise for *Eat for Energy*

"This book is required reading for anyone who wants a scientific road map out of lethargy and into full vitality. Ari Whitten has been my go-to reference for the true science of the human body for years—there's no one I trust more. No matter what kind of eating approach you currently follow, this book will give you dozens of new nutrition strategies to fully optimize your energy."

— **Susan Peirce Thompson, Ph.D.**, *New York Times* best-selling author of *Bright Line Eating*

"Ari Whitten shows us how to activate our own internal energy powerhouses—the mitochondria—to lose fatigue and gain clarity and energy. Ari's approach is innovative, compassionate, and most of all effective. Whether you're struggling with chronic fatigue, or simply want a bit more energy, I highly recommend *Eat for Energy*."

— **Izabella Wentz, PharmD**, *New York Times* best-selling author of *Hashimoto's Protocol*

"Nutrition is one of the five key foundations for turbocharging your energy production and mitochondrial function. Here is a science-based approach that will expertly guide you on how to do this!"

— **Jacob Teitelbaum, M.D.**, fibromyalgia specialist and author of the best-selling *From Fatigued to Fantastic!*

"If you're ready to have the energy of a child again and want the most cutting-edge methods to make it a reality, *Eat for Energy* will literally have you bouncing off the walls. Read it. Apply it. And reignite the energy stores within you!"

— **John Assaraf**, *New York Times* best-selling co-author of *The Answer* and CEO of NeuroGym

"Packed with practical, evidence-based advice, this book not only helps you understand what is going on in your body but empowers the reader to take what they learned to supercharge their life!"

— **Madiha Saeed, M.D.**, author of *The Holistic Rx* and *The Holistic Rx for Kids*, and creator of *The Holistic Kids' Show* podcast

"Learning how to optimize your child's mitochondrial function through Ari's proven approach will lay the foundations to both prevent and reverse chronic disease no matter what stage of health your child is currently in."

— **Elisa Song, M.D.**, integrative pediatrician and pediatric functional medicine expert, and founder of Healthy Kids Happy Kids

"Ari Whitten has done a masterful job of explaining the mechanisms of energy production and how you can learn to optimize your body's potential. This is a must-read book for anyone suffering from fatigue."

— **Datis Kharrzian, Ph.D., DHSc, DC, M.S., MMMSc, FACN**, Harvard Medical School researcher, Associate Clinical Professor at Loma Linda University School of Medicine

"Ari's book is for everyone who wants to learn and practice the what, when, where, why, and how to nourish oneself for vibrant life energy."

— **Theodore B. Achacoso, M.D.**, founding pioneer of Health Optimization Medicine and Practice Association and European double-board certified in Anti-Aging Medicine and Nutritional Medicine

"In *Eat for Energy*, Ari Whitten looks at almost a thousand scientific papers to provide you with the science behind the relationship between nutrition, mitochondria, and energy."

— **Evan H. Hirsch, M.D.**, chronic fatigue specialist, and author of *Fix Your Fatigue*

"Ari touches on imperative topics that are often overlooked, including skeletal muscle and protein. This book contains easy-to-follow science that can be utilized for daily actions to increase energy and improve body composition."

— **Dr. Gabrielle Lyon**, founder of the Institute for Muscle-Centric Medicine™

"*Eat for Energy* provides a clear blueprint that will take your life up a level and more. It is practical, informative, and easy to read."

— **Michael T. Murray, N.D.**, co-author of *Textbook of Natural Medicine*

"As a scientifically trained college holistic nutrition professor, finding adequate nutrition texts for my students has been impossible . . . until now. With Ari Whitten's long-needed *Eat for Energy*, the nutrition world finally has a text that is rooted in scientific honesty."

— **Lori Valentine Rose, Ph.D.**, CNP, board-certified holistic nutrition consultant, RH (AHG), NBC-HWC, FDN-P, and Hill College life sciences professor

"In a world that is overwhelming us with information, this book distills the most up-to-date and useful scientific data and creates a fully actionable blueprint for people that want to look and feel 20 years younger."

— **Ben Pakulski**, former Mr. Canada, IFBB pro bodybuilder, and founder of Muscle Intelligence and MI40

"In this comprehensive book, Ari walks you through what causes low energy and how to eat and live to increase energy."

— **Rajka Milanovic Galbraith, M.D.**

EAT
FOR
ENERGY

HOW TO BEAT FATIGUE, SUPERCHARGE YOUR MITOCHONDRIA AND UNLOCK ALL-DAY ENERGY

ARI WHITTEN

WITH ALEX LEAF, MS

HAY HOUSE

Carlsbad, California • New York City
London • Sydney • New Delhi

Published in the United Kingdom by:
Hay House UK Ltd, The Sixth Floor, Watson House,
54 Baker Street, London W1U 7BU
Tel: +44 (0)20 3927 7290; Fax: +44 (0)20 3927 7291; www.hayhouse.co.uk

Published in the United States of America by:
Hay House Inc., PO Box 5100, Carlsbad, CA 92018-5100
Tel: (1) 760 431 7695 or (800) 654 5126
Fax: (1) 760 431 6948 or (800) 650 5115; www.hayhouse.com

Published in Australia by:
Hay House Australia Ltd, 18/36 Ralph St, Alexandria NSW 2015
Tel: (61) 2 9669 4299; Fax: (61) 2 9669 4144; www.hayhouse.com.au

Published in India by:
Hay House Publishers India, Muskaan Complex, Plot No.3, B-2,
Vasant Kunj, New Delhi 110 070
Tel: (91) 11 4176 1620; Fax: (91) 11 4176 1630; www.hayhouse.co.in

A catalogue record for this book is available from the British Library.

Tradepaper ISBN: 978-1-78817-682-8
Hardback ISBN: 978-1-4019-6496-2
E-book ISBN: 978-1-4019-6501-3
Audiobook ISBN: 978-1-4019-6502-0

Printed and bound by CPI Group (UK) Ltd, Croydon, CR0 4YY

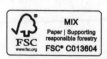

To my wife, Marcela, and my kids,
Mateo and Kaia, who inspire me to create a
more beautiful world for them to live in.

CONTENTS

INTRODUCTION

The Hidden Epidemic

Imagine that every day, for some odd reason, you stabbed yourself in the foot with a fork. Then you went to the hospital and all the doctor did was send you home with painkillers. You're not in pain anymore, but the next day you stab yourself in the foot again, so you go back to the doctor. More painkillers. The next day, the pattern repeats.

The obvious solution is to stop stabbing yourself in the foot rather than use painkillers to suppress the symptom.

It's the same idea with chronic fatigue. Your lack of energy is a symptom of something that is off inside your body, and every day, through the food and lifestyle choices you make, you are stabbing yourself—unintentionally, of course. And rather than simply pushing through the fatigue, or covering it up with stimulants, sugar, or caffeine, the smart solution is to address the underlying factors that control how the human body produces energy.

It isn't your fault that you haven't already been doing that. No one has taught you about the factors controlling human energy levels. No one has shown you the science behind why, and how, to give your body and brain the right nourishment they need. As a result, you're unknowingly making choices that sap you of energy and restrict your cells' ability to properly function. The solution is to learn the science of what controls and regulates your energy levels, so you can stop unknowingly making energy-destroying choices and start doing more of the things that build energy.

Yet, as a culture, we have normalized fatigue.

We think it's normal. Or worse, a badge of honor conferring status, as we even use our level of fatigue and low energy levels to virtue signal to others how important and busy we are. How often do you hear people say, "I'm so exhausted" or "I've just been slammed at work," meaning *I'm so ambitious and I'm such a go-getter, and so important at work that I don't get enough sleep.*

We are exhausted, stressed, burned out, anxious, depressed, and plagued with brain fog, memory loss, and poor concentration. We're constantly borrowing energy from tomorrow to pay for today as we drag ourselves through the day with caffeine, sugar, and stimulants. We have lost the core ingredient necessary to thrive in our relationships, our work, and our lives—energy.

I'm not just talking about people who have been medically diagnosed with chronic fatigue syndrome (or myalgic encephalomyelitis, ME/CFS), the most severe and worst-case scenario that affects about 1.5 percent of the world's population and about 5.4 million adults in the U.S., which is defined as more than six months of severe fatigue, combined with the presence of other symptoms like post-exertional malaise.[1]

I'm talking about the true fatigue epidemic that affects 50 to 100 times more people. In fact, fatigue falls on a spectrum running the gamut from the severe, debilitating ME/CFS to the far more common general state of daily low energy levels and lack of vitality that afflicts a huge percentage of the population.

Just how big a problem are we talking about? Consider this:

- In the National Safety Council's Fatigue in the Workplace report,[2] 76 percent of workers say they feel tired at work, 53 percent feel less productive, 44 percent have trouble focusing, and 27 percent have trouble making decisions because of fatigue.

- Of those who visit doctor's offices, about 40 percent complain of fatigue and one in five have chronic fatigue syndrome.[3]

- In probably the largest study to date, which assessed over 1 million adults, one out of three men and one out of two women report being easily fatigued.[4]

Of course, occasionally feeling a little tired or wanting to lie down and rest after a long day of hard physical and mental work is perfectly normal. But having near-constant low energy levels is most definitely not.

That's your body crying for help.

MY FATIGUE STORY

I've spent more than 20 years helping people fix their health problems using lifestyle, nutrition, and targeted supplements. Not only have I witnessed thousands of clients go from their couch to hiking mountains, but I've experienced the transformation myself.

What first inspired my obsession with the science of optimizing human energy was my own debilitating journey through chronic fatigue that no medical expert—conventional or alternative—was able to help me fix.

Years ago, I was a healthy, active, energetic 24-year-old in a brief stint of living and working on a communal farm in Israel when I contracted the Epstein-Barr virus and came down with a severe case of mononucleosis (also known as "glandular fever" or "the kissing disease"). I had no idea that I would spend nearly a year trying to recover my health, well-being, and energy. I went from loving my full-throttle life to being incapable of getting out of bed. My throat became so sore, swollen, and filled with pus that I couldn't eat anything but soup, and I rapidly lost more than 30 pounds of muscle mass. I lost all endurance and stamina to the point that small activities winded me and lost all my resilience such that I needed to lie in bed for 24 hours after even mild physical activity.

Like anyone, I wanted answers and I wanted to get better, so I went to see doctors—people with M.D.s after their names and years of experience. To my shock, no one knew what was causing my conditions. It took multiple doctors and visits to the emergency room before I was finally diagnosed with the Epstein-Barr virus (EBV). At first, I felt relieved knowing what was wreaking havoc on my health, only to quickly discover that the doctors had virtually nothing to offer—no treatments, no real help for people with mono.

Recovery took months, and I was left with severe fatigue that didn't improve. I felt like my life was passing me by, as I was unable to muster enough energy to engage in physical activities I love, like rock climbing, strength training, and surfing. I didn't have the energy to spend time with friends or to be with my girlfriend, or to have any semblance of a social life. And I was unable to do the physically demanding job I had at the time, working in the farm's fish ponds doing intense manual labor (often in over 100 degree heat). It felt like everything in my life was being taken away from me, because I just didn't have the energy to do it.

Unable to live like this or to wait any longer to regain my life, I turned to the alternative health community for help. Instantly, I was diagnosed with adrenal fatigue, and I finally had hope. I became obsessed with the adrenal fatigue hypothesis—the notion that chronic stress wears out our adrenal glands causing them to be unable to produce enough cortisol (a key stress hormone produced by the adrenal glands), resulting in fatigue and all sorts of other symptoms. I read every book and watched every video on the subject, many created by people I considered mentors and experts in natural health and functional medicine.

I was convinced I had adrenal fatigue and that I had a path to healing, but when I mentioned it to my conventional doctors, they brushed it off, telling me there was no such thing as adrenal fatigue and that it was pseudoscience. This frustrated me. *How could they dismiss this serious condition and have no way of helping people like me?* I was determined to prove the Western medical establishment wrong, so I devoted about a year to combing through and analyzing the full texts of hundreds of published studies, doing nothing day after day but digging through every piece of literature I could find related to fatigue and adrenal function/cortisol, to prove the adrenal fatigue theory.

Except . . . I couldn't prove it. Ultimately, I was beyond frustrated to discover that the body of scientific research on this doesn't support the idea that low cortisol or abnormal adrenal function was to blame for chronic fatigue. The vast majority of studies that tested adrenal function (and cortisol levels) in those with chronic fatigue conditions versus normal healthy people found no differences whatsoever in adrenal function or cortisol levels. Even though I didn't want to admit it, the research was clear that adrenal dysfunction and abnormal cortisol levels were not a valid explanation for chronic fatigue, because they were not even present in the vast majority of people with fatigue.

So there I was, stuck, without so much as a shred of hope that anyone had the answers to my chronic fatigue issues. The conventional medical community had nothing to offer me as I was suffering with fatigue, while most of the alternative/functional medical practitioners were still operating in a paradigm of energy that the science clearly did not support.

It was this moment that I realized: virtually no one in the medical establishment had really solved the human energy puzzle.

This revelation changed the course of my life.

After that point, I became utterly *obsessed* with making sense of the science of human energy. For *years*, I wanted to do nothing more than spend all day, every day digging into the scientific literature and piecing together an actual understanding—a true scientific framework—of the *real* factors that regulate and control human energy levels, why people get fatigued, and, most importantly, how to fix it.

This book is an extension of my decades studying, compiling research, and developing programs and protocols that can help anyone and everyone suffering on the fatigue spectrum regain their energy and life.

WHERE HUMAN ENERGY COMES FROM

Over the last decade, a considerable body of research has been conducted revealing the real cause of fatigue: *mitochondrial dysfunction*.

We have hundreds to thousands of mitochondria inside almost all of the trillions of cells in our body, and they literally produce virtually all the energy that each cell needs to perform its unique function. Mitochondria are often referred to as the "powerhouse of the cell." You can think of them as the battery or energy generators of our cells. When our mitochondria become dysfunctional or, more accurately, when they *turn down energy production* (for reasons we'll discuss in depth), then they cannot produce the energy that our cells need to do their jobs. Heart cells can't effectively pump blood, muscle cells can't effectively move your body, immune cells can't effectively fight infection, gut cells can't effectively digest food, gland cells can't produce hormones optimally, and neurons can't effectively power your brain functions.

This lack of efficient cellular energy production results in *you* feeling the symptom of fatigue, or chronically low energy levels.

The great news is that you can do something about it. In the last decade, science has uncovered critically important facets of how mitochondria function to power our cells, which factors shut down their energy production, and how to optimize them to help them regenerate, grow, and even how to build new mitochondria from scratch—thus allowing you to conquer your fatigue.

Eat for Energy is designed to help you better understand the real science behind your fatigue; the role your mitochondria play in producing and enhancing your energy; how your body works to regulate your energy levels; and how you can use nutritional strategies, targeted foods, and powerful supplements and compounds to supercharge your mitochondria, get rid of your fatigue, and experience all-day energy, every day.

Years ago I joined forces with several top health experts and renowned doctors with a singular goal in mind: to advance our understanding of the causes of fatigue and pioneer new protocols that help people overcome fatigue and live with abundant energy.

After many years of hard work, our team of experts developed a powerful, comprehensive, evidence-based system for energy optimization, *The Energy Blueprint*, which is quickly becoming recognized as the world's top program for people looking to overcome fatigue and increase their energy levels.

Over the last few years, we've reached over 2.5 million people through our free educational articles and podcasts, and over 200,000 people use *The Energy Blueprint* training programs, coaching services, and supplements. Our work provides our clients with hundreds of energy-building strategies and "biohacks," as well as premium energy-enhancing supplements to help them overcome fatigue and get their health, energy, and lives back.

Eat for Energy is the best nutritional wisdom that my team and I have uncovered, systematized, and refined over the last decade with thousands of our clients. In this book, I'll do what I do with all my clients and in all my programs: cut through the pseudoscience to illuminate the real causes of fatigue and how you can rewire your body (and mitochondria) to produce youthful levels of energy once again.

I've divided the book into two parts. Part I explores the real culprit of fatigue—poor mitochondrial function—and how to fix many of the biggest factors that affect our mitochondria, including:

- Circadian rhythm dysregulation and poor sleep
- Carrying too much body fat and too little muscle mass
- Poor gut and microbiome health
- Blood sugar dysregulation
- Nutritional toxicities and deficiencies
- Neurotransmitter and hormone imbalances

In these chapters, I explain the connection between these stressors and how they affect your mitochondria and energy levels, before diving into numerous diet and nutritional strategies you can use to improve the functioning of these systems, your mitochondria, and your energy.

You are not meant to try all the strategies included in a chapter at once. Instead, I recommend picking one strategy in a chapter, mastering that over a couple of weeks (or longer if needed), and then adding another strategy, mastering that, and then another, and so on. This is called *stacking strategies*. It's the slow and steady approach that allows you to really master new ways of eating for energy.

These chapters will give you a holistic understanding of energy and how every organ and system in your body is connected. It's critical to understand that when it comes to fatigue, issues are never localized. It's never just one thing that's wrong. For example, if you have poor gut or microbiome health, that issue doesn't stay in the gut. We now have thousands of studies on the gut-brain axis, the gut-immune axis, and the gut-mitochondria axis. So a problem in the gut will often quickly turn into brain problems, skin problems, immune problems, or energy problems. And this applies across the board to pretty much all systems of the body. Such is the interconnectedness of the systems of the human body.

Fortunately, this also works in the other direction. By optimizing your nutrition, circadian rhythm, sleep, gut health, body composition, brain health, and, in particular, your mitochondrial health, you can cause a cascade of positive effects that spread throughout all the systems of your body. Just as one example, we know that optimizing your circadian rhythm can simultaneously boost your energy levels, improve your brain function, help prevent cancer, improve exercise performance, improve your mood, and help you lose fat—all at the same time. This is how the body works—either our inputs are creating downward spirals of negative effects pulling us toward accelerated aging, disease, and fatigue, or positive upward spirals of disease prevention, youthful vitality, resilience, and energy.

Then in Part II, once you've put together an optimal foundation by getting your diet in order, I share specific foods, supplements, and compounds that you can add to the nutritional strategies outlined in the previous chapters to supercharge your mitochondria and increase your energy levels. So even if you're a health science nerd like me who has already spent 25 years studying natural health, and you're already dialed in on your nutrition and other lifestyle habits (exercise, sleep hygiene, circadian rhythm, stress management, hormesis, etc.), you're still going to get a ton of value in Part II of this book, where you'll get detailed guidance on how to optimize your supplement regimen to build a better brain and higher energy levels.

To be clear, we are not sharing some kind of new hyped-up bizarro diet that we're claiming is the new big thing. We're not sharing any one specific diet at all. We're sharing nutrition principles, strategies, and tactics that can be applied universally and paired with a wide variety of specific dietary choices, from veganism to the Mediterranean diet to paleo to keto. The nutritional strategies in this book are culled almost entirely from controlled interventions in humans and have been scientifically vetted numerous times to support their efficacy. I will be sharing this evidence liberally throughout the book and in the Endnotes because I never want anyone to simply take my word for it.

Most importantly, these powerful, science-based solutions go far beyond the typical advice you will likely get from your doctor or health coach or functional medicine practitioner. When it comes to the health of your mitochondria and overall energy levels, nutrition is arguably the biggest factor in the fatigue epidemic, but if you go to a conventional doctor, they typically won't even ask about your nutrition or consider using it as a tool.

It's also vitally important to know that it's not just an epidemic of fatigue we're dealing with in the Western world. We're also contending with alarming rates of:

- Cancer
- Heart disease
- Neurological diseases like Alzheimer's and Parkinson's

- Diabetes

- Obesity

These are modern lifestyle and civilization diseases, and a whopping 80 percent of the overall disease burden in the United States and throughout the West can be traced to nutrition and lifestyle factors.[5]

With that in mind, you should know that not only will the nutritional strategies in this book help you fix your energy levels but they will significantly reduce your risk for developing dozens of other damaging and deadly chronic diseases. It is not a big leap to say that by getting your nutrition on track, you will likely add years, if not decades, to your life. For many people, it can be the difference between dying from a heart attack at the age of 63 and living relatively healthy to 100 and beyond.

Every day I hear stories from clients who have reached bottom. They have sought help from conventional and alternative medical practitioners, only to be told there was little they could do to fix their energy.

It may sound like I'm trying to bash doctors or that I'm anti-doctors. I'm not. My goal is always to communicate the facts born of the research and studies. And you'd better believe that if I get shot, stabbed, have an acute life-threatening infection, lose a limb, or am faced with several other health scares, I will go to a conventional medical doctor because they do incredible work in these and many other areas.

Unfortunately, when it comes to fatigue and most other "diseases of civilization" caused by nutrition and lifestyle factors (which, again, comprise over 80 percent of the disease burden in the West), with a few exceptions, conventional medicine typically has little to offer.

And when it comes to functional medicine and natural health/wellness practitioners, while many offer us more than the conventional ones, it's hit or miss whether your physician understands the role that mitochondria play in our energy levels.

But fatigue is not a life sentence.

There is a way out.

Eat for Energy is for anyone suffering on the fatigue spectrum, from full blown and debilitating to a more subtle kind that follows you throughout the day. The strategies you are about to learn can help you maximize your physiology—allowing your body and brain to work as they were designed, so you can live at the peak of your energy, brain function, mood, and health.

Many of my clients find that when they implement these strategies, it's not just their energy levels that go up, but other transformative health benefits occur, such as better sleep; fat loss; lower blood pressure; more stable blood sugar levels; better brain functioning, including memory and concentration; and an increased feeling of motivation, happiness, patience, and being able to connect with their friends and family.

Energy matters.

It's time for you to live the life of your choosing.

PART I

RESTORE YOUR ENERGY

CHAPTER 1

MEET YOUR MITOCHONDRIA, YOUR ENERGY GENERATORS AND REGULATORS

When I first met Rea, she appeared to be the picture of health. In her mid-30s, she worked out five times a week, ate a mostly healthy diet rich in whole foods, and limited her sugar and processed carbs. But on the inside, over the last couple of years, her energy levels had steadily plummeted. Every morning, she struggled to get out of bed, despite sleeping for at least seven to eight hours. She didn't "get going" until after her first cup of coffee, and she had to keep guzzling the dark stuff all day. She had been to her primary care physician, but her test results came back normal, and she had spent a small fortune trying different healing modalities, from naturopaths to herbalism, homeopathy to acupuncture, and talk therapy to kinesiology. Nothing worked.

Similarly, my client Neal couldn't shake his anxiety or exhaustion. In his early 50s, Neal shared with me, "My energy levels are so low that I don't want to do anything or be around anyone, not even my wife or kids. I barely sleep four hours at a time, and it's increasingly hard to concentrate at work. Even though I don't want to, I snap at my employees. My anxiety is getting worse, and my doctor wants to increase my medication, but I'm worried.

What if nothing helps? What if I keep getting worse? What if there is no getting better?"

A third client, Jasmine, had strong stomach pains, bloating, irregular bowel movements, and an exhaustion that she could never shake. When we met, she shared pages of test results that doctors had run before diagnosing her with irritable bowel syndrome. She had also seen a naturopathic doctor, who had told Jasmine she had adrenal fatigue. Desperate for relief, Jasmine explained that she had tried hormone replacement therapy and integrated de-stressing activities like deep-breathing exercises and gentle yoga, and she had experimented with taking vitamin C, licorice root, and magnesium supplements. While she had noticed some small improvements with each treatment, nothing lasted. A single mother of two young boys, she tearfully confided, "I can live with the low energy and the stomach issues—I've had those forever—but my mental capacity feels off now, and that scares me because if I can't work or if I lose my job, then I can't provide for my sons."

Three people, all struggling with fatigue and a multitude of other health conditions that no doctor could explain or treat. On the surface, it may appear they had different illnesses, but deep inside their bodies they shared a common cause.

THE CRUX OF CHRONIC FATIGUE

At the most basic, biological level, fatigue is fundamentally an imbalance between energy supply and energy demand. You have chronically low energy levels when your cells do not get the energy supply they need, or the demands on them are too high—or both. This creates an *energy deficit*, which results in the symptom of fatigue.

While there are many contributing factors to this energy deficit, the single most important thing to understand is that the fatigue story centers around your *mitochondria*.

What are our mitochondria? Well, you might remember them from your biology courses in high school or college as the "powerhouse of the cell." Within almost *every* cell of our body, we have between 500 to 2,000 mitochondria whose job is to literally make the energy your cells need to work. Mitochondria take the oxygen you breathe and the food you eat (primarily carbs and fats) to create *adenosine triphosphate (ATP)*, the fuel used to power all cellular and metabolic processes.

Without mitochondria, your cells wouldn't have the ability to create the energy they need to function, meaning no process in the body can happen the way it was designed. It's no stretch to say that without mitochondria there is no life!

Fundamentally, low energy levels are simply the result of a chronic cellular energy deficit. Fatigue is the *symptom* that results when the mitochondria in the trillions of cells that make up your body—your muscles, your hormone-producing glands, your heart, your liver, your brain, etc.—are not producing enough energy to power their functions effectively.

And as we now know through dozens of studies involving people with chronic fatigue or other disease states in which fatigue is commonly present,[1] consistent associations between fatigue syndromes and mitochondrial dysfunction include:

- Deficits in carnitine, which is required to transport fat into mitochondria for use as an energy source

- Deficits in coenzyme Q10 (CoQ10), which is required to produce energy

- Lower concentrations of antioxidants and higher levels of oxidative stress

- Lower rates of ATP (cellular energy) production

- Reduced gene expression in functional pathways for energy production, such as those related to metabolism, protein transport, and mitochondrial morphology

The core idea is that lack of energy at the macro level (you) is caused by lack of energy at the micro level (in the trillions of cells that you are composed of). But the reasons *why* mitochondria fail to produce enough energy—which is critical to understand if you want to increase your energy—is an extremely complex story that has taken researchers decades to piece together, one that we'll unravel in depth in this book.

The vital questions are: What causes our cells to have a deficit of energy? And why do our mitochondria sometimes fail to produce enough of it?

And the answer is: *signals.*

The quality of mitochondria function is determined by the *signals* that your mitochondria are receiving about their environment—from the things you *do* or *don't do*. The signals from your environment are the critical factors that determine whether your mitochondria are performing at 20 percent or 100 percent of their capacity for energy production.

In the longer term, these signals also tell your cells to either increase or decrease the number and size of your mitochondria, which is a process that heavily affects not only your energy levels, but also your resistance to dozens of diseases, which heavily impacts your aging process and longevity.

If you want to beat fatigue and build a high-energy body, the big key is that you want to give your mitochondria the *signals* that allow them to function at as close to 100 percent of their capacity as possible.

SYMPTOMS OF MITOCHONDRIA BEING SHUT DOWN

- ▸ Brain fog
- ▸ Chronic inflammation
- ▸ Poor detoxification
- ▸ Poor stamina
- ▸ Poor mental and physical performance
- ▸ Chronic fatigue

Mitochondrial shutdown is the fundamental reason for chronic low energy levels.

So what are these environmental signals that are dictating how much energy your mitochondria are producing? To answer that, we must now turn to the work of the brilliant Robert Naviaux, M.D., Ph.D., who has been instrumental in advancing our knowledge of the causes of chronic fatigue, most notably the role of mitochondria in our energy levels.

A few years ago, Dr. Naviaux performed a ground-breaking "metabolomics" study where he and his team looked at over 600 metabolites (products of cell metabolism) from 63 biochemical pathways in people with chronic fatigue and found that, compared to healthy adults, a mind-blowing *80 percent of those metabolites were decreased,*[2] meaning that there were widespread systemic changes in metabolic function throughout their organs and cells of their whole body.

Interestingly, Dr. Naviaux described this downregulated metabolic state as chemically similar to a peculiar state of physiology called *dauer*, a state that worms enter as a survival mechanism when they are put in extremely harsh or toxic environmental conditions. These worms essentially shut down their metabolism to survive, keeping all their body's machinery working just enough to stay alive (but not really to function well), with the hope that they can switch on again when in a safer, less toxic environment.

In other words, Dr. Naviaux found that the biochemistry of a person with chronic fatigue suggests that their body is going into a hibernation-like mode and turning down the dial on energy production. Their body is keeping just enough of the machinery on to stay alive and continue functioning, but not enough to actually function with vitality and abundant energy.

The key takeaway:

Fatigue is a type of survival mechanism that switches on in response to signals that you're in a harsh environment.

MITOCHONDRIA AND THEIR DUAL ROLE

While mitochondria have long been known as the powerhouses or energy generators of our cells, they are generally talked about as though they are mindlessly taking the fats and carbs we eat and pumping out cellular energy. In reality, it turns out that they are much more than that.

Dr. Naviaux's work has shown that mitochondria actually have a second, newly discovered and critically important function beyond just their role in generating energy: cell defense.

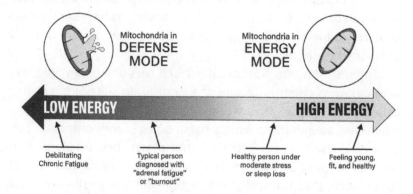

Mitochondria in **DEFENSE MODE** — Mitochondria in **ENERGY MODE**

LOW ENERGY — **HIGH ENERGY**

Debilitating Chronic Fatigue — Typical person diagnosed with "adrenal fatigue" or "burnout" — Healthy person under moderate stress or sleep loss — Feeling young, fit, and healthy

This is a remarkable discovery that has huge implications for our understanding of fatigue.

Dr. Naviaux's recent research has uncovered that our mito-chondria are not just energy generators—they are stress sensors *and* cell defenders. Mitochondria play a central role in protecting our cells from harm by initiating what Dr. Naviaux has termed the *cell danger response* (CDR).[3] In the words of Dr. Naviaux, "The cell danger response (CDR) is the evolutionarily conserved metabolic response that protects cells and hosts from harm. It is triggered by encounters with chemical, physical, or biological threats that exceed the cellular capacity for homeostasis. The resulting meta-bolic mismatch between available resources and functional capac-ity produces a cascade of changes in cellular [function]."[4]

This cascade of cellular changes typically results in symptoms like brain fog, poor mental and physical performance, chronic inflammation, poor detox, and most commonly, *fatigue*. And the newly discovered role of mitochondria in cellular defense actually has an enormous impact. It is, in fact, *the critical factor* in determining the amount of energy they generate. In Dr. Naviaux's words:

> *Mitochondria lie at the hub of the wheel of metabolism, coordinating over 500 different chemical reactions as they monitor and regulate the chemical milieu of the cell. It turns out that when mitochondria detect "danger" to the cell, they shift first into a stress mode, then fight mode that takes most of the energy-producing metabolic functions of mitochondria offline. . . . Energy production and cellular defense are two sides to the same coin. . . . Mitochondria cannot perform both energy and defense functions at 100% capacity at the same time.[5]*

Here is the big key to understanding what controls our energy levels: Our mitochondria perform dual roles—in both energy production and cell defense—and these functions are mutually exclusive. The more your body shifts into defense mode, the more it shifts out of energy mode.

Your mitochondria are exquisitely sensitive environmental sensors that are taking samples and testing your body's status, constantly asking, "Are we in a peaceful and safe environment where we should focus on producing abundant energy, or are we under attack or in a state of stress?"

Think of it like this: Imagine someone threw poisonous gas outside your house. It would be a terrible, lethal mistake to say, "Oh, no big deal, let's just resume function as normal, keep the windows open, and let in the fresh air, and maybe later, we can go for a walk outside." If you kept functioning normally, you'd die. If you want to survive, your immediate reaction needs to be to shut all the doors, close all the windows, and stay inside your house.

And that's exactly what your mitochondria do when they sense a threat.

When mitochondria sense danger, they lock the cells, so that nothing from the outside can get in, and they turn off normal cell functioning (like energy generation). As Dr. Naviaux explained:[6]

> All the air we breathe and all the nutrients we eat and drink are ultimately delivered to mitochondria to help us move, think, work, and play. Mitochondria continuously monitor the chemical environment of the cell and instantly respond to danger by changing their activities from healthy function (producing energy) to cellular defense. When cells go to war, they do what nations do when they go to war. When the CDR is activated, cells harden their borders, don't trust their neighbors, and restrict the exchange of resources with their neighbors.

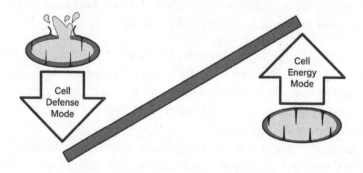

Remember, the more your mitochondria shift into the cell danger response, the more they shift out of energy production mode. And the more your mitochondria operate in cell defense, the worse you will feel.

Keep in mind, this is not black or white, where either you have youthful high energy levels or debilitating chronic fatigue syndrome. This is not an on-off switch—it's a dimmer switch. So the more that mitochondria are getting the right inputs, the more they operate in "peacetime metabolism," where they invest most of their resources into producing abundant energy. And to the extent that they are detecting threats, they pull back energy production and shift most of their efforts to cellular defense, or "wartime metabolism," which causes fatigue, either to a slight or severe degree.

How do mitochondria decide whether to produce lots of energy or shut down energy production? Simple: in response to what kind of environment they perceive themselves to be in.

If all of this seems abstract to you, let me ground this in your own personal experience so it makes more sense. Just think for a moment about the last time you got an infection like a severe flu or cold and felt really sick. What was one of the key symptoms? Probably fatigue.

Remember how your body felt really tired and like you had a lot less energy than you do normally? These are classic signs of your body engaging the cell danger response. The reason why you feel you have less energy is because your body has literally shut down a large portion of your body's energy-producing machinery.

This simple everyday phenomenon is actually the key to understanding fatigue.

In response to stress or danger signals (a harsh environment), the body survives better by lowering the dimmer switch on energy production and shifting resources toward cell defense. Seen in this context, we can quickly realize that fatigue is actually a powerful, adaptive, and intelligent survival mechanism in the context of a harsh environment. It's also an intelligent and adaptive response during times of excessive stress, overexertion, and when energy demands are beyond the body's ability to sustain, because it helps decrease the tendency to continue to overwork oneself, and helps shift bodily resources toward healing, defense, recovery, and cell regeneration.

When you're sick, overly stressed, or in an overexerted and sleep-deprived state, it's not pathological to be fatigued—it's *the natural result* of your body's efforts to shift its focus to healing and regeneration to get itself back to health.

This is fundamentally what fatigue is: your energy declines to the degree that your cells are being forced to defend against threats.

So if you want to know why you're fatigued and how to fix it, here's the key to etch into your mind:

Your energy levels are ultimately a reflection of what kind of environment your mitochondria perceive themselves to be in.

Thus the central goal of overcoming fatigue and getting your energy back is to give your mitochondria the right signals so they feel safe enough to turn energy production back on.

This requires us to first understand and identify the factors in our environment and lifestyle that are sending these signals to our mitochondria, so that we can fix the bad ones and increase the good ones.

> As you go about your daily life, take the time to ask yourself: *Are my mitochondria switched into high-energy mode or cell defense? And will this food choice enhance or deplete my mitochondria and energy levels?* By asking these questions, you will increase your awareness and ability to tune in to your body, which brings you and your actions around food into alignment with what your mitochondria need for your body to thrive.

THE CELL DANGER RESPONSE

Mitochondria are like the canary in the coal mine, as they are extraordinarily sensitive to virtually every type of threat, danger, or biological stressor you can imagine, including:

- Infections caused by viruses and bacteria
- Toxins like heavy metals, pesticides, and thousands of others
- Excess body fat
- Poor gut health like dysbiosis and/or leaky gut
- Physical injury or tissue damage (e.g., sunburns)
- Sleep deprivation and circadian rhythm disruption

- Psychological and emotional stress and trauma
- Nutrient deficiencies
- Overexertion and overexercising
- Poor diet

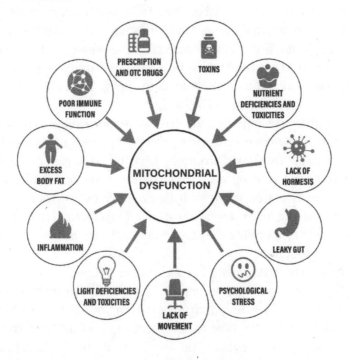

How can mitochondria possibly be able to detect such a wide variety of different types of stressors?

The answer lies in the fact that virtually every type of stressor ultimately converges into just a few cellular mechanisms of harm—mostly inflammation, oxidative stress, and cellular damage. Virtually every type of stressor stresses or damages our cells through one or more of these pathways. For example, poor diet, poor microbiome health, sleep deprivation, overexercising, carrying excess body fat, and being exposed to mercury can all lead to increased levels of inflammation. Inflammatory cytokines, the molecules of inflammation in our body, can be *directly sensed* by mitochondria, which interpret them as a "danger signal."

Oxidative stress is basically the opposite of antioxidants, where oxidants or "free radicals" in the cells increase to excessive levels and cause damage to the cell.

Most biological stressors lead to oxidative stress. This oxidative stress can also be directly sensed by our mitochondria.

When cells are damaged, they leak certain compounds into the bloodstream that act as "danger signals" that can be directly sensed by mitochondria in other cells. The presence of these molecules signals that the body is being stressed or damaged and are what really drive the mitochondria to engage the CDR—to switch out of energy mode into defense mode.

Regardless of whether the stressor is poor diet, exposure to toxins like mercury or arsenic, sleep deprivation, excess body fat, circadian rhythm disruption, high blood sugar, psychological stress, or anything else, these stressors are translated in the body into increased levels of inflammatory cytokines, increased oxidative stress, and markers of cellular damage. In turn, the mitochondria shift more into defense mode and turn down the dial on energy production.

This is the fundamental cause of your fatigue.

To get more energy, you must *decrease* the threats by decreasing the stressors sending danger signals to your mitochondria.

You can take the most expensive drugs and undergo the fanciest medical treatments in the world, but if you don't put in the time and energy to eliminate or significantly reduce the CDR triggers in your environment and lifestyle, your efforts are not likely to get you very far.

NUTRITION TO THE RESCUE

Starting with nutrition and creating new strategies were the foundation I used to help Rea, Neal, and Jasmine overcome their exhaustion. Like I do with all my clients, I encouraged them to focus for four to six weeks on revamping their diets by picking one stressor and beginning the work of eliminating its negative effects. For Rea, we focused on getting her circadian rhythm regulated.

This included having her eat more of her calories earlier in the day, consuming her food within a 10- to 12-hour window, and stopping her caffeine consumption by noon. Within three weeks, Rea noticed she was sleeping for longer periods, fell asleep faster, and felt more energetic.

She then went to work on her brain functioning, adding fish or seafood twice a week to her diet, and incorporating one to two servings of berries and two to four of leafy green vegetables into her daily diet. After another three weeks, Rea reported her sleep had improved further, she could concentrate for longer periods, and her energy was steadily improving.

For Neal, we started with his body composition, working to reduce his body fat and increase his lean muscle mass. Neal had about 80 pounds of fat mass to lose, so we focused on increasing his protein intake, making sure he ate at least 30 grams with every meal and/or snack. And he had to eat two meals per day that were prepared from scratch and/or contained only minimally processed ingredients that he could find in nature.

Initially Neal didn't believe body composition was the solution, but I encouraged him to try eating this way for just two weeks, keeping track of his energy and moods. To his surprise, not only did he lose 10 pounds in those weeks but he also reported feeling less tired, irritable, and anxious. That two-week sprint gave him the confidence to go for another two weeks, using the same strategies and adding another: consuming more fibrous vegetables with one to two meals per day. When we met at the six-week mark, Neal had lost a little over 20 pounds and was feeling better than he had in years. We talked about increasing his protein intake per meal to 35 to 40 grams and gradually adding strategies to improve his sleep, such as closing his window of eating, and increasing meal consistency and decreasing frequency.

As I had with Rea and Neal, I suggested that Jasmine pick the stressor that produced other uncomfortable conditions. For her, that meant focusing on her gut health. Because it had plagued Jasmine for so long, we started by slowly repopulating her gut with natural probiotics that she consumed with one meal per day, and she experimented with the supplement glutamine, taking 15 grams per day. These were the only strategies she used for four weeks. Jasmine reported moderate improvements, so we added more strategies, including consuming cooked and cooled starches at one or more meals per day, and consuming fibrous vegetables with two meals per day.

Jasmine used these strategies for another four weeks. By the two-month mark, she reported more noticeable improvements. It still was not 100 percent, but her energy was headed in the right direction and her gut health and bowel movements seemed to stabilize. Because gut health can take time to fix, she continued working on her gut for another month before we moved on to tackling her next stressor, brain health.

Rea, Neal, and Jasmine all noticed marked improvements simply by working to reduce one stressor at a time and using one or two nutritional strategies for two to four weeks before adding other strategies or moving on to tackle another stressor.

What Rea, Neal, and Jasmine have experienced is what I want for you too.

Thankfully, you can address the most common CDR triggers using nutrition alone.

Every day, what you eat is either an opportunity to nourish your mitochondria or to hurt them, and to give them signals that either sabotage or build your energy levels. Without the right nutritional strategies, you will not have the right foundation to generate the energy you need to live the life of your choosing.

This entire book takes you through the most common CDR triggers and the key nutritional strategies you can use today to enhance your energy.

Circadian dysregulation and sleep disruption, carrying too much body fat and too little muscle mass, poor gut health and dysbiosis and leaky gut, insulin resistance and blood sugar dysregulation, poor neuron functioning, key hormone and neurotransmitter imbalances, and nutrient toxicities and deficiencies are CDR triggers intimately tied to mitochondrial health and energy levels. It is through each of these that your diet can improve your vitality. As we go through each chapter, I'll talk about how different triggers relate to your mitochondria and how you can use nutrition and targeted supplementation to lessen the stressors and to heal and build more and stronger mitochondria.

I want to encourage you to embrace a new perspective on your fatigue. It's easy to feel frustrated with our bodies, to get impatient, and to beat up on ourselves when we lack energy. It's easy to start hating the fatigue and wanting to "fight against it." We tend to harshly judge ourselves—whether it's conscious or not.

Here's the thing: Most of us aren't taught how to optimize our energy. We haven't been taught the factors that go into enhancing our energy levels. Most doctors in the conventional medicine world don't talk about mitochondria, and it's hit or miss in the functional medicine field too.

I invite you to go easy on yourself. Right now, that is all that matters. What you decide to do with the information in this book is what counts.

And that fatigue that's "plagued" you? Instead of hating it, what if you saw it for the amazing survival mechanism that it was designed to be? Because that fatigue is the by-product of your mitochondria working hard to keep your cells and all your organs and muscles *alive* in the midst of a toxic environment that's bursting with threats and stressors. Try thanking and honoring your mitochondria for doing their job, for keeping you safe, for alerting you to the danger that you've been living under.

You can fix the signals.

You can reduce the threats and stressors to the point where your mitochondria deem it's safe to turn on energy production again and dial back the CDR.

You can build and strengthen your mitochondria, and even create more of them from scratch via a process called mitochondrial biogenesis, so that when a threat comes knocking again—because it will—they are strong, resilient, and energetic enough to handle it.

CHAPTER 2

REWIRING YOUR ENERGY CLOCK

Megan fought back tears. She never felt rested, and at 43, she thought she was failing everyone.

"I can't remember the last time I had a good night's sleep," she admitted during our first coaching session. Megan had tried all kinds of sleep hygiene hacks. She used blackout shades on her bedroom windows, diligently shut off screens an hour before bed, and spent 15 to 20 minutes journaling, meditating, or sitting quietly before turning in.

Nothing seemed to work.

Every morning when her alarm buzzed at 5:45 A.M., she had to drag herself from bed having logged maybe five hours of sleep. She didn't have the energy or patience for her three kids. Her brain felt foggy, her memory suffered, and she struggled to stay alert—all problems that made her job as a paralegal more stressful and difficult. Megan also didn't feel connected to her husband, but she didn't have the energy to work on their relationship.

"I feel like there's something deeply wrong with me and that I'll never fix it," Megan said to me.

UNLOCKING THE MYSTERIES OF YOUR CIRCADIAN RHYTHM

In the Western world, especially in the United States, we have a sleep problem.

According to the American Academy of Sleep Medicine and the Sleep Research Society, we need seven to eight hours of sleep per night. Anything less is bad for our health and linked to worse cardiovascular, metabolic, and mental health; decreased immune function and physical performance; and pain. It also increases the risks of dying.[1]

But nearly 30 percent of American adults sleep less than six hours per night.[2] That's over 75 million adults. One in three adults also complain of difficulty falling asleep, difficulty staying asleep, or not getting restorative sleep.[3] Sleeping has become such a challenge that 20 percent of Americans take at least one medication to help them sleep.[4]

It's not that people don't want to sleep; it's that they can't. And the reason is that they suffer from a dysfunction in their biological clocks also known as *circadian rhythm dysregulation*.

Your circadian rhythm is the key to enjoying a healthy and vibrant life. A large and rapidly growing body of research has discovered that the circadian rhythm is a key controller of mood, motivation, body fat, metabolism, hormonal rhythms, neurotransmitter balance, cellular regeneration, sleep quality, and the health of your mitochondria—all of which have a huge impact on your energy.

An optimized circadian rhythm means that you experience:

- Deep and undisturbed sleep (no midnight wakeups or tossing and turning)
- No insomnia
- A quiet and peaceful mind
- Improved mood

- Better brain function, including clarity, focus, and creativity

- Reduced risk of heart disease, diabetes, and cancer

- Bursts of energy and increased levels of energy all day

Many of my clients who live with disrupted circadian rhythms often suffer from other illnesses that make their fatigue worse. Circadian dysregulation is possibly one of the best-researched causes of modern chronic disease, so much so that an international team of researchers has proposed changing the term *metabolic syndrome*—which is a group of conditions including high blood pressure, high blood lipids, high blood sugar, and excess body fat—to *circadian syndrome*.[5]

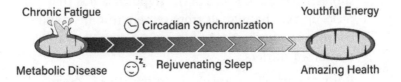

Studies have also revealed that some of the most common health conditions have clear circadian links too, including:

- Obesity[6]

- Type 2 diabetes[7]

- Cardiovascular diseases[8,9]

- Neurodegenerative diseases[10,11]

- Psychiatric disorders[12,13]

- Chronic, low-grade inflammation[14]

- Oxidative stress[15]

- Mitochondrial dysfunction[16]

- Cancer[17]

To understand how your circadian rhythm may have become disrupted, we must go back in time. The world may look vastly different from the one our grandparents and great-great-great grandparents lived in, but one thing has remained constant: every 24 hours, the sun rises and sets.

While modern living may have caused us to forget our connection to the 24-hour sun cycle, our biology hasn't. The sun rising and falling cues a symphony of hormonal, neuronal, and behavioral responses that govern our metabolism and appetite, stress levels, risks of developing a disease, aging, sleep/wake cycles, and energy levels.

The link between the outer world of light and darkness and the inner world of our biochemistry is our circadian clock or circadian rhythm. Our circadian rhythm consists of two parts:[18]

- **Brain clock.** This is the master clock located in the suprachiasmatic nucleus of the hypothalamus that picks up external signals from our environment and coordinates our body's responses via hormones and neurotransmitters.

- **Body clocks.** These are clocks in our tissues, organs, fat cells, gastrointestinal tract, and muscle tissue that regulate processes occurring at the cellular level.

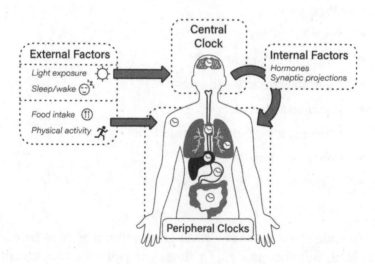

Our brain and body clocks work together to synchronize our biology to the external world through a process called *entrainment*. Much as we set the hands of a watch to establish its time, our biological clocks are set, or entrained, by external or environmental factors called *zeitgebers* (German for "time givers"). Some of the most powerful zeitgebers include light, temperature, physical activity, drinking, and eating.

The zeitgebers affect different clocks. Light, for example, is a potent zeitgeber of the central clock in the brain, but it has no effect on other clocks like the skin.[19] Similarly, eating is a strong zeitgeber for digestive organs like the liver and pancreas, but it has a lesser effect on the master clock.[20]

Despite the different effects, our brain clock and body clocks constantly communicate with each other. And it's this constant communication between our brain clock and body clocks that creates our circadian system, which oversees our sleep/wake cycles and energy levels. In fact, sleep and energy are two sides of a coin connected via the circadian system.[21] Our circadian rhythms are the primary determinant of how well we sleep, controlling how much sleep we get, its quality, and what kind of cellular regeneration processes happen—or don't—because of how deeply we sleep.

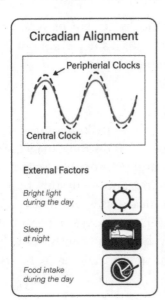
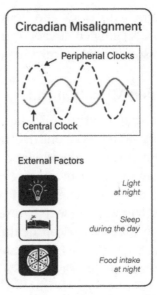

Our challenge is that we live in a world fundamentally mismatched to the signals that our brain clock and body clocks were designed for. Biologically, the human body is designed to live in tune with the rising and setting of the sun. We're designed to wake at dawn and to sleep at night. We're not designed to be indoors almost all day and then to stare at different artificial light sources after the sun sets. We're designed to eat early in the day when the sun is high and to stop as it gets dark for a fasting cycle, not to consume big meals or snack into the night.

Divorcing our lives from the natural 24-hour light/dark cycle sends the wrong signals to our brain clock and body clocks, causing them to become misaligned and resulting in *circadian dysregulation*. Circadian dysregulation leads to poor sleep; your body doesn't know when to shut down and go into rest mode or when to stay pumped with energy to remain alert and awake. But poor sleep also leads to circadian dysregulation so, very quickly, this becomes a vicious cycle where the two play off each other, driving us more deeply into a pit of daily fatigue and suffering.

THE CIRCADIAN RHYTHM–MITOCHONDRIA LINK

When our brain clock and body clocks get out of sync and we battle a dysregulated circadian rhythm, it's depleting our energy levels in specific biological and cellular ways.

Weakened Mitochondria

Our circadian rhythm plays a vital role in keeping our energy producers—our mitochondria—healthy and strong. In fact, studies show that circadian dysregulation and poor-quality sleep directly contribute to fatigue by causing mitochondrial dysfunction.[22]

In a study on genetically identical twins, researchers found that the twin who got less than seven hours of sleep per night and who reported worse sleep quality had significantly fewer mitochondria than the twin who slept more than seven hours and who enjoyed quality sleep.[23]

Not only do circadian rhythms impact mitochondrial function but mitochondrial function impacts circadian rhythms in a metabolic cross talk. That is, circadian dysregulation and mitochondrial function can be addressed at each end of the spectrum. As one improves, the other will as well. This is how we turn spirals of poor sleep and low energy levels into deep sleep and high energy levels.

Our mitochondria also have their own daily rhythms that rely on their own circadian rhythm to regulate, including oxygen consumption and energy production. When that's disrupted, our mitochondria can't perform to their optimal levels. In studies where mice were genetically altered to lack key circadian genes, researchers discovered extensive damage to mitochondria that negatively affected their functioning including:

- Reduced oxygen consumption and energy production[24,25,26,27,28]

- Less fat oxidization and usage as an energy source[29]

- Less pronounced and fragmented changes in morphology[30,31,32]

- Disrupted mitochondrial protein acetylation[33]

- Increased oxidative stress within mitochondria[34]

- Less mitochondrial resilience to oxidative stress-induced damage[35]

- Impaired mitochondrial autophagy, called *mitophagy*[36]

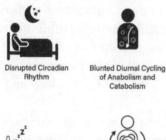

Disrupted Circadian Rhythm

Blunted Diurnal Cycling of Anabolism and Catabolism

Impaired Mitophagy

Low Energy and Lifespan

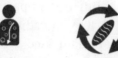

Optimal Circadian Rhythm

Optimal Diurnal Cycling of Anabolism and Catabolism

Enhanced Mitophagy

High Energy and Lifespan

While all mitochondria impairments can wreck energy levels, mitophagy deserves special attention.

Mitophagy evolved as a key mechanism for keeping a healthy pool of mitochondria in our cells, by eliminating mitochondria that are damaged and dysfunctional,[37] then regenerating more mitochondria from the healthier, stronger ones. Mitophagy is necessary to prevent the accumulation of old and damaged mitochondria that contribute to oxidative stress, crushed energy levels, and metabolic disease.

As you might guess, mitophagy takes place during sleep. And if you don't get enough sleep, your body cannot get rid of the damaged mitochondria, and then you're functioning today on yesterday's poorly functioning and damaged mitochondria. And if that trend continues over months and years, chronically low energy is the unsurprising and logical result.

Reduced Melatonin

Melatonin is commonly called *the sleep hormone* because it helps us do just that. When there is minimal or no light, our master clock in the brain picks up the lack of blue light waves and sends a message to the pineal gland (also in the brain) to secrete melatonin.

Staying up late and spending less time sleeping result in less time for our brain and body to be bathed in melatonin. But even more importantly, a disrupted circadian rhythm can also profoundly suppress our body's production of melatonin at night, by upward of 70 percent! Besides being a "sleep hormone," melatonin is also a powerful *energy hormone*: not in the sense of providing an immediate energy boost when it's present, but indirectly because it is arguably the most important hormone when it comes to mitochondrial health. Melatonin has antioxidant properties that help protect our mitochondria from oxidants and the highly toxic free radicals,[38] which, when in excess, damage our mitochondria, eventually leading to decreased energy production.

To keep our mitochondria healthy and our cells functioning, our bodies eliminate free radicals through the use of antioxidants like vitamin C and glutathione and minerals including zinc and copper. But while most antioxidants can only neutralize one free radical at a time, melatonin can simultaneously neutralize multiple free radicals and works synergistically when combined with other antioxidants.[39,40] Plus, if a melatonin is lost to a free radical, then three other antioxidants will emerge to take its place.[41]

Amazingly enough, melatonin also increases the production and activity of other antioxidant enzymes like glutathione peroxidase, superoxide dismutase, and catalase.[42] It also has the special ability to easily pass through cell membranes and reach inside our mitochondria to provide antioxidant protection to the mitochondria, even more than vitamin E and vitamin C.[43] Furthermore, melatonin is as good as, or better than, fabricated antioxidants in protecting against mitochondrial oxidative stress.[44,45] These factors and more[46] have led some researchers to call melatonin the true mitochondrial-targeted antioxidant.[47,48,49]

Hindering Toxic Cleanup in the Brain

Every day, your brain produces toxic waste products from normal processes like thinking and coordinating bodily movements. Deep sleep allows your brain to clean and clear itself of these waste products using a process called *glymphatic drainage*.[50] The depth and quality of your sleep is vital to allowing the glymphatic system to work efficiently.

When circadian dysregulation and sleep disruption prevent our glymphatic system from functioning properly,[51] these toxins accumulate in our brain, which can lead to neuroinflammation, a known cause of chronically low energy levels.[52] Toxins also directly and indirectly shut down energy production by our mitochondria.

Hormonal Dysregulation

A dysregulated circadian rhythm invariably leads to hormonal havoc. That's a huge problem since hormones are directly and indirectly involved in energy production. For example, your *thyroid hormone* is essential for metabolism, heat production, and growth. Some of the most common and debilitating symptoms of having an underactive thyroid gland (hypothyroidism) are chronic fatigue, body aches and weakness, weight gain, chills, and constipation.

We've known for decades that thyroid hormone metabolism exhibits a circadian rhythm, with the lowest levels occurring during the day and the highest levels at night.[53,54] Yet this natural oscillation from low to high gets demolished by sleep disruption.[55] That's not good for your metabolism or your energy.

Circadian disruptions also impact the release of *human growth hormone*, which is critical for releasing energy reserves in fat and glycogen and promoting cellular growth and healing. Human growth hormone increases significantly during slow-wave (deep) sleep compared with light and REM (Rapid Eye Movement) sleep,[56] so if you struggle to get into deep sleep, your growth hormone levels will be lower, which can contribute to lower energy levels. In fact, adults with chronic fatigue syndrome only release half the growth hormone that non-fatigued adults do.[57]

Finally, there is *cortisol*, a stress hormone that peaks each morning to get us up and going. While the majority of chronic psychological and physical stressors do not cause any detectable decrease in cortisol levels, even when present for several decades,[58] there is no doubt that having blunted cortisol levels or chronically elevated cortisol levels causes fatigue, either through not transmitting its signal (too low levels) or causing the body to become habituated to its signal (too high levels).[59]

This is where things get interesting for you night owls. Several studies have shown that staying up late and sleeping in can cause morning cortisol levels to be reduced massively below normal.[60,61,62,63]

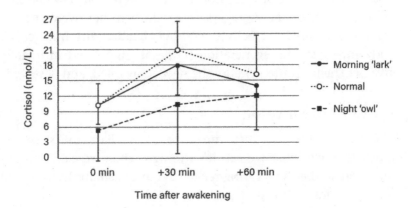

Several studies have also shown that disrupted and poor-quality sleep will cause a lower peak in morning cortisol,[64,65,66] one of which showed a dramatic 24 to 43 percent reduction,[67] enough to get one diagnosed with "adrenal fatigue."

CIRCADIAN RHYTHM REBOOT

It takes effort and intention to take control of our environment and behaviors to bring our brain clock and body clocks back in sync and as close to the natural 24-hour light/dark cycle as we can. Sleep hygiene, like using blackout curtains to keep the bedroom dark, taking a hot shower or bath an hour before sleep to jump-start a temperature change in our body, shutting off devices and screens an hour before bed or using blue (and green) light-blocking glasses, or journaling or meditating for 20 minutes before bed can profoundly help rewire our clocks and reset our circadian rhythm.

So can nutrition.

With Megan, I wanted her to continue her sleep hygiene habits: using blackout shades, turning off screens at least one hour before bed, journaling or meditating for 20 minutes before sleeping, and taking a warm shower or bath at night. While those alone weren't enough to get Megan's sleep on track, I knew that if we layered on a few nutritional strategies, we could help her overcome her insomnia, rewire her clocks to reset her circadian rhythm, get her body into rest-and-regeneration mode at night, and ultimately give her the unlimited energy she needed, wanted, and deserved.

Use Chrono-Nutrition

The primary way our diet impacts our circadian clocks isn't so much through what we eat; it's through when we eat. Chrono-nutrition studies how eating relates to our circadian rhythm, and it involves four main strategies:[68]

1. Window of eating
2. Clock time of eating
3. Stacking more calories earlier in the day
4. Consistency of eating

1. Window of Eating

Every human (and animal, for that matter) alternates between feeding and fasting, and these cycles are dominant synchronizing signals for our peripheral clocks.

In the Western world, we've been taught that we need to eat three meals per day: breakfast, lunch, and dinner. You may also hear recommendations to add in a snack or two in the midmorning and afternoon, leading to the societal norm of eating five to six times per day.

When the U.S. government asked over 62,000 adults about their eating habits, 60 percent said they ate three meals per day, while 90 percent said they eat at least one snack per day and 67 percent said they eat two or more snacks per day.[69] However, when Satchin Panda, Ph.D., an expert in the field of circadian rhythm research and the author of *The Circadian Code*, studied this issue, he found some surprising results. For three weeks Panda had adults use a smartphone app to track their food intake. He found that the least frequent eaters ate an average of 3.3 times per day, while the most frequent eaters ate on average a whopping 10.5 times per day.[70]

Most importantly, less than 10 percent of the participants in Panda's study ate all their food within a 12-hour window, and a staggering 85 percent had a window of eating (the time from your first to your last bite of food) of a whopping 13 to 16 hours per day.

This means that the body clocks in your organs, tissues, and muscles are constantly getting signals to stay active and digest food. Let's imagine that you start eating at 7:00 A.M. and you continue until shortly before bed at 11 P.M. Remember that your body clocks constantly communicate with your brain clock, so our brain clock will also get the signal that our bodies need to stay awake.

When I had Megan track her eating windows for one week, we discovered that most days, she ate for 14 to 16 hours. To reduce Megan's eating window, we used a tool called *time-restricted feeding* (TRF). This is an eating pattern that involves shortening the window to 10 hours or less every day and fasting for at least 14 hours before eating again.

By confining our food intake to only a portion of the day and allowing for a lengthened fasting period overnight, we allow for something vital to happen for optimizing our energy levels: we sync the body clocks and brain clock so that our circadian rhythm optimizes our metabolic health and produces abundant energy. This strategy is one of the fundamental aspects of a healthy circadian rhythm.[71]

We have a lot of data in animals showing that TRF prevents the development of cardiometabolic diseases,[72] and an ever-growing body of research in humans is beginning to find similar benefits.[73,74,75] There's also research showing that it helps keep mitochondria youthful in the face of nutrient overload (and remember: most of the population has constant nutrient overload).[76]

In fact, several studies show that eating all our food within a 6- to 10-hour window regulates our circadian rhythms, which also leads to improvements in body composition, glycemic control, insulin sensitivity, oxidative stress, and energy levels.[77,78,79,80] This is without changing any of the foods that we would normally eat.

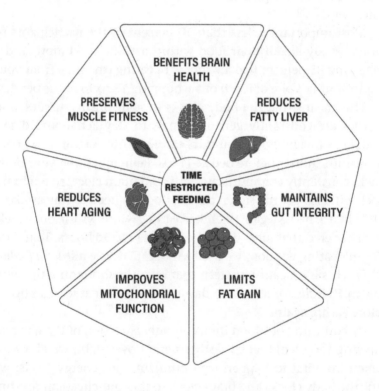

With Megan, getting her to a 10-hour eating window was our goal, but I had her aim for a 12-hour TRF window first. I often recommend 12 hours with my coaching clients to start, because it's an attainable goal that most people can sustain over the long haul that doesn't require drastic adjustments.

I encouraged Megan to pick 7 A.M. to 7 P.M., 8 A.M. to 8 P.M., or 9 A.M. to 9 P.M. Megan chose 7 A.M. to 7 P.M. She was sure she did not want to eat past dinnertime, which was usually 6 to 7 P.M., so this would let her eat breakfast as early as 7 A.M. to stay on track but give her the option of pushing it back for an even tighter TRF window if she could manage that.

I suggested Megan try this for a month and if she felt great and wanted to try closing the window again, then she could. "There is no rush," I emphasized. "If you feel fantastic eating in a twelve-hour window, then stick with it."

I always encourage my clients to experiment with windows between 8 and 12 hours to see how their bodies feel and what best fits into their lifestyles. Any variation works, so pick one that is relatively easy.

Some of the most popular eating windows my clients use include:

- 8 A.M. to 6 P.M.

- 9 A.M. to 6 P.M.

- 9 A.M. to 5 P.M.

However, there are cases where someone simply cannot eat breakfast early in the day and therefore opts to use a TRF window later in the day, such as 12 P.M. to 8 P.M. While not ideal, it is certainly a viable strategy for those who need to make the best of their situation. Stressing over morning meals is the last thing we want for those who have a tight morning schedule, so be sure to pick a TRF window that you can enjoy sticking with.

Finally, I want to be clear that TRF is not intermittent fasting and doesn't require anything extreme like eating just once per day. TRF is a daily practice rather than an intermittent one, and it doesn't restrict how much we eat, since we can still consume two to four meals in a 6- to 10-hour eating window. Comparatively, intermittent fasting involves going for more than a day (24-plus hours) without eating several times per week or month and thereby inherently involves dietary restriction.

2. Clock Time of Eating

In the United States, the average American eats less than 25 percent of their daily calories before noon, 37.5 percent after 6:00 P.M., and 12 percent after 9:00 P.M.[81] This means we're consuming almost 50 percent of our calories at night, which is a problem because it kills our energy levels.

Our gastrointestinal tract is lined with enteroendocrine cells that provide an endless supply of neurotransmitters, peptides, and hormones when we eat. Metabolic health and energy levels depend on these gastrointestinal signals being matched to the appropriate signals put out by the brain during the day.[82]

At night, these signals change, and the later we eat, the more these signals become disrupted, our body clocks and brain clock misalign, and our sleep suffers. One study with animals showed that altering the timing of their food intake by having them eat when they should have been sleeping potentially decoupled the circadian rhythm of their liver and other body clocks from their brains.[83,84]

We see similar detriments from inappropriate eating times in night shift workers, who demonstrate significantly greater rates of obesity and metabolic dysfunction than non-shift workers.[85,86] This isn't the same as professions that involve carcinogen exposure, like asbestos workers or farmers who spray pesticides. Yet shift work is the *only* profession to be classified as a carcinogen in and of itself.[87]

Research also shows that eating at night can cause fat gain, which affects our energy levels. When mice are fed diets that are meant to cause obesity, but their eating is confined only to hours when they are meant to be awake and active (versus giving them access to food day and night), they do not develop metabolic dysfunction (fat gain) and circadian dysregulation.[88,89,90]

When it comes to regulating our circadian rhythm and improving our sleep, research reveals that altering when we eat makes a stark difference in realigning our circadian rhythm, improving sleep, maintaining a healthy weight, and boosting energy.

3. Stacking More Calories Earlier in the Day

On the flip side of killing your energy levels by eating too much at night, there may be energy benefits, such as improved metabolic health and flexibility, in eating most of your food earlier in the day, at breakfast and lunch.[91]

One study found that eating most of our calories in the morning with a big breakfast and lunch leads to greater fat oxidation and reduced appetite compared to a more even spread of calories throughout the day.[92] Data also shows that eating a large breakfast and lunch, compared to a more even spread of food throughout the day, enhances circadian gene expression and amplifies the natural circadian rhythms of hormones like cortisol, making it have a higher peak in the morning and drop at night.[93]

Eating more food earlier in the day primes your body to give you a natural energy boost upon waking each morning. I wanted Megan to consume more calories earlier in the day, so I challenged her to eat a bigger breakfast and lunch, a small snack midafternoon, and then a light dinner.

Because Megan had a hectic life and kids who needed wrangling, I didn't want to overwhelm her with a strict "you must do this seven days a week, forever" approach. Instead, I suggested she aim to eat like this three times a week, for a month, and then reassess.

While ideally we want to aim to eat most of our food every day at breakfast and lunch, I also know that life stresses and daily schedules can get in the way of our best intentions. If eating most of your food early in the day is too stressful, then don't worry about it for now. Focus on the other, less stressful changes that are within your reach.

4. Consistency of Eating

The last piece of our chrono-nutrition puzzle is to practice consistency with our eating schedule. Our circadian system works to predict events, learns to anticipate mealtimes, and adjusts the body's metabolic responses and hormones accordingly.[94]

For instance, one study found that regular breakfast eaters who skipped breakfast had worse glycemic control at lunch, while those who habitually skipped breakfast had no metabolic issues.[95]

Like many working parents, Megan often grabbed food when she could, typically on the go and without a set schedule. I challenged her to create a traditional schedule with three meals and a snack. She put mealtimes into her calendar to remind her to eat, and also to help her prioritize and shift how she thought about meals.

Again, I know that it's not always easy sticking to a schedule. Life does get in the way. Still, bringing more consistency to eating at the same time every day can go a long way in helping optimize our circadian rhythm. The goal isn't to be perfect, but to establish new habits.

Targeted Nutrient Mix

There's an ever-growing body of evidence investigating how different macronutrients (protein, carbohydrate, and fat) impact sleep. Dr. Marie-Pierre St-Onge from the Institute of Human Nutrition and Department of Medicine at Columbia University reviewed 11 clinical studies regarding how different diets impacted sleep and made several important observations:[96]

- Higher-carbohydrate diets tend to shift slow-wave (deep) sleep toward REM and reduce the amount of time it takes to fall asleep each night.

- Higher-protein diets tend to reduce nightly awakenings.

- Eating digestible carbohydrates within an hour of going to sleep disrupts sleep quality compared to eating those carbohydrates four hours before.

- Skipping dinner or eating earlier in the day doesn't negatively impact sleep.

These findings show us the importance of blending when we eat with what we eat for our sleep quality and circadian rhythms. Generally, eating a higher-protein diet with slow-digesting carbohydrates like whole grains, legumes, and vegetables around lunch or dinner, but not within several hours of going to sleep, should allow for the deepest and most rejuvenating sleep.

Megan regularly consumed proteins such as chicken and ground turkey, and fish like salmon and cod. The biggest change for her was ensuring she ate protein at every meal, especially dinner. With three kids, sometimes dinners were quick and easy— pasta or cheese quesadillas with flour tortillas. I encouraged Megan to see her nutrient mix as a fun challenge rather than a frustrating one. For lunches and dinners, I suggested she try quick, easy, and light recipes that were also kid-friendly, including steak, baked fries, and tomato salad; Mexican-style chicken soup; pulled chicken and curry-roasted mixed vegetables served over baby spinach with raisins, cilantro, and a mint-lime yogurt dressing; and chicken sausage, veggies, and creamy polenta.

Finally, Megan and I also talked about alcohol. While not a huge drinker, she would have a glass, sometimes two, after the kids went to bed a few times a week. While alcohol can help us unwind, it can mess with our sleep. Both acute and chronic consumption of alcohol, even at "social drinking" amounts (about two to seven drinks per week, whether each beverage is 12 ounces of beer, 5 ounces of wine, 1.5 shots, or some combination), reduces melatonin levels by 15 to 40 percent, with higher doses of alcohol having a stronger inhibitory effect.[97,98,99] Alcohol also greatly reduces sleep quality and increases sleep disruptions.[100]

I recommended to Megan that she should remove alcohol entirely, but if she didn't want such a sharp cutoff, she should try to keep it to one drink, two tops, once a week. I would recommend the same to you. If you're struggling with sleep and circadian rhythm dysregulation, then I recommend removing alcohol entirely. If you are going to have a drink, try to have it earlier in the evening.

Kicking the Caffeine Dependency

In our brain there's a molecule called *adenosine* that makes us tired. It binds to its own (adenosine) receptors in the brain, which transmits a signaling of sleepiness that builds up as more and more adenosine binds throughout the day. When we ingest caffeine, it binds to the receptors and blocks adenosine from binding and doing its job,[101] which causes us to feel more awake, alert, and energized.[102] Caffeine works because it prolongs the time until we become tired. The caffeine needs to wear off before adenosine can start binding its receptors again.

Caffeine provides a short-term energy boost that can be useful under the right circumstances, such as when you want to increase your physical strength and improve your endurance for a workout session.[103,104,105,106]

But caffeine's effects can turn problematic when used in the afternoon and evening because it interferes with sleep quality. In one study, sleep disturbances were increased when caffeine was ingested as far out as six hours before going to sleep, with the detriments growing the closer to bedtime caffeine was ingested.[107] Studies have found that caffeine's half-life—which is how long it remains active in our systems—ranges from three and one-half to eight hours, depending on the person.[108]

In addition, it takes only several days of caffeine use to build up a tolerance to its effects,[109,110] meaning that you will gradually need to consume more caffeine to get the same energy boost. This also means your energy levels dip without caffeine and your mental and physical performance declines.

As Megan and I worked together, we dramatically curtailed her caffeine use. Typically, she would have a cup as soon as she finished her morning jog, then two more before lunch, and then she'd have a fourth and sometimes a fifth in the afternoon, sometimes as late as 4 to 4:30 P.M. I had Megan slowly kick the caffeine habit by first stopping its consumption by 2 P.M. She did this for a week, and then over the following two weeks, I had her slowly cut back from four to five cups down to two to three. Then I had her attempt taking days off from drinking it, beginning on the weekend. Caffeine withdrawal and the accompanying headaches are a real thing, so you want to slowly wean yourself from any dependency.

My best advice based on the science: use caffeine sporadically for targeted purposes like just before a workout session several times per week or if you have an important meeting or project that depends on mental alertness. If you enjoy caffeine, it is important that you also pay attention to when you have your last cup. The worse your sleep, the earlier I recommend you stop consuming caffeine. Typically, I recommend stopping between noon and 4 P.M. The more fatigue you feel and the more severe your sleep issues, the sooner you should halt the caffeine intake.

MAKING THE CHANGES STICK

Megan spent two months implementing these nutritional strategies. Some days she didn't hit her goals, but she did notice her sleep improving little by little, and she started stringing together better nights with more consistency. As a result, Megan felt like she had energy to show up with more vitality, clarity, and focus of mind, and she had an increased capacity to connect with her kids, husband, and coworkers.

For many of my clients, it only took a week for them to start realizing benefits, but for others, it took up to a month, sometimes two. This is not set-it-and-forget-it. It's about adopting new patterns and ways of eating, and different nutritional habits that will rewire your brain and body clocks to support your circadian rhythm alignment throughout your life. And not only will these strategies boost energy levels but they will have the widespread positive side effects of lowering your risk of dozens of diseases, including heart disease, diabetes, obesity, neurological disease, and cancer.

ACTION LIST

It's time to rewire your brain and body clocks so you enjoy better sleep and more energy. The action items I've gathered will help you start this journey. I've ranked the nutritional strategies in the order that has produced the most effective results for my clients. If you want to start at the first nutritional strategy and work your way through the others one at a time, do it. You can also choose where to start, so if you want to work on limiting your caffeine intake first, then do that.

To help you more easily incorporate new strategies into your daily life, I've divided each action into multiple steps. Stay on each step for *at least two weeks*. But if the step or the strategy still feels uncomfortable, or you want to continue integrating it into your daily routine, then stay until it feels comfortable and you're ready to progress. Once you've reached your desired level of progress with one strategy, move on to the next. Keep repeating this process for as long as you need.

Whatever nutritional strategy you start with, keep a journal and note your sleep patterns. Each morning, grade your sleep quality and morning energy levels on a scale from 1 to 10. Track any changes and use these daily sleep and energy grades to help analyze your progress.

- ☐ **Confine your food and caloric beverage intake to a time-restricted window.**
  - ☐ Consume all your calories within 12 to 14 hours.
  - ☐ Consume all your calories within 10 to 12 hours.
  - ☐ Consume all your calories within 6 to 10 hours.

☐ **Do not eat or consume caloric beverages at night or close to bed.**

    ☐ Stop eating before 10 P.M.

    ☐ Stop eating before 9 P.M.

    ☐ Stop eating before 8 P.M.

    ☐ Stop eating before 7 P.M.

☐ **Consume most of your calories in the morning and afternoon (e.g., breakfast and lunch).**

    ☐ Consume roughly 30 percent of your calories before 3 P.M.

    ☐ Consume roughly 50 percent of your calories before 3 P.M.

    ☐ Consume roughly 70 percent of your calories before 3 P.M.

☐ **Be consistent with your mealtimes.**

    ☐ Eat 1 meal at the same time each day.

    ☐ Eat 2 meals at the same time each day.

    ☐ Eat all meals at the same time each day.

☐ **Limit your intake of rapidly digestible carbohydrates at dinner.**

    ☐ Do not consume rapidly digested carbohydrates at dinner 2 to 3 days per week.

    ☐ Do not consume rapidly digested carbohydrates at dinner 4 to 5 days per week.

    ☐ Do not consume rapidly digested carbohydrates at dinner more than once per week.

☐ **Limit your intake of alcohol.**

    ☐ Drink no more than one drink per night 2 to 3 days per week.

    ☐ Drink no more than one drink per night 4 to 5 days per week.

    ☐ Drink no more than one drink per night 6-plus days per week.

☐ **Reduce caffeine consumption in the afternoon and evening.**

    ☐ Stop drinking caffeine past 4 P.M.

    ☐ Stop drinking caffeine past 2 P.M.

    ☐ Stop drinking caffeine past 12 P.M.

CHAPTER 3

BURN FAT, BUILD MUSCLE, BOOST ENERGY

Talking about weight is hard.

It leaves many people feeling ashamed, frustrated, and uncomfortable. When we carry extra fat—whether that's a little or a lot—we know it. We feel it.

One of the most discouraging realizations that I often hear from my clients is that they have diet hopped for years, going from paleo to calorie counting to low fat to low carb. They see results at first, but nothing lasts. They have no idea what to do next, and they *still* struggle with extra fat and feeling fatigued.

This was Christina's story. When I first met her, she had just turned 38 and had spent the past year trying to regain her health and energy. She was working through food addiction recovery, and on managing anxiety and depression with a therapist. She had lost about 10 pounds through counting calories.

Christina knew she had made many positive strides in one year, and she had improved her overall health and well-being, but she hadn't solved the mystery of her fatigue and energy crashes. She would have unlimited energy and feel upbeat and happy for a day or two, but then she would crash and be in a slump for a week, sometimes two or more.

"There are days that are so oppressive that I am pretty much non-functioning and bedridden—or at least, I want to be, but I can't because of work and my family obligations," she told me.

She felt the most frustration with her weight and its effect on her moods. She wanted to lose about 30 pounds, but it was hard.

After her first child was born, Christina gained about 20 pounds but took it off relatively quickly through diet and exercise. Her struggles really began after the birth of her second child. Not only did she put on about 25 pounds during the pregnancy, but after the birth, she began yo-yoing.

"I tried every diet from calorie counting to low carb, and I would lose the weight, but then I'd add it back with an extra five or ten, once fifteen pounds," Christina said. "I want to lose more weight, but I'm also terrified that if I do, I won't keep it off. I'm also so tired that I don't feel like I have the energy to stay the course, but deep down, I really do want to feel better in my body and have more energy."

Christina paused, taking a deep breath. "I just don't know how to do this."

UNLOCKING THE MYSTERIES OF YOUR BODY COMPOSITION

Christina articulated so well the weight issue that challenges millions of us today. In the United States, it's estimated that *one in three* adults is obese while another *one in three* is overweight, meaning that two of every three adults do not have a healthy body weight.[1] (The World Health Organization and most other health authorities define obesity as having a body mass index (BMI) greater than or equal to 30 and being overweight as greater than or equal to 25.)

I knew the key to addressing Christina's low energy rested with improving her *body composition*, which consists of two things:

- **Lean mass** (our muscle tissue, bones, and water)

- **Fat mass** (fat stored in our bodies)

While there is no clear-cut definition on what represents a healthy balance between lean mass and fat mass, we know that carrying too much fat and having low muscle mass are both harmful to our overall health and energy levels.

Body composition is the real issue facing our world. If we combine more accurate measurements of body composition with markers of metabolic health, then some researchers have proposed that *90 percent* of adults in the U.S. are "overfat," meaning they carry enough fat that it is harming them.[2]

Before we go further, I want to be clear: if you're struggling with excess body fat, please know there is nothing *wrong* with you.

Our world is fundamentally *obesogenic*, meaning that just by existing today, the default destiny for most people (over 70 percent) is to be overweight. It is more typical to carry more body fat than it is to live at one's optimal body composition. In our modern obesogenic environment, carrying around extra fat is a natural by-product of the way our environment overrides our evolutionary programming.

At the same time, our society also has a propensity to shame and judge people who carry more body fat. That is the last thing I want to do. My aim is to help you *shift* your perspective around your body, fat, and muscle mass. This is about *empowering* you with easy-to-implement nutritional strategies that will help you lose body fat, gain lean muscle, and maintain an optimal and healthy body composition so you feel energized instead of chronically slow and fatigued.

As you read this chapter, I want you hold this thought:

You are not fighting some enemy that is your current body. Rather, you are healing the temple that your body represents.

THE BODY COMPOSITION–ENERGY LINK

While there is absolutely nothing wrong with you if your body composition is off, there are health risks in addition to low energy levels that come from carrying excess fat and/or too little lean muscle mass.

Obesity is associated with an increased risk for having 18 comorbid diseases, including:[3]

- Type 2 diabetes
- High blood pressure
- Strokes
- Heart failure
- Osteoarthritis
- A variety of cancers

RISK OF HAVING A CO-MORBIDITY WHEN OBESE RELATIVE TO BEING NORMAL-WEIGHT
Meta-analysis of 89 studies

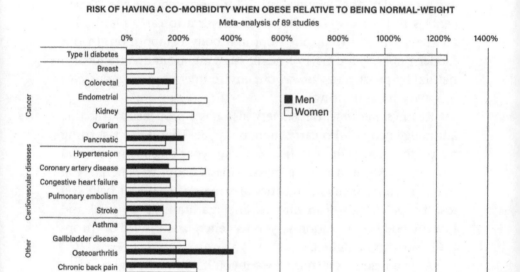

Globally, obesity accounts for 5 percent of all deaths, and nearly half of people who are obese die directly from it.[4] The top killer is cardiovascular disease, accounting for 40 percent of all obesity deaths, followed by type 2 diabetes at 10 percent, cancer at 5 percent, and chronic kidney disease at 5 percent.

There are also heavy financial costs to obesity. The growing health burden of carrying excess fat is one of the most well recognized in the world, estimated to cost about $2 trillion, or 2.8 percent of the global gross domestic product.[5] That's equivalent to the global impact from smoking; or armed violence, war, and terrorism; or the combined costs of drug use, workplace risks, household air pollution, child and mother undernutrition, and unsafe sex.

If we look at just the U.S., the annual health care cost for obesity is $340 billion, which represents 28 percent of all health care spending,[6] and people dealing with obesity often spend 42 percent more on direct health care costs than normal-weight adults.[7]

There are also numerous studies that have looked at how quality of life changes with body composition. One meta-analysis of eight studies and over 43,000 adults found that as weight goes up, physical health–related quality of life goes down.[8]

And when it comes to energy levels, research has found that obesity is associated with a *40 percent greater* chance of being fatigued and 7 to 12 percent less vitality than being at a normal weight.[9,10]

None of these stats are shared with disdain, disgust, or dislike. "Fighting obesity"—as many in the health and wellness sector have called it—has led to extensive collateral damage, like unhealthy preoccupations with food, eating disorders, self-hatred, stress, and all the health consequences that result.

But that's why we aren't fighting obesity; we are nourishing our temple by returning it to a healthy body composition.

There is an enormous difference between self-hate and simply acknowledging that your body composition is increasing your risk of disease, lowering your quality of life, and negatively affecting your energy levels. It's just a fact because there are real changes happening within your body that have led you away from optimal health and energy.

Chronic Low-Grade Inflammation

We evolved the ability to store fat as a protective mechanism against "energy poisoning" during times of overeating and to provide us with an energy reservoir that could be used during times of fasting and famine. However, there are limits on our ability to store fat safely.

As the fat cells take in more energy, they expand in size. But much as a balloon can hold only so much air before it pops, so too can fat cells hold only so much fat before they die. When you carry around too much body fat, your fat cells become overwhelmed, dysfunctional, and inflammatory—all effects caused by fat cells trying to prevent their deaths. This results in chronic, low-grade inflammation that can cause fatigue in three major ways:[11]

1. Altering neurotransmitter and reward pathways in the brain

2. Causing mitochondrial dysfunction

3. Disrupting sleep and circadian rhythms

When there is inflammation in our body, it responds by lowering our energy levels so that we *rest and recover*. Inflammation is a sign that something isn't right in our bodies and our bodies need to conserve energy so that everything goes into fighting that infection or healing that wound. Specific molecules are sent to stop neurotransmitters like dopamine and serotonin from doing their jobs, which include regulating our mood, physical activity, motivation, and anxiety.[12,13,14] During our evolutionary history, we would only need to rest and recover from an illness or injury. Today, it occurs *around the clock*, thanks to the low-grade inflammation pervading much of modern society.[15,16]

Think about what happens when you are sick. You feel tired, you lack motivation to do anything physical or mental, you may feel depressed, or your brain feels fuzzy or lacks focus; these symptoms are collectively called sickness behavior.[17]

A mountain of data also shows us that chronic, low-grade inflammation leads to mitochondrial dysfunction and reduced energy production,[18,19,20] which is bad news, because our bodies need our mitochondria pumping out more energy to support the overactive immune system.[21,22]

Dr. Tamara Lacourt of the University of Texas MD Anderson Cancer Center recently proposed that chronic fatigue is caused and maintained by this chronic inflammation–induced imbalance between cellular energy availability and the needs of the body.[23]

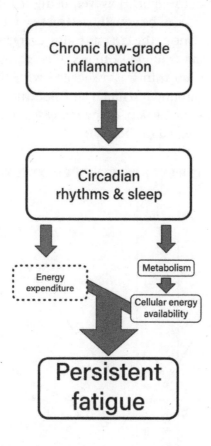

Dr. Lacourt noted another contributing factor: circadian and sleep disruption. Excess body fat is related to poor-quality sleep, including greater sleep disturbances and shorter sleep durations.[24] Sleep loss and circadian disruption can also cause low-grade inflammation or amplify any inflammation that is already present in the body, thereby intensifying inflammation-induced fatigue.[25,26]

Too Little Muscle Mass

Obesity and being overweight get the lion's share of attention when we talk about weight. However, being *too thin* and having *too little muscle mass* can be equally destructive for our bodies and our energy levels. One of the largest studies ever conducted, which aggregated the data from 189 other studies across 32 countries, found that being too thin was associated with the same risk of dying as carrying around too much fat.[27] Specifically, as a person's BMI fell below 20, their risk of dying increased to the same extent as if their BMI increased to above 30.

ABSOLUTE RISK OF DYING IN THE NEXT 35 YEARS (%)

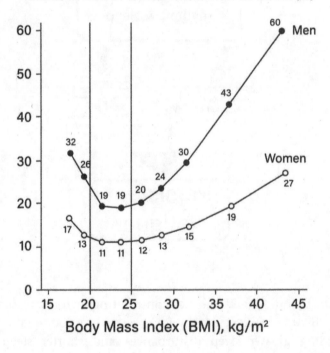

In the study the risk of death increased as BMI fell below 20, correlating to a body fat percentage of 15 percent in men and 25 percent in women.[28]

To be clear, the risks associated with being too thin are owed to a lack of muscle mass, strength, and functionality, which increases our susceptibility to injury and death, and not to lower fat mass levels, which is why healthy athletes and active adults may have lower body fat levels.

Our muscles are a key regulator of metabolism and vital for the prevention of many chronic diseases.[29,30] Yet a tremendous proportion of the population meets the definition for *sarcopenia*, a condition characterized by low levels of muscle mass that cause weakness and impaired physical function.[31] In the U.S., sarcopenia afflicts more than half of adults aged over 50 years, 20 to 35 percent of middle-aged adults, and roughly 1 in 10 young adults.[32]

PREVALENCE OF SARCOPENIA IN THE U.S.

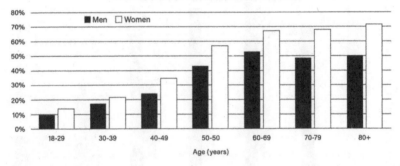

Age (years)

You need muscle to move your body and to sustain a healthy metabolism. If you have low amounts of muscle tissue, you're going to tire more quickly and have a harder time getting through the day because your mitochondria aren't producing the energy your body needs. Ultimately, impaired physical function and muscle weakness are strongly related to fatigue,[33] and having more muscle mass is associated with less fatigue severity.[34]

NOURISHING THE TEMPLE

The path to a healthy body composition and regaining energy is straightforward: lose fat and build lean muscle.

Several studies have shown that modest weight loss improves quality of life and physical function.[35,36,37] When researchers look at how the extent of weight loss impacts quality of life, improvements increase as the extent of weight loss increases.[38,39]

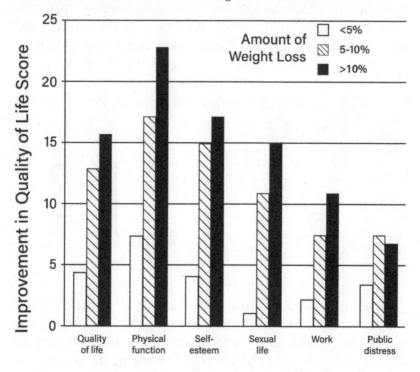

When someone with obesity adheres to a 10-week weight loss diet, general and mental health, physical function, vitality, bodily pain, and social function all improve.[40]

Many of my clients tell me they struggle to lose weight. But that's not entirely true. They know how to lose weight and have done it multiple times. It's maintaining the weight loss that's hard.

Most people who embark on fat loss journeys make it about six months before they reach a weight loss plateau and the weight starts returning.[41] It doesn't matter whether they start exercising, begin a new diet, use meal replacements, drastically cut calories, or take advantage of weight loss drugs.

This was Christina's major struggle. "I think you do know how to lose excess fat," I gently told her. "Taking off ten pounds in a year . . . that's a phenomenal start. Working with a food addiction therapist? Brilliant! And kudos to you for taking that step. Now we are going to build off that work and ultimately make the changes stick. We're not going to focus on weight loss, but on creating a new body composition that centers on *fat loss and muscle gain*. This isn't about a fad or overly restrictive diet. It's about giving you the right nutritional tools that will help improve how you feel in your body, boost your energy levels, and yes, likely change the number on the scale too."

Before diving into the nutritional strategies that I wanted Christina to use daily, I also challenged her to reframe her weight loss journey to a *fat loss journey*.

The two words—weight and fat—often get used interchangeably, but there is a huge difference in what they represent. Your body weight, that number you see on the scale, includes all parts of you—fat, muscle, bone, water, etc. When you embark on a weight loss journey, what you really desire is fat loss. As you build muscle, especially if you are strength training, the number on the scale may not go down at all—it could even go up—but your body composition will be better and your health, well-being, and energy will improve. On the other hand, if your body weight goes down due to muscle loss, it's not healthy or desirable.

The focus should be on losing excess fat and gaining lean muscle. You can set a fat loss goal, say losing 25 or more pounds, and you can use a scale as a tool, checking in to ensure you're headed in the right direction toward a healthier body composition. I also encourage you to use other tools to help gauge your fat loss journey and body composition. When we lose fat, our body reshapes itself, so notice how your clothes fit around your waist, hips, arms, and legs. Also, pay attention to your energy levels like if you wake up feeling more energized and can go longer during the day without feeling like you need a nap. Note your moods and how you feel, including being happier, more patient, or more peaceful. These are all important indicators that you're moving toward a healthier body composition.

Eat Enough Protein

Want to kick-start fat loss and optimize energy? Then make protein your best friend. Protein is the *only* macronutrient (carbs and fats are the others) that supports lean muscle growth, maintenance, and repair.

High-protein diets also tend to squash hunger better than carbs or fats.[42] When our bodies digest or break down protein, amino acids are left, which get absorbed by different organs, muscles, and tissues throughout the body and are used for various functions, including the satiety centers of the brain that help regulate our appetites. Amino acids also help reduce the pleasure response (also found in the brain) that we get when we eat, leaving us less motivated to consume more food.

As a final benefit, protein requires the most energy of the three macronutrients to digest relative to the energy it provides.[43] We call this *diet-induced thermogenesis*.

When it comes to dropping excess fat, there have been numerous investigations on this subject and the role that protein plays. For example, in 2012 Thomas Wycherley from the University of South Australia published a meta-analysis aggregating data from 23 interventions. He found that consuming 1.1 to 1.6 g/kg (0.5 to 0.7 g/lb) of protein led to more fat loss, less muscle loss, greater satiety, and a lesser reduction in metabolic rate compared to eating less protein each day.[44] Furthermore, a meta-analysis was done of 20 studies looking exclusively at adults over 50 years old.[45] Again, consuming 1.1 to 1.6 g/kg (0.5 to 0.7 g/lb) of protein led to more fat loss and less muscle loss compared to eating less protein. In fact, 80 percent of the higher-protein group lost more than 70 percent of their weight as fat mass, compared to only 50 percent of the lower protein group.

Finally, a meta-analysis involving 74 studies found that eating a diet higher in protein has been found to significantly reduce several cardiometabolic risk factors, including waist circumference, blood pressure, and triglyceride levels, while also increasing satiety.[46]

The Ultimate Protein Guide

When I talk about increasing your protein, I'm not suggesting throwing back pounds of fatty bacon or sausage.

At first, when you're just starting your fat loss journey, and if you aren't physically active (which is okay, for now), you want to aim to eat about 1.1 to 1.6 g/kg (0.5 to 0.7 g/lb) of protein every day. If you eat three meals per day, then this is obtainable by having 3 ounces of cooked meat at each meal plus 0.5 to 1 cup of cooked beans. Of course, dairy and soy products, eggs, and grains also supply protein. You want to aim for higher protein, not high fat. Options include chicken; turkey; grass-fed beef or bison; fish, including tuna, snapper, and salmon; dairy products like hard and soft cheeses (in moderation) or plain yogurt; seeds; nuts, including nut butters like peanut or almond; beans; and some grains.

Once you've reached a healthier body mass and weight, and are more physically active, then you'll want to up that protein intake to about 1.6 to 2.2 g/kg (0.7 to 1.0 g/lb) per day.[47,48] This will help with repairing muscle damage from working out (this isn't a bad thing but what builds strength) and maintaining your muscles.[49]

Eat Protein at Every Meal

It's not just that we want to eat enough protein every day; it's that we want to eat it at *every meal*. Eating protein at every meal is critical because it stimulates *muscle protein synthesis* (MPS), a naturally occurring process in which protein in our muscles is produced to help repair any tissue damage, which leads to stronger and leaner muscle mass.

To figure out how much protein we need to eat per meal, Dr. Stuart Phillips from McMaster University in Ontario, Canada, aggregated the data of six studies and found that most young adults could maximize MPS with 0.4 g/kg of whey protein, while older adults (50-plus years) required upward of 0.6 g/kg.[50] To put that in perspective, it equates to a 176 lb (or 80 kg) young adult eating 32 grams, or an older adult eating 48 grams of protein per meal.

As you consider how much protein to eat with each meal, a solid rule is to aim for a minimum of 0.4 to 0.6 g/kg. You can certainly eat more protein, especially as you age.

Aging tends to cause our muscles to become less responsive to the anabolic effects of eating,[51] which is why older adults need more protein to max out the MPS signal at every meal.

But even if we maximize muscle protein synthesis, we need additional protein so that protein synthesis in other areas of the body, like the gut and immune cells, will work properly.

For Christina, I knew upping her protein intake would be a huge factor in kick-starting more fat loss and building leaner muscle. Her initial weight was about 165 lbs (or 75 kg), so our goal was getting Christina to eat about 120 grams of protein per day (aiming for 1.6 g/kg).

To keep it simple, her target was to eat *at least 30 grams of protein with every meal.*

I didn't want Christina to be overly restrictive in her protein sources, but instead to choose foods she enjoyed eating. For breakfast, Christina would eat a pumpkin spirulina bowl with crunchy clove granola. Because she had young kids, she also often made baked egg dishes loaded with vegetables and topped with a little cheese that she could quickly reheat in the morning. Lunch was often a big salad with protein, and dinner would be snapper filets over cauliflower mash and crispy kale, wild salmon over brown rice, or pulled chicken with roasted vegetable salad, topped with raisins and cilantro.

Whether they are animal or plant-based, it doesn't matter what protein sources you use; just make sure you incorporate them into every meal. Pick ones that you know you'll eat, that are easy (and fun) to prepare, that fit into your budget and schedule, and that you're likely to stick with.

When cooking meats, poultry, and seafood, you want to use gentle cooking methods such as steaming, boiling, braising, baking, or pressure cooking. This is because potentially harmful chemicals form when these foods are cooked with more aggressive methods such as grilling over an open flame, broiling, and smoking.

Another trick—regardless of the cooking method you use—is to cook with spices, herbs, ginger, garlic, and turmeric, or to use marinades made with olive oil, lemon juice, and/or vinegar. These ingredients can inhibit harmful chemical compounds and sometimes prevent them from forming.

Protein for Vegetarians and Vegans

So far we've mostly discussed animal protein, but I know many people eat a vegetarian or vegan diet or rely more heavily on plant foods. This is not a judgment about what diet is better. I'm for the one that helps you feel the best and promotes optimal health.

However, vegetarians and vegans still do need to pay attention to where they get their protein.[52] Most plant sources of protein, such as legumes and grains, come with quite a few calories for the protein they provide. If you're trying to restrict calories (to some degree, not severely), then this can be problematic. You may overeat, thus destroying any fat loss benefits the higher protein can provide and possibly gaining more fat.

The other challenge facing plant-based diets is that humans simply don't digest protein nutrients from whole plants as well as we do from animals. Animal-based proteins consistently demonstrate a digestibility rate higher than 90 percent, whereas proteins from the best plant-based sources (legumes and grains) show a digestibility rate of 60 to 80 percent.[53]

The lower digestibility in plants is due to compounds called *antinutrients* that prevent protein digestion and absorption, such as trypsin inhibitors, phytates, and tannins.[54] While cooking does reduce antinutrient concentrations, it doesn't eliminate them

entirely. None of this means that antinutrients and the plants containing them are harmful (in fact, there is much research showing
so-called "antinutrients" like phytic acid are actually very *beneficial* to health), only that the protein isn't as available for our bodies to digest as is the protein found in animal products.

If you are vegan, eat a heavily plant-based diet, or are struggling to eat enough protein while on a mixed diet that includes
animal products, consider using plant-based protein powders.[55] In
the case of plant-based protein powders, the protein is extracted
from plants and doesn't supply a lot of extra calories from carbohydrates or fats that would occur in whole plants. Plus, the
processing methods used to create plant-based protein powders
destroy antinutrients and increase the protein's bioavailability to
levels seen in animal products. They are easy to consume and can
be mixed into smoothies or other foods like oatmeal or yogurt, or
just taken straight with water.

DIGESTIBILITY OF PROTEIN FROM PLANT- AND ANIMAL-BASED PROTEIN POWDERS

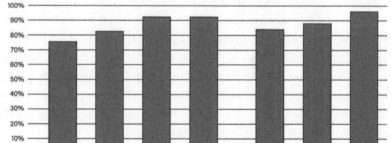

However, if you're looking to get your protein from whole
plants, then consider prioritizing high-protein sources like a variety of soy products (edamame, tempeh, tofu, etc.) and cooked
legumes such as lentils, split peas, and your favorite type of bean.

Other modest protein sources include cooked grains such as amaranth, quinoa, oat bran, wild rice, oatmeal, and buckwheat.

Load Up on Fibrous Vegetables

Now that we've increased your protein intake, it's time to talk about vegetables. Yes, you still need them. Not only are they a rich source of nutrition but they are also full of fiber and water, which can help keep your appetite in check[56] by stretching your stomach and delaying its emptying.[57]

Research shows that simply eating a salad at the start of a meal can reduce caloric intake for the entire meal because people eat less of the higher-calorie foods.[58] It's not an insignificant amount either—11 percent fewer calories. Quite simply, the salad takes up room in the stomach, so you reach satiation more quickly.

The *volumetrics diet* is based on the satiating properties of high-fiber, high-water foods. When overweight women were told to follow this diet by eating more fruits and vegetables while reducing fat, they experienced less hunger and 23 percent more weight loss than the control group who had only been instructed to eat less fat-rich food.[59]

Fibrous Vegetables				
Artichokes	Cabbage	Dandelion greens	Mushrooms	Spinach
Arugula	Cauliflower	Eggplant	Mustard greens	Summer squash
Asparagus	Celery	Garlic	Okra	Tomatoes
Beet greens	Chard	Green beans	Onions	Turnip greens
Bok choy	Chives	Kale	Pea sprouts	Watercress
Broccoli	Collard greens	Leek	Peppers	Zucchini

Christina's diet already included lots of vegetables, and lunch was typically a big salad. For her, this was a simple shift. I suggested she just add more fibrous vegetables and not stress about the "right ones" but rather have fun trying some new ones. I suggested she pick vegetables that were easy to get at her local grocery store and that would be simple to prepare. None of these strategies need be expensive or time consuming, so opt for starting with the "low-hanging fruit," adding the sources that are easiest and affordable.

You want to eat a big helping of fibrous vegetables at each meal. You can make smoothies and juices too, but they can't be a replacement for the whole-food form.

Eat Whole Foods

A diet based around high-protein foods and vegetables feeds perfectly into the next dietary strategy for optimizing your body composition: eating a diet based around whole, minimally processed foods. I know: this idea has been around forever. But a tremendous amount of research supports its importance.

When it comes to the obesity epidemic, overeating is the biggest driver. And what do we tend to overeat? Processed foods like doughnuts, pastries, ice cream, and pizza. Why? Because they taste good. As they were designed to.

Every time we crunch a chip or pop a pretzel into our mouths, we're biting into hyper-palatable calorie bombs that are rich in sugar, refined grains, fat, salt, and flavorings. It isn't far-fetched to say that we no longer eat to live; we live to eat.

Of all the research on animals done to date, feeding them a cafeteria diet, where they have access to a seemingly endless variety of food flavors, has been proven the most surefire way to fatten them. The animals simply can't stop eating; they don't get full.

This diet promotes voluntary hyperphagia (aka overeating) that results in rapid weight gain, increased fat mass, and metabolic disturbances such as insulin resistance and glucose intolerance.[60] The cafeteria diet also engages hedonic feeding, or eating for pleasure, which produces long-lasting neuronal alterations that favor body fat gain.[61]

When researchers put overweight men and women on a bland liquid diet within the research center at Columbia University, they started losing weight rapidly.[62] Even though they could eat as much as they wanted, they ate almost nothing, no more than 500 calories per day, on average—all without hunger.

A Word about "Processed"

The definition of "processed" food can be confusing. I've seen some people immediately default to "anything processed is bad," but that's not entirely true. For example, technically both dough-nuts and spirulina are "processed." However, they have vastly different effects on the body. Spirulina is a blue-green algae powder supplement that contains nutrients such as vitamins E and B, anti-oxidants, and beta-carotene, and it's used to fight fatigue, stimulate the immune system, and help people lose weight. Doughnuts, on the other hand, are possibly one of the worst foods you could regularly eat.

Almost all beneficial supplements are highly "processed," but they may be—and often are—perfectly compatible with health or even extremely beneficial to improving our well-being.

In another study, for two weeks participants ate a diet based on processed foods and then for two weeks ate unprocessed foods, or vice versa, with each diet divided across three daily meals plus snacks. The diets were matched for their calorie density and macronutrient content, and the participants were instructed to eat as much as they wanted. When the researchers looked at what occurred during each diet period for both groups, they found that participants eating the processed diet gained two pounds, while participants on the unprocessed diet lost two pounds. The researchers determined calorie intake to be the determining factor in the differences. When folks were on the processed diet, they ate significantly more calories—about 500 extra per day, on average—than when they were on the unprocessed diet.

Yet despite this difference in calorie intake, there weren't any differences between the diets in feelings of hunger or fullness, meaning that the processed diet required more food and calories to achieve the same level of satiety as the unprocessed group.[63]

To get an accurate read on what Christina was eating, I had her track what she ate for a week. She was already using a restricted-calorie diet, so this was easy information to collect. While she did not rely heavily on processed foods, Christina did turn to quick, mostly processed, zero or 100-calorie snack foods once or twice per day.

Although these foods were technically low in calories, they weren't high in nutritious value either, so I wanted to flip that. On Christina's next shopping trip, I suggested that she stock up on snack-size vegetable packs of carrots, celery, cauliflower, broccoli, or snap peas and experiment with different dips like hummus, guacamole, black or white bean spread, tomato salsa, or nut butters. I also suggested she start using one cup of Greek yogurt or cottage cheese topped with some berries or other fruit as snacks. Both yogurt and cottage cheese offer protein punches that would help her meet her goals and satiate her between meals. Protein bars and jerky can also be viable alternatives, as long as they are not loaded with sugar or additives.

Stop Grazing

When it comes to shedding excess fat and building lean muscle, science tells us that eating two to three, or three to four meals per day (depending on your eating window) offers you the most benefit. That's because eating meals with a break in between stimulates muscle growth.

Research has shown that consuming protein every three hours is better at stimulating muscle protein synthesis throughout the day than consuming smaller amounts of protein every hour and a half or larger amounts every six hours.[64]

This is contrary to the belief in some health, fitness, and wellness circles that the best way to eat for fat loss or muscle gain is five to seven small meals per day.

It can take up to five hours for us to digest a large meal, so a good goal is to try to eat every three to five hours depending on your eating window. This works out to two to three meals in a six- to eight-hour eating window, or three to four meals within an eight- to ten-hour window.

Christina tended to eat smaller meals throughout the day, often on the run. Wanting to get her into more structured meals, we started with a ten-hour time-restricted feeding window that had four meals every three to four hours.

This took some getting used to for Christina, so I suggested that if she got hungry between meals, she should add an extra snack in the morning and/or afternoon. This will vary from person to person. If you're used to grazing, it can take a couple of weeks for your body to acclimate to a different schedule, so just be consistent, stick with it, and gradually move yourself toward eating just meals.

If you're eating enough protein at every meal and loading up on fibrous vegetables, then that should also help get you from meal to meal. If you're still ravenous a couple of hours after a meal, then review your meals to make sure you're getting adequate nutrients, especially protein.

Increase Your Energy Flux

You've probably heard the saying *eat less, move more*.

But eating less food can be hard, especially if you're inactive or have a small physique and are already working with a reduced calorie budget. In this instance, eating less food means that you run a greater risk of not getting all the nutrients you need to be healthy and energized.

So let's change the saying to: *eat more, move more*.

This is the basis of *energy flux*, which is the sum of the energy we burn daily, plus the energy we get from food. Studies show that the people who are best able to maintain significant amounts of fat loss do so by maintaining a higher energy flux.[65]

Consider these scenarios:

- 3,000 calories out − 2,500 calories in = 500-calorie deficit

- 2,000 calories out − 1,500 calories in = 500-calorie deficit

Both scenarios have the same daily energy deficit of 500 calories, but the first scenario has a *higher* energy flux (5,500 vs. 3,500 calories). Maintaining a high energy flux does wonders for fat loss because it increases your resting metabolic rate (RMR), reduces your appetite, and lowers the chances that you will overconsume food.

When we start losing fat, hormone concentrations change, as do gut peptides, body weight, and nervous system activity. Although you want to lose fat, your body reads the loss as something "bad," so it slows down your RMR. As your body attempts to regain the weight you lost, your appetite will increase while your energy level will decrease. However, several studies have shown that increasing energy flux can help stop your RMR from slowing down in response to dieting.[66,67,68,69] In one study, obese adults lost 7 percent of their body weight over several months and then spent three weeks staying at their reduced body weight while in either a high- or low-flux state.[70] Participants in the high-flux condition burned an extra 500 calories each day through exercise while also eating an extra 500 calories to make up for it. Not only were their RMR and fat oxidation greater but hunger was lower too.

I know that moving more can be difficult when you don't have a lot of energy. This was a challenge for Christina, who had very little "extra" to give in her life. At first we worked on Christina keeping it simple, adding a 20- to 30-minute walk three to four times per week. Christina found it easier to split her time, so she would go for a 15-minute walk at lunch and then another when she got home or after dinner. Sometimes Christina's husband would watch the kids while she got some "Christina time," but it soon became a family outing, with her husband and kids joining.

For Christina, walking was the perfect activity, but you may decide you want to add more physical activity like strength or resistance training, yoga, hiking, biking, swimming, or jogging to your daily routine (if you haven't already). Research also shows exercise boosts our energy levels.[71] And when you take individuals with chronic pain and have them start a resistance training program, they fatigue less easily, their strength increases, they have less pain, and they feel healthier.[72]

Because increasing our energy flux and being physically active can boost fat loss and improve lean muscle mass, it's something I strongly support for your overall health benefits—physical, mental, and emotional. However, if you're extremely fatigued and/or your schedule or life keeps you hopping from the moment you wake to the time you close your eyes, adding physical activity may be difficult. That's okay. You can look for small areas where you can add extra steps, like parking farther away from a store entrance or walking up and down your stairs more often at home.

And if reaching high energy flux doesn't work now, then focus on supplying your body with the right nutrients—that's something anyone can do at any time in their lives and at any fatigue level on their energy-enhancing journey. It's all about gradually building up the *eat more, move more* mindset.

Ditch the "Perfect" Diet

Christina was committed to increasing her protein intake and believed it was achievable. But she also wanted to know what the best diet was for losing fat.

Like many people, Christina had tried all the top diets and found early success with each, but nothing stuck. I told Christina what I told everyone: "I don't care what diet you follow. You can use keto, paleo, a mixed balance of animal protein and plants, Mediterranean, low-fat omnivorous, low glycemic, vegetarian, or vegan—they all work as long as you stick with making sure you're

eating enough protein, and at every meal, and you're eating minimally processed, real food, mostly plants."

My advice isn't based on anecdotal evidence but actual findings from Dr. David Katz and his colleagues at Yale School of Medicine. Dr. Katz conducted one of the most important studies in the
history of nutritional science, noteworthy for its breadth, depth,
diversity of methods, and consistency of findings.

In "Can We Say What Diet Is Best for Health?" Dr. Katz and his
team reviewed hundreds of scientific studies on the health effects
of different dietary patterns, including mixed balance, low fat,
low carb, low glycemic, Mediterranean, paleo, and vegetarian and
vegan.[73] While they concluded there are not enough head-to-head
dietary trials comparing the different diets to make any determi-
nation of what is the healthiest, they did find that the healthiest
diets consisted of:

- Minimally processed foods and foods direct
  from nature

- Mostly plants

- Animal products from animals that ate as natural a
  diet as possible, as would be found in wild settings
  (e.g., wild caught fish, pastured cattle and poultry,
  and milk and eggs from pastured animals)

I could tell Christina was taken aback by what I said. When
you're used to following a specific diet, it can feel scary to have
fewer restrictions. But once you eat this way for a few weeks, and
then a few months, you can gradually retrain your mind to not
fear food.

MAKING THE CHANGES STICK

After about two months of using these nutritional strategies,
Christina lost about 1.5 pounds per week, for a total of 12 pounds.
She had exceeded her initial movement goal and was walking five

to six times per week for 30 to 45 minutes. Then she was ready to add resistance training into weekly movement. She didn't have much experience in this area, so I encouraged her to join a local gym that was welcoming, encouraging, and inclusive of people at all stages of their body composition journey and experience, and to work with a professional who would help create a program and teach her the proper form.

Overall Christina found incorporating the nutritional strategies easy, but she wasn't used to eating as much protein, nor was she used to eating three to four times per day. It took more meal planning and prep to ensure Christina ate enough protein. For her, it helped to pick one night to plan all her meals for the week rather than decide what she was eating each day.

There was also a psychological shift she had to make as she increased her food intake. "Slow and steady, that is the secret," I told Christina. "I know you want to see the number on the scale continue going down, *and* this is about creating healthier eating habits that will stay with you for the long haul."

As you incorporate some of the nutritional strategies in this chapter, keep in mind that you are not a victim of the circumstances that have led to an unhealthy body composition. You can choose to change at any moment.

You have the power.

Your health and body composition are in your hands. You have the control over how your life plays out from this moment forward.

Meet yourself where you are. Give yourself time. Fuel your temple with lots of protein, minimally processed whole foods, and fibrous vegetables, and add physical activity into your daily life as you can. You can implement positive, lasting change, and it will affect your energy levels for the better.

ACTION LIST

The following checklist will help you start on your energy healing journey through losing fat and building muscle. Like last time, pick one to two items to work into your life today that you feel you can start implementing immediately. After a couple of weeks, or when those actions become habitual, level up or pick one or two more.

If you find you can work more than two into your lifestyle, that's fine. Just don't overwhelm yourself. Your body composition can't change in a day. Take your time.

Each task has a primary goal with three to four smaller stepping-stone goals beneath it. Establishing new habits often requires baby steps in the right direction. Start with the first stepping-stone and work your way down before checking off the primary goal box.

- ☐ **Ensure that your diet is providing you with adequate protein daily.**
  - ☐ Calculate your ideal protein intake and eat it 1 to 2 days per week.
  - ☐ Eat sufficient protein 3 to 4 days per week.
  - ☐ Eat sufficient protein 5 to 6 days per week.
  - ☐ Eat sufficient protein every day.

- ☐ **Eat sufficient protein at every meal.**
  - ☐ Calculate your ideal protein intake per meal and eat at least that amount at 1 meal per day.
  - ☐ Eat sufficient protein at 2 meals per day.
  - ☐ Eat sufficient protein at every meal.

- ☐ **Minimize snacking and reduce your meal frequency.**
  - ☐ Eat 2 to 4 meals per day plus 2 to 3 snacks (including caloric beverages).
  - ☐ Eat 2 to 4 meals per day plus 1 to 2 snacks (including caloric beverages).

☐ Eat 2 to 4 meals per day with zero snacking (including caloric beverages).

☐ **Eat a diet based on mostly whole foods.**

 ☐ Eat 1 meal per day that is prepared from scratch and/or contains only minimally processed ingredients that you could find in nature.

 ☐ Eat 2 meals per day that are prepared from scratch and/or contain only minimally processed ingredients that you could find in nature.

 ☐ On 3 to 4 days per week, eat only meals that are prepared from scratch and/or contain only minimally processed ingredients that you could find in nature.

 ☐ On 5 to 6 days per week, eat only meals that are prepared from scratch and/or contain only minimally processed ingredients that you could find in nature.

☐ **Eat a diet based on fibrous vegetables.**

 ☐ Consume fibrous vegetables with 1 meal per day.

 ☐ Consume fibrous vegetables with 2 meals per day.

 ☐ Consume fibrous vegetables with every meal.

CHAPTER 4

REBUILDING THE GUT BARRIER TO KEEP FATIGUE AT BAY

Think about how your stomach feels.

Do you struggle with diarrhea? Constipation? Nausea? Do certain foods send it screeching?

If you said yes to any of these questions, welcome to the world of poor gut health. It's a world most of us live in but few people think about, yet the connection between odd stomach ailments and fatigue is very real.

When Nick first joined my program, he told me, "After I hit my thirties, my health started to decline precipitously. I had energy problems, joint issues, depression, and skin problems, to name a few. I relied on caffeine strategically spaced throughout the day just to keep going, but even that isn't working any longer."

Nick said he had made every reasonable effort to improve his health—a variety of diets, supplements, and exercise strategies. He got some results from each, but he confessed, "I feel less sick, but I'm nowhere near feeling optimal or healthy."

When I dug more deeply into Nick's background, I discovered that throughout his life he had cycled through bouts of constipation and loose stools, felt bloated and became gassy after most meals, and most days, had a low-level stomach discomfort. He had assumed these issues were normal, but in fact they were a sign that his gut had been compromised and needed healing.

UNLOCKING THE MYSTERIES OF YOUR GUT MICROBIOME

"All disease begins in the gut," said the ancient Greek physician and philosopher Hippocrates 2,500 years ago. While I don't 100 percent agree with this statement—disease can begin in other places and then can cause gut issues, thus creating a vicious cycle of dysfunction—Hippocrates was onto something.

Today we have a large body of research demonstrating a link between our gut health and the health of various organ systems throughout the body, including:

- Brain[1]
- Liver[2]
- Muscles[3]
- Fat cells[4]
- Bones[5]
- Joints[6]
- Lungs[7]

Studies also show that when our gut health becomes compromised, it can lead to other serious chronic issues,[8] such as:

- Obesity[9]
- Diabetes[10,11]
- Cardiovascular diseases[12]
- Neurodegenerative diseases[13]
- Frailty with aging[14]

The health of your gut has everything to do with the health of your *gut microbiome*, which is made up of trillions of microorganisms—viruses, microbes, and (mostly) bacteria—living in your digestive system. Within your large intestine alone exist about 40 trillion microorganisms—a number roughly equal to every cell in your body—most of which are bacteria.[15]

A healthy microbiome provides for three primary functions:[16]

1. Providing an abundance of metabolic pathways that ultimately foster a stable, mutually beneficial relationship (i.e., does a bunch of biochemistry that benefits us)

2. Self-regulating its growth and preventing the colonization of pathogens (i.e., lots of different bacteria don't let any one group outgrow the others and develop a stronghold)

3. Resisting harm and returning to a healthy state after exposure to harm (i.e., isn't excessively perturbed in response to pathogen or toxicant exposure and recovers to its previous healthy state after antibiotic exposure)

Although everyone has their own personal blend of bacteria due to genetics, lifestyle, and the environment,[17] it's the microbial *diversity* that determines the health of our microbiome. We categorize the organisms as good (beneficial) or bad (pathogenic).

The beneficial organisms play critical roles in helping us remain healthy, improving our metabolism and nutrient production, and educating our immune system. These bacteria help us break down the food we eat into the vitamins, minerals, and macronutrients that our mitochondria use to create the ATP that fuels our organs, muscles, and tissues. Everyone has some harmful pathogens (bacterial and viral) living in their microbiome. As long as the microbiome stays healthy, the harmful pathogens are kept in check by the beneficial bacteria that compete for resources.

But when something upsets the wondrous microbiome diversity—whether a toxin or toxicant (such as most pollutants, endocrine disruptors, heavy metal contaminants, etc.), life stress, antibiotics, or not enough fiber—that balance can become disrupted and the bad bacteria can multiply in number beyond what the beneficial bacteria can keep in check. As the bad bacteria increase in number, they take over, colonizing the microbiome and leading to a cascade of health issues and fatigue.

THE GUT-MITOCHONDRIA LINK

Researchers are finding links between the health of our microbiomes and energy levels, particularly with regard to chronic fatigue syndrome.[18] And it has become clear that people with chronic fatigue have:

- Lower microbial diversity
- Fewer bacteria known to pump out beneficial metabolites like short-chain fatty acids (SCFAs), needed to make ATP
- More bacteria known to release harmful inflammatory metabolites like endotoxins

In fact, the researchers found that a computer program could predict *with 90 percent accuracy* whether someone had chronic fatigue syndrome based exclusively on their microbiome composition and the concentration of inflammatory molecules in their blood.

Leaky Gut and Inflammation

Gut dysbiosis is the state of bacteria imbalance in our microbiome that has been linked to a very problematic condition known as *leaky gut* (intestinal permeability).

When healthy bacteria decrease and harmful bacteria surge, the harmful ones produce more inflammatory, carcinogenic, and genotoxic molecules than the microbiome and immune system can handle, which creates inflammation and dysfunction of our intestinal lining[19,20]—the barrier between our gut, bloodstream, and the rest of our body.

Our digestive system works synergistically with our microbiome to break down the food we eat into the nutrients we need to function, like vitamins and minerals. When those molecules are small enough, they pass through our gut lining and get absorbed into our bloodstream. These molecules then get delivered to the trillions of cells where our mitochondria are waiting for them.

Our gut lining acts as a protective barrier to keep foreign molecules out of our bloodstream: those harmful bacteria, viruses, microbes, undigested food molecules, toxic by-products generated by harmful bacteria, and other compounds that live in the gut and should stay in the gut (or get sent on for elimination).

When we lose microbial diversity, our gut lining can develop holes or cracks: hence the name leaky gut. When this happens, foreign molecules can leak through the gut lining, get absorbed into our bloodstream, and be carried to various organs, tissues, and cells in our body.

Our immune system—our threat detector and bodily defender—then kicks into high gear to try to eliminate them. A natural by-product of this immune response is inflammation, meaning that having a leaky gut becomes another source of chronic low-grade inflammation,[21,22] damaging your mitochondria and leading to their dysfunction and reduced energy output.

The riled-up immune system also explains why leaky gut has been so strongly linked to the development and perpetuation of autoimmune diseases including:[23,24,25]

- Crohn's disease
- Ulcerative colitis
- Type 1 diabetes
- Celiac disease
- Multiple sclerosis
- Hashimoto's thyroiditis

Autoimmunity involves an overactive immune system. So if you have a leaky gut and foreign molecules have been passing through your gut lining and getting absorbed into your bloodstream causing constant inflammation for years, then the link between poor gut health and autoimmune disease becomes very clear to see.

Intestinal Mucosal Barrier Breakdown

One of the most important components of the gut barrier is a thick layer of mucus rich in immune cells and antimicrobial peptides, which help protect against bacteria, fungi, viruses, and parasites. This mucus layer acts as a barrier between our gut bacteria and gut lining, and it prevents the uncontrolled absorption of pro-inflammatory endotoxins and antigens[26,27]—which stimulate harmful inflammatory responses.

Despite being a barrier against gut microbes, the mucosal layer relies quite heavily on them for proper development. For example, sterilization of the gut (e.g., killing off the microbiome) leads to a thinned and weakened mucus lining,[28] which can be reversed upon colonization with a healthy microbiome.[29]

A similar observation has been made when, instead of no microbiome, one has the wrong type of microbiome. The carbohydrate-rich mucus lining provides a valuable food source for many types of bacteria that exist within our microbiome.[30,31] Normally, bacteria eating the mucus layer isn't problematic—our body replenishes any lost mucus throughout the day.

But this becomes an issue when the microbes eat the mucus layer at a faster rate than our body can produce it. When our microbiome is unbalanced, or if we're not eating the right foods to sustain our microbes, they will turn to this mucus membrane to fortify themselves. This contributes to intestinal inflammation and leaky gut.[32,33] It also reduces the abundance of bacteria like *Bifidobacterium*, which help build up a strong mucus lining.[34]

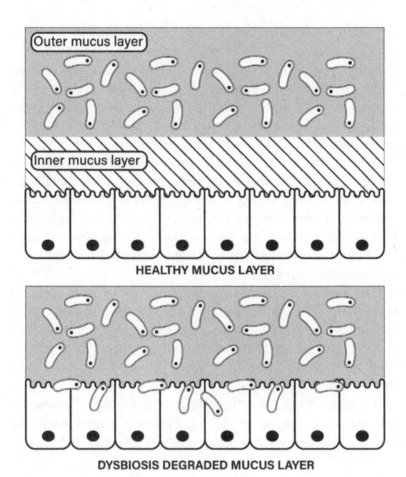

HEALTHY MUCUS LAYER

DYSBIOSIS DEGRADED MUCUS LAYER

Short-Chain Fatty Acids Shortage

When we lack beneficial bacteria, our gut cannot produce important energy-related metabolites such as acetate, propionate, and butyrate (all short-chain fatty acids) or urolithin A.

SCFAs help regulate a variety of processes and systems in the body that have beneficial effects on our metabolism, appetite, body composition, and immune function.[35] They are some of the best sources for energy production, better than other fatty acids.[36] SCFAs such as butyrate can freely enter mitochondria without the need for chaperone proteins or transporters. They simply waltz into the mitochondria and stimulate the processes necessary for energy production.[37] This is particularly helpful when the mitochondria are dysfunctional, which is often the case with chronic fatigue. In particular, butyrate increases mitochondrial energy production and the ability to use fat as an energy source within the liver and skeletal muscle, leading to protection against the development of fatty liver and insulin resistance.[38,39,40]

Within the gut SCFAs also nourish our intestinal cells, regulate the activation of anticancer genes and cell death signals, and help maintain the integrity of our intestinal barrier. Studies show that without a microbiome, intestinal cells suffer from mitochondrial dysfunction and are starved of energy, but when cells are provided with only pure butyrate, mitochondria are restored to near-normal function.[41]

The microbiome produces an abundance of molecules, and while SCFAs are the most plentiful and important for our health and energy, urolithin A also deserves special mention. Urolithin A is produced by beneficial bacteria in the gut when they metabolize ellagitannin phytochemicals present in certain fruits, berries, and nuts, particularly pomegranates.[42]

Urolithin A is a powerful inducer of mitophagy, helping prevent the accumulation of old and damaged mitochondria that contribute to oxidative stress, metabolic disease, and reduced energy levels.

Excessive Endotoxin Absorption

When certain bacteria die, they release endotoxins, which are incredibly inflammatory molecules. When endotoxins seep through your gut lining and get absorbed into your bloodstream, they cause a ton of damage. For example, the endotoxin lipopolysaccharide (LPS) is the most prominent "alarm molecule" sensed by our immune system as an early warning for infection. When LPS gets into the bloodstream, it causes a powerful immune response, even if an infection never materializes.[43,44] This results in a lot of inflammation—and if it's happening constantly, then you're getting hit by massive amounts of it.

Endotoxins are also powerful disrupters of mitochondrial function.[45] When mitochondria get exposed to endotoxins like LPS, it increases oxidative stress, disrupts mitochondrial membrane stability, causes DNA fragmentation and cell death, and strongly inhibits energy production.[46,47,48,49] One study showed that chronic fatigue patients have significantly elevated blood concentrations of bacterial endotoxins.[50]

GUT HEALTH ISSUES

- Increased gut permeability
- Dysbiosis in the gut

LEAD TO...

MINOR PHYSIOLOGICAL CHANGES

- Increased endotoxin absorption
- Leaky gut
- Immune over-activation and elevated markers of inflammation

RESULTING IN...

MAJOR PHYSIOLOGICAL CHANGES

- Mitochondrial dysfunction/shut down
- Toxin accumulation
- Cellular damage
- Leaky blood-brain barrier
- Hormonal disruption
- Neurotransmitter imbalances

WHICH ULTIMATELY CAUSE...

EXTERNAL SYMPTOMS AND EFFECTS

- Lethargy and fatigue
- Brain fog and poor cognitive function
- Mood changes
- Heightened anxiety
- Increased risk of depression
- Poor sleep

Essential Nutrient Deficiencies

Food is fuel. Literally. Our digestive system breaks down what we eat into the vitamins, minerals, and macronutrients we need to survive, and our mitochondria need them to make energy. But when we're struggling with dysbiosis and leaky gut, it can predispose us to nutrient deficiencies through several ways:[51]

- Avoidance of certain foods or food groups because they cause discomfort
- Increased nutrient losses from conditions such as diarrhea
- Reduced nutrient absorption from a damaged or inflamed intestinal tract
- Increased nutrient requirements for intestinal repair
- Increased nutrient excretion from medications used to alleviate intestinal discomfort and symptoms

Studies have found that adults with chronic fatigue syndrome tend to have lower levels of vitamins and minerals including vitamin D, vitamin E, and magnesium[52]—all critically important for optimal cellular energy production. None of this is to say that you personally have nutrient absorption problems, only that it is a possible (and common) link between poor gut health and fatigue.

REBUILDING YOUR GUT WITH NUTRITION

In my experience, everyone with severe chronic fatigue has some gut rebuilding to do. Gut issues are that prevalent. The good news is that what you eat, along with other nutritional strategies, can help you make significant strides toward repairing and restoring your microbiome diversity. In fact, studies have shown that using nutrition and supplementation to repair the gut of chronic fatigue patients often results in dramatically improved energy levels.[53]

As you incorporate new foods, pay close attention to how your body responds to certain foods. Notice if what you eat makes you feel bloated or gassy, gives you an upset stomach, or causes any gastrointestinal upset. If you can, release any expectation as to how your body will react and adopt an experimental attitude where you're open to trying new foods, assessing the results, and tweaking, as necessary.

Enjoy More Prebiotic Fibers

Fiber is your friend.

It's not that your organs or tissues need it; it's for your beneficial bacteria. They feast on it. Fiber is what strengthens them, multiplies their numbers, and allows them to do the hard work of digesting food and eliminating waste.

But most of us, especially in the Western world, are not feeding our beneficial bacteria—we're starving them, and in turn destroying the rich diversity we need in our microbiome. The average American barely consumes *16 grams* of fiber on a typical day.[54] This is a dramatic drop from the fiber consumption of our Paleolithic ancestors, who are estimated to have eaten a daily average of *45 grams* (with variations depending on season and geographical location).[55]

In modern times, indigenous societies have vastly more microbial diversity than other human cultures, where there is a clear trend toward reduced microbiome diversity as diets become more and more Westernized. This is due in large part to the drastically different intake of plants.[56]

The Western diet is abysmally low in the fruits and vegetables that provide the *prebiotic fibers* and *phytochemicals* that are key to growing beneficial bacteria. This has massive consequences for our gut health, our risk of numerous diseases, and our energy levels.

The solution is clear: eat more fiber, especially prebiotic fibers.

These are most beneficial for the gut, stimulating the growth and proliferation of exclusively beneficial bacteria that produce energy-enhancing SCFAs and other molecules critically important for mitochondrial health like urolithin A. One study found that men and women who increased their fiber intake from an average of 18 grams per day up to 30 grams per day for two weeks saw an increased concentration of the beneficial bacteria genus *Bifidobacterium* by over threefold.[57] While different kinds of prebiotic fibers stimulate the growth of different beneficial bacteria, most offer similar health benefits, like improving metabolic health, stimulating satiety, enhancing immune function, and strengthening gut barrier integrity.[58,59,60]

Best Sources of Prebiotic Fiber		
Absolute Best	Great	Good
Artichokes	Cardoon	Endive
Jerusalem artichokes	Leeks	Spaghetti squash
Salsify	Peppers	Pumpkin
Onions	Carrots	Zucchini
		Brussels sprouts
		Cauliflower

Common food sources of inulin and FOS prebiotics.[61]

Because of their high-water, high-fiber content and low calorie density, you should be able to incorporate a generous serving of fibrous vegetables into your diet no matter what diet you're following.

If you have poor gut health and currently eat a low-fiber diet, then you may only see a modest improvement in the beginning. As you introduce more fiber into your microbiome, it can result in gastrointestinal discomfort including gas and bloating. But as your beneficial bacteria begin multiplying and growing stronger, those symptoms should gradually diminish.

With Nick, we first looked at how much fiber he was eating daily. He tracked it for five days and found that on average he ate between 14 and 20 grams. While that was well in line with what typical Americans consume, he needed to significantly increase it.

The current Dietary Reference Intake guideline for fiber is 30 to 38 grams per day for men and 21 to 26 grams per day for women.[62]

I wanted Nick to gradually work up to his target intake over the course of the month. Nick was a meat-and-potatoes guy who went light on the greens, so we focused on finding easy and palate-pleasing ways to incorporate more fiber into his diet. Often, Nick skipped breakfast, but I advised that he add egg casseroles or egg scrambles into the mix. This would allow him to throw in lots of prebiotic-rich vegetables like onions, peppers, leeks, and zucchini. For lunches and dinners, we added giant salads, stir-fries, and sheet-pan meals. Nick would roast chicken, onions, broccoli, carrots, cauliflower, brussels sprouts, and parsnips in the oven. It was a simple, healthy, and quick way for him to prep multiple meals for the week.

Resistant Starches

When you think about starch and starchy foods, you may think about carbohydrates and higher blood sugar. However, not all starch is created equal. One of the best prebiotic fibers are *resistant starches*, which resist digestion.

This incredibly beneficial type of prebiotic fiber has been linked to greater microbial diversity in the gut, enhanced butyrate production, and improved bowel function.[63,64] A meta-analysis of studies in animals and humans with inflammatory bowel disease reported that supplementing with resistant starch significantly improved gut integrity and reduced clinical symptom severity.[65]

There are currently five known types of resistant starch, and all can be found in nature or made through cooking except for resistant starch type IV, which is synthetically created.

Resistant starch type I escapes absorption simply because our digestive enzymes can't reach it, usually because it's trapped within a fibrous cell wall. The best source is minimally processed whole grains, particularly if eaten raw or toasted rather than boiled or simmered since the combination of heat and moisture breaks down the fibrous cell walls.

For example, the resistant starch content of uncooked oats is around 7 percent, or 7 grams per 100 grams of uncooked oats.[66] Yet with cooking, it drops down to just 1 percent due to the swelling of starch granules and destruction of the fibrous cell walls that were preventing digestive enzymes from reaching the starch. To enjoy the benefits of resistant starch in oatmeal, consider eating it in its raw form as muesli or sprinkled over yogurt.

Resistant Starches		
Resistant Starch	**Description**	**Food Sources**
Type I	Physically inaccessible	Minimally processed whole grains
Type II	Uncooked amylose	Raw potatoes and green bananas
Type III	Retrograde	Cooked and cooled starches like potatoes and rice
Type IV	Chemically modified	Synthetic; not found in nature
Type V	Amylose-lipid complex	High-amylose starches cooked in the presence of fat, such as stir-fried rice

Resistant starch type II is similar to type I, except that instead of being confined within a cell wall, it's packed together so tightly that our digestive enzymes can't penetrate it to break it down. Foods high in this type of resistant starch tend to be high in amylose (a type of starch molecule) and uncooked since cooking causes the starch to alter structure and become more digestible. The best examples are raw potatoes and green bananas, which are almost entirely composed of resistant starch type 2 (as you can tell from that distinctive "chalky" taste).

While we certainly don't expect you to eat raw potatoes and green bananas, numerous studies have documented gut and health benefits from adding a couple of tablespoons of green banana starch or potato starch to the diet.[67,68,69,70] Specifically, there were consistent increases in butyrate-producing bacteria, reductions in pathogenic bacteria, and increases in SCFA production. Try experimenting by adding these starch powders into a smoothie or yogurt, or sprinkle them on anything you will not then cook.

Resistant starch type III is the saving grace of cooking. While cooking destroys certain types of resistant starch and makes most of it accessible for digestion and absorption by our enzymes, if you let cooked starch cool in the fridge, it will form resistant starch type III, also called *retrograde starch*. The cooled starch molecules will rearrange back into a type that our enzymes cannot access.

Retrograde starch will form in nearly every carbohydrate-rich food you cook and cool, but the best example is the humble spud. A cooked and cooled potato is roughly 4 to 5 percent resistant starch by weight,[71] so if you let a medium baked russet potato cool in the fridge overnight, the next day it will give you nearly 10 grams of prebiotic fiber. (Just don't reheat it too much, as that causes the resistant starch to break back down into normal digestible starch.)

Resistant starch type IV is a synthetic starch that can't be obtained naturally in the diet. Still, if you find and use it as a supplement, just 10 grams per day has been shown to increase the concentration of numerous beneficial butyrate-producing gut bacteria, as well as improve glycemic control, blood lipids, and inflammatory markers.[72]

Resistant starch type V forms when starch is cooked in the presence of fatty acids, especially saturated fatty acids, and then allowed to cool.[73] One study found that cooking a half cup of rice with just a teaspoon of coconut oil and then letting it chill in the fridge for 12 hours overnight increased the resistant starch content tenfold.[74] In fact, so much of its starch became resistant to digestion that its calorie content was cut in half!

In addition to having Nick add more prebiotic vegetables to his diet, we focused on resistant starches. For those stir-fries Nick made, I advised him to make the rice the night before. Nick liked cooking in batches, so he would make 3 to 4 cups of white rice and toss in 1 to 2 teaspoons of coconut oil. Then the next day, he would sauté a vegetable medley, add an animal protein, and then mix it with the premade rice.

Nick loved potatoes, so the only change we made was in preparation. I had him bake them and let them cool in the refrigerator overnight to bump the resistant starch content.

Lean into Fermented Foods

Natural probiotics supply millions to billions of beneficial bacteria (such as *Lactobacillus* and *Bifidobacterium*) that colonize our gut, produce SCFAs, stop harmful pathogenic bacteria from taking over, and interact with our immune system to enhance its ability to fight infections.[75,76,77]

You can introduce an assortment of beneficial microbes into your gut by eating and drinking fermented foods including:

- Yogurt
- Cheese
- Kimchi
- Sauerkraut
- Tempeh
- Miso
- Kefir
- Kombucha

If you don't want to eat fermented foods, you can consider a supplement. Numerous studies have shown that supplementing with probiotics can help turn a dysregulated microbiome into a healthy one.[78] These probiotic supplements are no different from what we would obtain with a generous serving of fermented food.

For Nick, we looked at ways he could add fermented foods into his diet. Yogurt and cheese became staple snacks, and Nick experimented with kimchi and sauerkraut too. For the first couple of weeks, the fermented foods mixed with the higher prebiotic vegetable intake proved too much for Nick's system, so we took out the fermented foods and focused only on upping his prebiotic and resistant starches.

I love fermented foods and my digestive system processes them fine, but some of my clients report a lot of discomfort and negative reactions to them. Let me be clear: you *do not* need to eat fermented foods for optimal gut health.

My best advice is to try them for a week and monitor how you feel. Start with smaller servings, like ¼ to ½ cup, and see how your body reacts. If you experience a lot of discomfort—gas, bloating—then reduce the amount for a few days and see if that makes a difference. If you still have negative reactions, then take fermented foods out entirely and focus on eating more prebiotic fruits and vegetables. It could be that you need to rebuild more microbiome diversity before you can add fermented foods into the mix.

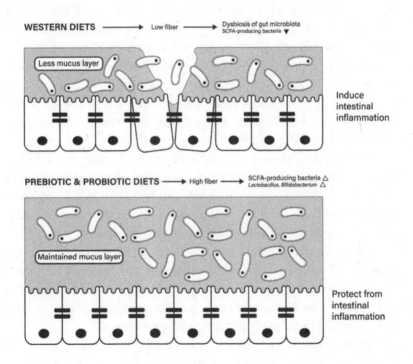

When More Fiber Isn't Enough

In a perfect world, you would increase your fiber and within a couple of months, your gut microbiome would be healthier, your mitochondria stronger, and your energy levels improved.

But life isn't always perfect.

For some people, switching to a high-fiber diet worsens their gastrointestinal symptoms, including gas, bloating, stomach pain, constipation, or diarrhea. This is because some of the fiber-rich foods like garlic, onions, fruits, leeks, cauliflower, brussels sprouts, wheat, legumes, and grains are FODMAPs (fermentable oligosaccharides, disaccharides, monosaccharides, and polyols).

When some bacteria feed on FODMAPs, they produce a gas that leads to stomach discomfort and many other uncomfortable symptoms. Therefore many people go on an elimination or low-carbohydrate diet[79]—also known as a low-FODMAP diet.

However, a low-FODMAP diet doesn't address the root cause of dysbiosis; it simply starves the bacteria of food so they can't produce gas. In the short term, people may feel better on a low-FODMAP diet, but they are likely doing long-term damage to the health of their microbiome.[80]

To reverse dysbiosis, we need to eat a diversity of fiber-rich plants—possibly supplementing with fermented foods—which will create a robust and healthy microbiome. This is the only solution to digestive issues that treats the root cause of the problems rather than simply masking symptoms of discomfort.

For some people, this may be difficult to achieve given the digestive distress this strategy causes. If this is your situation, please don't give up. It may be tempting to opt for a low-fiber diet, but instead I encourage you to seek out a health care professional who may offer you more guidance and assistance.

Most people in this situation need a personalized protocol to repair, regrow, and restore their gut health. This may include needing to use short-term antibiotics or herbal antimicrobials to first kill off some of the harmful, pathogenic bacteria before repopulating the gut by eating more prebiotic fibers and fermented and other probiotic foods, and/or taking a probiotic supplement.

MAKING THE CHANGES STICK

When I spoke with Nick about six weeks after his initial diet adjustments, he was surprised that adding more fiber to his diet was easier than he had expected. As I had recommended, he focused on just increasing his prebiotic vegetable and fruit intake for the first two weeks. Initially Nick noticed an increase in gas, bloating, and stomach cramps, but he experienced a significant reduction around week two.

At this time, he added about ½ to ¾ cup of fermented foods—mostly kimchi or sauerkraut—or yogurt mixed with blueberries, raspberries, strawberries, or an apple (with the peel since that's where the most fiber is). Again, he noticed an uptick in gas, bloating, and cramps, but since he'd been through it before, he had expected this. After another week, the stomach discomfort was still there, so he reduced his serving size, figuring that he just needed to give his microbiome more time to regrow.

Nick was spot-on in playing with portion sizes, listening to his gut, and taking a very thoughtful approach to rebuilding his microbiome. Six weeks in, he was eating about 45 to 50 grams of fiber daily, and he noticed an increase in energy and a dramatic decrease in his stomach conditions. "You don't realize how bad you really feel until you start feeling better," Nick said. "I have regular bowel movements and a lot less gastric distress, and I didn't realize how self-conscious those conditions had made me."

In our last coaching session, I left Nick with a final message: "Fiber is your lifelong friend. This is not a strategy that you want to kick to the curb now that your symptoms are improving. You need to constantly feed your microbiome. Those beneficial bacteria depend on you. Feed them the right nutrients, and they will help feed your mitochondria."

Gut issues are some of the most pervasive health challenges facing people living in our modern world, especially in the West. We must be diligent about taking care of our microbiomes and supporting their diversity. No matter how long you've lived with gut issues, you can course correct, and when you do, your overall health and energy will improve.

ACTION LIST

The following checklist will help you start on your energy healing journey through healing your gut and building a strong microbiome. I recommend that you pick one or two items that feel attainable and try them for at least two weeks or until it feels comfortable.

You may find you are able to implement more than two challenges. That's perfectly fine, but do not overwhelm yourself. Your microbiome won't get rebuilt in a night, so take your time and make sure these changes stick before moving on to the next.

As in other chapters, you'll notice that each challenge has a primary goal with three to four smaller stepping-stones. That's intentional, as establishing new habits often requires baby steps in the right direction. Start with the first stepping-stone and work your way down before checking off the primary goal.

During this time you may notice an increase in gastrointestinal discomfort, but that should subside as your microbiome becomes repopulated again. If the symptoms become too uncomfortable, then reduce the portion size, return to the previous level, or drop one of the challenges.

- ☐ **Eat a diet based on fibrous vegetables.**
  - ☐ Consume fibrous vegetables with 1 meal per day.
  - ☐ Consume fibrous vegetables with 2 meals per day.
  - ☐ Consume fibrous vegetables with every meal.

- ☐ **Incorporate prebiotic vegetables into your diet.**
  - ☐ Eat "great" or "good" sources of prebiotic vegetables with 1 meal per day.
  - ☐ Eat "great" or "good" sources with 2 meals per day.
  - ☐ Eat "great" or "good" sources with every meal.
  - ☐ The above, plus adding an "absolute best" source at 1 or more meals.

☐ **Incorporate resistant starch into your diet (Note: you do not need to use all of these; pick whichever is most convenient for you given your dietary preferences).**

   ☐ Consume raw, minimally processed whole grains at 1 or more meals.

   ☐ Consume green banana or potato starch at 1 or more meals.

   ☐ Consume cooked and cooled starches at 1 or more meals.

   ☐ Consume cooked and cooled rice that was cooked with coconut oil.

☐ **Repopulate your gut with natural probiotics (Note: most important if you are coming from a historically low-fiber diet).**

   ☐ Consume fermented foods with 1 meal per day.

   ☐ Consume fermented foods with 2 meals per day.

   ☐ Consume fermented foods with every meal.

CHAPTER 5

CONTROLLING BLOOD SUGAR SWINGS TO STABILIZE ENERGY

"How did this happen and why now?" Bill said, sounding confused. During our first session, Bill told me that his doctor had just diagnosed him as prediabetic and suggested he take a prescription drug to help control his blood sugar levels—otherwise, Bill was on the fast track to developing type 2 diabetes.

In his mid-60s, Bill had recently become a grandfather for the first time. "I want to be around for my granddaughter and do fun things with her, and I'm scared that this is a sign that I'm on the downhill slope of life."

Adding to Bill's fears was the fact that his father had also developed type 2 diabetes later in his life and eventually died from heart disease. (Type 2 diabetes significantly increases the risk of developing heart conditions.)

Bill didn't want to become his father, but he wasn't sure he wanted to take the medication his doctor had prescribed either.

While Bill's prediabetes diagnosis was his greatest health concern, he had additional worries that drove him to seek me out. "I get so tired after a meal that I want to lie down, and all day long I feel like I go from being energized to fighting to stay awake," Bill explained.

I sympathized with Bill. Anytime we receive a major diagnosis or the medical community doesn't have a label for what's happening to us, it's frightening. It's also discouraging when we don't know what's causing our fatigue or medical condition. However, in Bill's case we knew exactly what needed fixing: his blood sugar levels.

UNLOCKING THE MYSTERIES OF BLOOD SUGAR

The human body needs blood sugar, specifically glucose, to survive.

Our mitochondria use it (along with fats, and amino acids from protein) to make ATP for our cells. However, some organs, such as your brain, use glucose as the main fuel source and need a steady supply of it to properly function. Glucose comes from carbohydrates. When carbs are digested, they break down into glucose, which then passes through your gut lining, gets absorbed into your bloodstream, and is delivered to the cells throughout your body for energy production or for storage and use later.

After you eat, blood sugar levels naturally rise. Then they fall and reach their lowest marks right before your next meal. This rising and falling is normal, but there is a range that is tightly regulated and controlled. If glucose levels fall too low, you may slip into a coma and die. If levels rise too high for too long, then you can damage blood vessels, nerves, and organs.

We need glucose, just not too much and not too little.

Millions of people, however, have what's called *poor glycemic control*, meaning their bodies have lost the ability to stabilize their blood sugar levels, which causes serious ramifications for their health, wellness, and energy levels.

In the United States, about *42 percent of adults* have been diagnosed as prediabetic or diabetic; roughly 30 percent are diagnosed as prediabetic while another 12 percent have full-blown diabetes, most of which is type 2 diabetes.[1] Type 2 diabetes occurs when the body has chronically high blood sugar levels that never decline into a healthy range. This is called *hyperglycemia*.

Prediabetes or diabetes is a serious health condition that goes beyond feeling fatigue. A meta-analysis of 97 studies involving over 820,000 adults shows that having diabetes increases your risk of dying from *any cause by 80 percent* and by a variety of other causes by upward of threefold, even after adjusting for other risk factors such as blood lipids, inflammation, age, and BMI.[2]

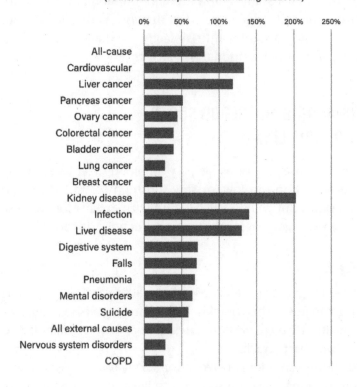

RISK OF DYING FROM VARIOUS CAUSES IF YOU HAVE TYPE 2 DIABETES
(% increase compared to not having diabetes)

A diabetic diagnosis is also expensive, costing the U.S. about $327 billion every year, or roughly $1 for every $7 spent on health care.[3] On a personal level, if you have diabetes, you can expect to pay more than double for health care than what someone without diabetes pays yearly: $16,752 for someone with diabetes and $7,151 for someone without.[4]

And for people who would not be considered diabetic based on established diagnostic criteria, having glucose levels that elevate too much after eating is still a health risk. The risk of developing or dying from cardiovascular diseases increases as glycemic control worsens, even within ranges that are considered normal within the medical community.[5]

The last and most critical issue around blood glucose control is *glycemic variability*, which refers to swings from high to low throughout the day. Studies show glycemic variability is a primary determinant of daily glucose average in those with and without diabetes,[6] and it is a significant risk factor for diabetes complications independent of traditional risk factors.[7,8]

UNDERSTANDING THE BLOOD SUGAR– MITOCHONDRIA LINK

Since your cells use glucose as fuel, if your blood sugar levels swing up and down, drop too low, or stay too high for too long, you will feel fatigue. But you will also get hit with exhaustion because unstable blood sugar levels affect your mitochondria too.

Hypoglycemia

When blood sugar levels fall too low, it's called *hypoglycemia*. This condition can hit rather quickly and is an established cause of sudden death through seizures, respiratory arrest (inability to breathe), and heart attacks.[9]

Since dying isn't advantageous for survival as a species, evolution put in some powerful stopgaps to keep hypoglycemia from happening. The liver, for example, constantly pumps out glucose to keep our blood levels stable throughout the day, and our adrenal glands are quick to hit us with an adrenaline rush if our blood glucose falls too low.

While clinical hypoglycemia that requires medical attention doesn't occur often, don't let this fool you into thinking low blood glucose problems don't exist. Roughly one in three adults experience symptoms of hypoglycemia after eating,[10] and this number can be as high as three out of four adults with diabetes, usually because of their antidiabetic medications.[11,12]

This is called *reactive hypoglycemia*, when your blood sugar drops too low two to five hours after eating. It's caused by a variety of factors such as accelerated emptying of the stomach, exaggerated gut hormone secretion, a delayed and exaggerated insulin response, insulin resistance that leads to compensatory hyperinsulinemia, or hypothyroidism.[13,14]

If you're still running low on blood sugar after eating, the amount of available energy for muscles, tissues, and organs such as the brain is reduced. Neurons in the human brain have the highest energy demand, requiring continuous delivery of glucose from the blood.[15] But while the brain only accounts for 2 percent of our body weight, it consumes *20 percent of glucose-derived energy*, making it the main consumer of glucose.

If your blood sugar dips too low, particularly after eating, then you may feel:

- Fatigue
- Shakiness
- Dizziness
- Confusion
- Moodiness
- Anxiety

Some people experience the symptoms of reactive hypoglycemia without having hypoglycemia.[16] This is called *idiopathic postprandial syndrome*, and there is currently no established reason why it occurs (*idiopathic* means "unknown cause").

The best explanation is that all the hormones involved in regulating blood glucose are successful in maintaining normal glucose levels but require exaggerated concentrations to do so.[17] For example, a delayed insulin response that would typically result in hypoglycemia is met with a powerful adrenaline rush that prevents hypoglycemia but still causes sweats and shakiness.

Not only will you feel fatigue because your cells literally do not have the fuel they need to burn but your mitochondria will also take a beating. When you have a hypoglycemic episode or hypoglycemic symptoms, it causes mitochondrial dysfunction. When blood sugar levels fall too low, this increases oxidative stress, which sends our mitochondria into cellular defense mode, thus reducing energy production even further.[18]

Hyperglycemia

Just as we don't want blood sugar levels to fall too low, we don't want them to remain too high for too long either. That's called hyperglycemia, and symptoms include:

- Fatigue
- Increased thirst and/or hunger
- Blurred vision
- Frequent urination
- Headache

Not only can chronic hyperglycemia lead to prediabetes and then full-blown diabetes, but hyperglycemia is a potent source of oxidative stress within the body, even when occurring only intermittently, like after meals.[19,20] This damages the mitochondria and causes deficits in energy production.[21,22,23]

In another blow to our energy levels, the oxidative stress caused by post-meal glucose spikes stimulates the immune system to secrete inflammatory signaling molecules.[24] This not only causes fatigue through the "sickness behavior" mentioned earlier but also leads to neuroinflammation that can ultimately cause neurodegenerative disorders and cognitive dysfunction.[25]

Blood sugar spikes also suppress orexin signaling within the brain.[26] Orexin is a neurotransmitter involved in wakefulness and the desire to be physically active. If you have low orexin levels due to poor glycemic control, you're going to be much more tired and fatigued.

So regardless of your personal health, having poor glycemic control can sap your energy levels. Both post-meal glucose spikes and reactive hypoglycemia cause oxidative stress and mitochondrial dysfunction, particularly within the brain.

If you have diabetes, where elevated blood glucose is chronic, then your energy levels will only continue dwindling. Chronic fatigue is a common problem in those with type 2 diabetes, affecting roughly *two out of every three* adults with the condition and being the second-most regularly complained about symptom.[27]

Even for diabetics who have adequately controlled their blood glucose levels, fatigue persists—that's understandable given that mitochondrial dysfunction is an intrinsic component of type 2 diabetes.[28,29]

If you're living with type 2 diabetes, it tanks energy levels not only through its physiological effects but also through psychological and lifestyle factors.[30] Some practitioners have coined the phrase *diabetes fatigue syndrome* as a means of establishing diabetes-induced fatigue as its own entity separate from other causes of chronic fatigue.[31]

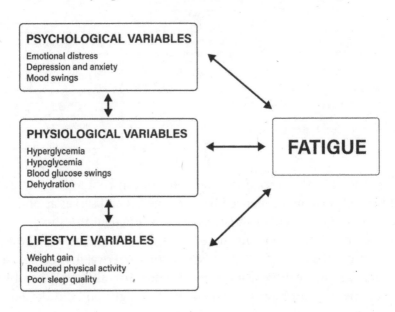

Exceeding Your Personal Fat Threshold

We all have an optimal range of body fat mass that we need to stay within for our metabolic systems to function normally. Once we've exceeded the upper range of what's called our *personal fat threshold*, our metabolic system can become dysfunctional, which can lead to type 2 diabetes.[32]

To keep safe, our bodies store fat underneath the skin. This subcutaneous fat sucks up the excess glucose and fat that aren't needed by our organs and muscles and gives them a safe place of storage for later use during times of fasting and famine. As the fat cells take in more energy, they expand in size like a balloon filling with air. But balloons can hold only so much air before they pop. When the fat cells reach a "critical threshold" in their size, they shut themselves off from the energy supply to preserve their own life and secrete molecules that lead to the formation of new fat cells that can take up more energy.[33]

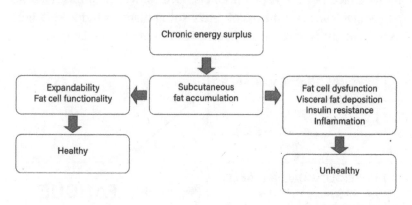

The ability to create new fat cells and distribute the energy burden is heavily influenced by our genetics and serves as one of the fundamental characteristics of the personal fat threshold. The more fat cells we have, the more fat we can gain before metabolic abnormalities occur.[34,35,36] This is why some overweight people are metabolically healthy, while others are not. This also explains why some people can have a "normal" body weight but still develop type 2 diabetes—it's because they have exceeded their personal fat threshold.

Metabolic dysfunction occurs when fat cells become too large and become insulin resistant in order to preserve their own life.[37] If no other fat cells can be recruited to take up the excess glucose, then the body tries to overcome the fat cells' insulin resistance by pumping out more insulin. It works, but it causes a damaging amount of fat storage in fat cells that results in oxidative stress, inflammation, and insurmountable insulin resistance.

At this point, the fat cells are dysfunctional.[38] The oxidative stress and inflammation of the fat cells lead to the secretion of pro-inflammatory signaling molecules that give rise to systemic inflammation. The insurmountable insulin resistance leads to the leakage of fatty acids into circulation that are inappropriately stored in our skeletal muscles, liver, and pancreas (ectopic fat).[39] Both systemic inflammation and ectopic fat can each lead to systemic insulin resistance, which causes metabolic dysfunction.

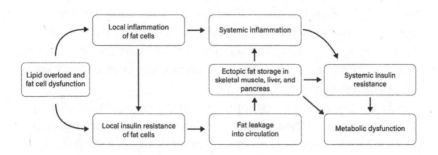

Insulin resistance and metabolic dysfunction ultimately leave the body immensely fatigued, and if allowed to persist for prolonged periods of time, can ultimately reach the apex—developing into type 2 diabetes.

STRATEGIES FOR STABILIZING BLOOD SUGAR LEVELS

If you want optimal energy and good health, then you want stable blood sugar levels throughout the day and night. That means minimizing huge blood sugar spikes, preventing large dips after a meal, and avoiding chronic hyperglycemia, which can put you on the path toward type 2 diabetes.

When it comes to improving your blood sugar levels and glycemic control, it's all about food. Blood sugar levels are directly connected to two things: (1) what you choose to eat and (2) your body fat.

As you learn about the following nutritional strategies, I want you to focus on regaining your power to control your blood sugar levels. It does reside with you and the choices you make for your diet. Diet alone can reregulate your levels and can even reverse prediabetes and type 2 diabetes diagnoses. (Yes, you really can change the course of this disease.)

Some of the nutritional strategies I detail in this chapter will probably be familiar to you—that's because they are the same strategies that help rewire your energy clocks and induce fat loss. In this chapter, I share the science-backed evidence on why you want to consider deploying these tactics to control blood sugar spikes and drops.

Don't hesitate to revisit previous chapters, especially Chapters 2 and 3. Circadian dysregulation and excess fat mass often go hand in hand with blood sugar issues, so embarking on a sleep recovery and/or fat loss journey will likely improve your glycemic control, especially if you have prediabetes, type 2 diabetes, or some other form of metabolic dysfunction.

For those people in the non-diabetic category, blood sugar issues may still be the cause of your fatigue. My best advice is to always stay regular on your blood work. When working with your doctor, make sure to check your fasting glucose, HbA1c, and fasting insulin. The glucose/insulin response to an oral glucose tolerance test can also be helpful for determining glycemic control.

Finally, pay attention to how you feel after a meal. Food is energy, so ideally you should feel energized after eating instead of lethargic or sleepy. While post-meal energy levels are connected to more than just blood sugar levels, blood sugar is one of the primary determinants and influences. And if you often feel fatigued post-meal, then you will want to pay close attention to this chapter.

Reversing Type 2 Diabetes

Did you know that it is possible to reverse type 2 diabetes in just a *few weeks*?

Over the last decade, numerous studies have shown that diet alone can reverse type 2 diabetes. It all comes down to losing enough body fat so you no longer exceed your personal fat threshold.

Roy Taylor, the man who first developed the personal fat threshold concept, has spearheaded these investigations.[40,41,42] In his proof-of-concept Counterpoint study,[43] a group of overweight and obese individuals who had type 2 diabetes for less than four years were fed a 600-calorie liquid diet for eight weeks while they simultaneously stopped taking all their diabetes medications.

The results were as follows:

- The participants lost an average of 34 pounds, or roughly 15 percent of their starting body weight, with 83 percent coming from their body fat.

- Skeletal muscle insulin sensitivity and ability to uptake glucose from the bloodstream was increased by 68 percent.

- Liver fat declined by 70 percent, completely resolving those who had a fatty liver diagnosis when the study began. This was accompanied by a 72 percent increase in the liver's insulin sensitivity and a 34 percent reduction in the liver's glucose output.

- Pancreatic fat dropped by 23 percent, leading to a normalization of the insulin response when eating carbohydrates.

- Fasting glucose levels fell by 40 percent, fasting insulin was cut in half, and HbA1c was reduced from 7.4 percent to 6 percent.

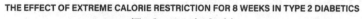

THE EFFECT OF EXTREME CALORIE RESTRICTION FOR 8 WEEKS IN TYPE 2 DIABETICS
(The Counterpoint Study)

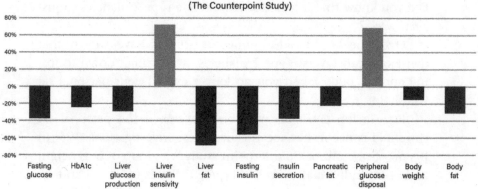

In eight weeks of extreme dieting, participants reversed their diagnosis of type 2 diabetes. In a follow-up study, Taylor had participants diagnosed with type 2 diabetes again do a 600-calorie diet for eight weeks, which was followed by a slow reintroduction of regular food over the course of six months.[44] Taylor found that as long as participants kept off the weight they had lost, the type 2 diabetes reversal persisted. These individuals also ate more calories and carbohydrates without any problems.

However, not everyone reversed their diabetes despite losing significant amounts of weight. While 87 percent of those who had type 2 diabetes for less than four years responded well to the fat loss intervention, only 50 percent of those who had diabetes for longer than four years were successful. One possible reason is that the longer you live with diabetes, the more pancreatic damage is likely to occur. Too much pancreatic damage and dysfunction may prevent reversal of diabetes despite fat loss. Furthermore, if you've had diabetes (or other diseases) for years and it's caused substantial damage (e.g., cell death) in certain tissues and organs or glands of your body like the pancreas, then it's likely that you will not *completely* reverse a type 2 diabetes diagnosis.

Whether or not they were able to reverse their type 2 diabetes diagnoses, by losing fat and keeping it off, all of the participants in the study still experienced marked health improvements, including healthier body compositions, the restoration of insulin sensitivity, and normalization of liver fat and liver functioning.

Taylor confirmed his findings in his later, yearlong DiRECT study,[45] which showed that the chances of reversing diabetes increased proportionally to the amount of fat loss—only 7 percent of participants who lost fewer than 12 pounds successfully reversed their type 2 diabetes compared to a staggering 86 percent of participants who lost more than 33 pounds.

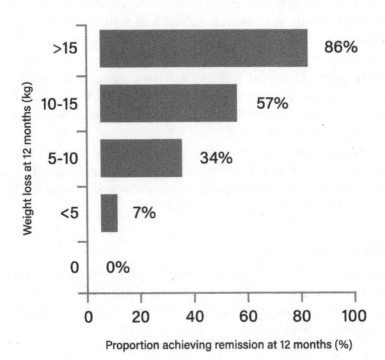

Some people reversed their diabetes when losing as little as 10 pounds because they had less weight to lose than others. Remember that type 2 diabetes is connected to exceeding our personal fat threshold, which is unique to each person. The amount of fat loss required for reversing type 2 diabetes will depend on the starting point, assuming that one's pancreas can resume normal functionality and insulin secretion.[46]

I'm not sharing this because I want to discourage or disappoint you. Losing fat will always have health benefits, and it's a journey that I encourage all my clients to take if they need to. However, I'm also not in the business of overhyping strategies. My goal is to provide you with the information you need to make the best choices for your health.

If you have type 2 diabetes, the takeaway is one of hope and optimism. You can reverse this diagnosis through fat loss. And for those people who have lived with this disease for many years, while you may not reverse it entirely, you can still make huge improvements in your overall health and well-being by reducing fat mass.

And no, you do not need to go to the extreme the Counterbalance participants did to kick-start the process. The only factor that matters is fat loss. You don't need to starve yourself on very-low-calorie diets or follow any specific diet to reverse diabetes.

You just need to lose fat.

And for those of you who may have pancreatic damage, there is hope. Studies show that the pancreas can heal and regenerate if given some time and the opportunity to do so by maintaining fat loss over the long haul.[47,48]

Switch to a Low-Carb Diet

It's normal and expected to have your blood glucose increase after eating carbohydrates, just as it's normal and expected to see blood increases in lipids after eating dietary fat and in amino acids after eating dietary protein.

However, if you are struggling to keep your blood glucose levels low, then eating fewer carbohydrates can be incredibly therapeutic—especially for prediabetic and diabetic people. Numerous studies and meta-analyses suggest that low-carbohydrate diets are more effective than moderate- or high-carbohydrate diets at lowering average blood glucose levels (HbA1c), reducing diabetes medication requirements, and putting type 2 diabetes into remission.[49,50]

The American Diabetes Association and the European Association for the Study of Diabetes endorse low-carbohydrate diets for addressing the elevated blood glucose levels seen in type 2 diabetes.[51,52] However, they rightly point out that overall diet quality still matters.

In particular, these organizations acknowledge that reducing overall carbohydrate intake is most effective for improving glycemic control and blood sugar levels, no matter the eating pattern or diet. Ketogenic, vegetarian, Mediterranean, or paleo diets can all work, provided you eat enough fibrous vegetables, fermented foods, and prebiotic fibers to maintain gut health.

If you opt for a low-carb diet, you will want to cut out carbohydrates and starches that cause blood sugar levels to spike, including cereal grains, breads, breakfast cereals, rice, pasta, most fruit, starchy tubers like potatoes and carrots, corn, and most beans and legumes.

Other foods, like cow's milk and most dairy, berries, and soy products, can be eaten in moderation, while meats, seafood, eggs, Greek yogurt, nuts and seeds, and fibrous, non-starchy vegetables such as tomatoes, eggplant, cabbage, and spinach can be eaten without restrictions.

Low-Carbohydrate Diet		
No Restrictions	**Monitor Intake**	**Avoid**
Meats and seafood Eggs Cheese Greek yogurt Nuts and seeds Fats and oils Fibrous vegetables Protein powders	Milk and most dairy Berries Soy products	Cereal grains Starchy tubers Most fruit Most beans and legumes

Bill's prediabetes diagnosis told me that he was at a weight that was over his personal fat threshold. While I didn't know for certain what Bill's magic number was, I could look at how much extra fat mass he carried and direct him to reduce that number.

Bill was a big guy. A former football linebacker who had played college ball, he had spent his career working as a construction foreman. It was a physically demanding job, so Bill figured that he burned enough calories to be lenient with his diet. A few times a week, he would have a burger and fries, pizza, a ham sandwich with chips, or spaghetti and meatballs with garlic bread on the side. He was also prone to late-night snacking.

Bill had about 25 to 35 pounds of excess fat mass, and just looking at his diet, I knew he would see marked and fast changes just by moving to a low-carb diet. But I also knew that given Bill's typical eating patterns, some of these changes might be hard for him to sustain.

Wanting to set up Bill for success, I suggested he start by eating one meal that replaces foods on the "avoid" list with those from the "no restriction" list. "Do this for two weeks, and then I want you to aim for two meals per day that contain only foods from the 'no restriction' list," I told Bill. "Then in a month, we're going for three meals."

My hope was that by gradually transitioning him to a low-carb diet, Bill would stop craving the carb-laden foods, start seeing progress with losing fat, and see some—albeit a little—energy improvement. These small steps in the right direction were aimed at motivating Bill and priming his body and mind to embrace these small, relatively easy changes.

I'm also very realistic and know that psychologically when we tell ourselves we can't have a certain food, it's all we focus on and crave. Switching to a low-carb diet can feel shocking to our system, and not always in a good way. A gradual change can make the difference between weight regain and a sustainable fat mass reduction that lasts.

"Remember, this isn't calorie counting, so you can eat as much as you need to satisfy your hunger from the 'no restriction' list," I told Bill.

Low-carb diets may seem restrictive, but the choices you have are endless. You get to eat as much animal protein and fish, fresh vegetables, healthy fats, Greek yogurt, and certain other dairy as you like. If your diet contains a lot of carbohydrates and starchy vegetables, then you will likely see some fast results from going low carb in terms of fat loss and energy improvement. Your blood sugar levels will also improve quite drastically in a matter of weeks.

But as important as low-carbohydrate diets can be, they do not inherently address the cause of type 2 diabetes, which is excess fat mass. If someone isn't actively losing fat mass, then a low-carbohydrate diet can reduce blood sugar levels, but it will not reverse the disease processes. Some people may lose fat mass through a low-carbohydrate diet, but if that isn't happening, then other fat loss tools will need to be added.

Embrace Time-Restricted Feeding

If you're struggling with glycemic control, then you'll want to look closely at how late you eat and how you sleep. There are often links between circadian misalignment and dysregulation and poor glycemic control.[53] Circadian dysregulation disrupts glucose metabolism, which occurs through direct mechanisms, such as impaired pancreatic and fat cell functioning, and indirect mechanisms including dysregulation of the gut microbiome, immune and endocrine systems, and satiety signaling.[54,55,56]

If you're not getting seven to eight hours of sleep each night, it can affect your body's ability to use insulin and absorb glucose. For instance, getting just five hours of sleep reduces insulin sensitivity—which decreases the body's ability to absorb and use glucose for energy—by 23 percent. That number doubles to 47 percent for people who sleep in short bursts combined with staying up all night and going to sleep around 9:00 A.M.,[57] as might happen with shiftworkers, for example.

Numerous studies have found that sleeping for less than five to six hours per night is also associated with an increased risk of developing type 2 diabetes and that these short sleep durations reduce glycemic control and insulin sensitivity.[58] Poor sleep quality can be due to actual sleep duration, as well as fragmented sleep, sleep apnea, and circadian rhythm disruption.

In fact, one meta-analysis found that difficulty initiating sleep was associated with a 55 percent increased risk of developing type 2 diabetes, while difficulty maintaining sleep was linked to a 72 percent increased risk.[59] The risk of developing diabetes associated with getting too little sleep (≤five hours per day) or having poor sleep quality was greater than that of being sedentary.

One factor that keeps people awake is when they eat. In humans, a plethora of evidence shows that many anabolic rhythms—when the body uses the energy our mitochondria produce—peak in the morning or early afternoon, and that glucose tolerance is worse in the evening and at night, which is when most people consume a high percentage of their daily food.[60] We've known since at least the 1970s that even if you have normal glucose tolerance in the morning, you may still be more likely to be metabolically equivalent to someone with prediabetes in the evening.[61,62]

In healthy men and women, eating a meal at 8:00 P.M. leads to a 29 percent greater peak glucose response, 86 percent larger total glucose response, and 66 percent more time spent in hyperglycemia than eating the exact same meal at 8:00 A.M., even after both meals are preceded by a 12-hour fast.[63]

If you're struggling with a disrupted circadian rhythm and/or you typically eat late into the evening, then you'll want to consider using time-restricted feeding (TRF). This will help you better control your blood sugar levels. One study involving men with prediabetes found that eating three meals within a six-hour TRF window benefited glycemic control, insulin sensitivity, blood pressure, and oxidative stress compared to eating those same three meals within a 12-hour window.[64]

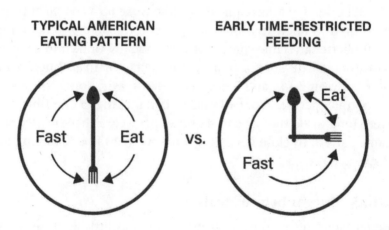

Similarly, a study in people with type 2 diabetes reported that eating two meals within a 10-hour TRF window resulted in significant reductions in body weight and improvements in glycemic control and insulin sensitivity compared to eating six meals per day across a longer eating window.[65]

Whether you choose to eat most of your food in the morning or evening will depend on your preferences. Although there's data showing that people with type 2 diabetes have better blood sugar control with a big breakfast compared to a big dinner,[66] there's also data showing that blood sugar control improves with skipping breakfast over several weeks.[67]

The body's circadian rhythms are heavily influenced by the timing of food intake, so it makes sense that it will "learn" about our regular mealtimes and adjust its internal clocks accordingly. That's why regular breakfast skippers don't show the same negative effects of skipping breakfast that we see in regular breakfast eaters who skip.[68]

If you're using TRF, just make sure you stay consistent with mealtimes throughout the day, whether you start your window of eating at 8 A.M. or at 11 A.M. Having erratic and spontaneous eating times is a surefire way to cause blood glucose swings, insulin resistance, and poor energy levels throughout the day.[69,70]

Bill often fell asleep quickly, but he woke up a couple of times each night. I knew that improving his sleep could also help him attain better glycemic control, so we gradually worked to get him to a 10-hour TRF. For one month, Bill tried to eat in a 12-hour window between 7 A.M. and 7 P.M. He started slowly, doing this about three times per week for two weeks, then moving to four times per week for a week, then five to six times per week. Then he used the same pattern to close his eating window to 10 hours, aiming for 8 A.M. to 6 P.M.

Drink Vinegar before Meals

Better blood sugar control can be yours in as little as 10 seconds. The trick? Start every meal with a shot of vinegar.

A meta-analysis of studies looking at how vinegar impacts blood glucose control found that having 1 to 2 tablespoons before eating reduced the overall post-meal blood glucose response by 11 percent and the overall insulin response by 16 percent.[71] What's more, it didn't matter if you had diabetes or were otherwise healthy—vinegar benefited glycemic control in everyone.

These benefits are likely owed to the defining characteristic of vinegar that makes it tart and acidic: its acetic acid content.[72] Studies have shown that acetic acid slows digestion and inhibits our digestive enzymes that break down starch and sugar.[73,74,75,76] These effects will cause a slower and less pronounced increase in blood sugar levels after eating.

More importantly, acetic acid increases the expression of AMPK (AMP-activated protein kinase) and GLUT4 (glucose transporter type 4), which are proteins that increase glucose uptake and use in the body.[77,78] Consuming vinegar increases carbohydrate storage in our muscles as glycogen,[79] even in people with type 2 diabetes.[80] Additionally, vinegar has been shown to stimulate vasodilation (the dilation of blood vessels, which decreases blood pressure) and to increase blood flow to skeletal muscle,[81,82] both of which are considered important components of insulin-mediated glucose uptake.[83]

If you are going to eat a meal that contains some carbohydrates, then consuming 1 to 2 tablespoons of vinegar is an easy way to increase your insulin sensitivity to the incoming glucose load.

Any vinegar will work, although apple cider and red wine vinegars tend to taste better. You will often see apple cider vinegars advertised as raw (unpasteurized) and unfiltered, thereby preserving "the mother." This is simply a nontoxic slime composed of yeast and acetic acid bacteria that forms during the fermentation process that creates vinegar.

The mother of vinegar appears to be a major source of bioactive compounds and antioxidant activity in vinegar, as well as minerals such as potassium, magnesium, calcium, and iron.[84] It remains to be determined whether consuming the mother has any discernible effect on health, but if you have the choice, it seems prudent to opt for it.

This doesn't have to be a literal shot of vinegar. You can mix it with water to dilute it, or you can use it as a salad dressing. Mix 1 to 2 tablespoons of vinegar such as red wine or apple cider with olive oil and toss it over a salad or over vegetables. This is how I had Bill incorporate vinegar into his diet. Admittedly, he didn't use it before every meal, but he aimed to have a salad one to two times per day and chose to eat it first to get that vinegar into his system.

Eat Your Veggies First

We can make a huge impact on our blood glucose control by changing the order in which we eat our food during a meal. Several studies in people with type 2 diabetes or prediabetes,[85,86,87,88] as well as healthy folk,[89] have found that eating fibrous vegetables at the beginning of a meal, before eating starchy carbohydrates, reduces blood glucose and insulin levels by 20 to 70 percent and 25 to 50 percent, respectively.

And if life gets in the way and prevents you from eating them with every meal, the same benefits are observed with just eating protein before any carbohydrates.[90] The theme is to simply eat your sources of carbohydrate (grains, legumes, tubers, etc.) last in the meal.

These glycemic benefits can also have a long-term effect. In one randomized, controlled trial involving adults with type 2 diabetes, taking the advice to eat veggies first and carbohydrates last in each meal was significantly more effective at lowering HbA1c than having them follow the standard American Diabetes Association advice of using a diabetic exchange food list.[91]

The benefits were seen in as little as one month and lasted for at least two years, when the researchers stopped collecting data. Overall, HbA1c from this little trick was slashed from 8.3 percent to 6.8 percent—just from altering the order in which the same foods within a meal were eaten. Essentially, the participants moved from full-blown diabetes to the lower cutoff of a diagnosis (>6.5 percent is diabetes, 5.7 to 6.4 percent is considered prediabetes, and 4 to 5.6 percent is considered healthy).

Another study, in elderly adults with type 2 diabetes, reported similar findings: eating high-carbohydrate foods last within a meal significantly lowers post-meal blood glucose levels, blood glucose swings throughout the day (meaning more stable energy levels), HbA1c, and fasting glucose.[92]

I wanted Bill to keep it simple. Whenever he could, he was to eat his fibrous vegetables first, and if he didn't have any in a meal (which is not ideal, by the way), which sometimes happened during breakfast, then he was to go for the protein, always leaving the carbohydrates like rice and bread for last (that is, if he were eating them, because we still had him focused on eating a low-carbohydrate diet).

Cinnamon

There are approximately 250 species of cinnamon, but cassia cinnamon is probably what you have in your cabinet. It is the most common cinnamon in the world, and studies have shown it can benefit glycemic control. For example, a meta-analysis of those with type 2 diabetes reported that eating 1 to 6 grams (¼ to 1 teaspoon) of cinnamon per day significantly lowered fasting blood glucose by an average of 24 mg/dL (1.3 mmol/L), which corresponded to 12 to 17 percent for the group.[93] Even if you don't have type 2 diabetes, you can benefit from some cinnamon. In overweight adults, adding a teaspoon of cassia cinnamon to oatmeal or farina porridge was shown to lower the glycemic and insulin responses, suggesting enhanced insulin sensitivity.[94,95]

In healthy adults, consuming 1, 3, and 6 grams per day of cassia cinnamon over 40 days has been shown to reduce post-meal blood glucose levels, with the greatest effect seen with 3 and 6 grams (an 11 to 13 percent reduction).[96] Another study reported that 5 grams of cinnamon taken during a glucose tolerance test reduced the post-meal glucose response by 13 percent and improved insulin sensitivity compared to a placebo.[97]

The reason cinnamon works to control blood sugar is that it facilitates glucose uptake from the blood into tissues like our muscles.[98]

Bill wasn't a huge cinnamon fan, so I didn't push this for him. When working with clients, I seek the path of least resistance and find what nutritional approaches, including specific foods, resonate the most. This is a great reminder that not all the strategies you come across will be right for you, and that's okay. Take the ones that excite you, and when you're feeling adventurous, I urge you to go outside your comfort zone to try something new. If you try something and it doesn't work, then let it go and move on. There are plenty of strategies to experiment with, and you will find the best ones that work well for you.

If, unlike Bill, you like cinnamon, then I urge you to incorporate it into your diet. Use it as a spice for your chicken or ground beef or sprinkle it onto Greek yogurt—about a teaspoon (5 grams) per day should do it.

MAKING THE CHANGES STICK

Bill had just been diagnosed as prediabetic, so I knew there was a strong chance that he could reverse it simply by moving to a low-carb diet, incorporating a salad with vinegar before each meal, and eating his vegetables first followed by protein.

"Our focus will be on helping you shed some fat mass so you can move back into your personal fat threshold," I told Bill. "You don't need to count calories. Just focus on removing carbs—especially breads, pastas, and rice—while increasing your healthy, wholesome vegetables, and let's cut out the late-night snacking."

The last thing I ever want to do is to overwhelm my clients with too many nutritional strategies, so I held off on introducing other tips on improving body composition. Incorporating too many changes can make them unsustainable, and sometimes our bodies don't welcome or respond well to multiple changes. Minor changes really do add up over time.

In one month, Bill was down about 10 pounds, and he was excited. He felt his energy levels were rebounding, although he still got fatigued, especially in the afternoon. At this point it seemed that Bill was ready to add more nutritional strategies, especially on fat loss and returning to a healthier body composition, so I had him increase his protein per meal and ideally add a 15-minute walk after every meal. Knowing that sometimes it wouldn't be possible, I told Bill to at least walk after his heaviest meal.

Three months later, Bill was down another 25 pounds, for a total fat loss of 35 pounds in four months. Overall, Bill said he hadn't felt this good or energized since he was in his 20s. He felt less irritable and moody. He was sleeping better, and when he went for a follow-up exam with his doctor, his blood results showed that he no longer met the diagnosis for prediabetes. This was fantastic news for Bill and what I hope for with all my clients struggling with blood sugar and/or a prediabetes/diabetes diagnosis.

Bill reached his goal, but his race wasn't done; it was just starting.

Bill now had to maintain his fat loss to stay within his personal fat threshold if he wanted to keep diabetes at bay. While he had gone on a rather restrictive low-carb diet, he wanted to slowly reintroduce some foods like the occasional bread or pasta. I tell my clients that reintroducing foods is a personal preference. Some people can eat certain foods in moderation, while for others, it's all or nothing and that "all" can tip the scales into an unhealthy place.

There's no right answer other than to be aware of your habits. If you can eat the occasional slice of bread or serving of pasta or ice cream without overindulging, then do it. But if that one serving is the entire loaf, box, or carton, then perhaps removing it from your diet is the healthier choice. Overall, though, I support a balanced diet that you can sustain over the long haul that keeps your blood sugar in check and your energy strong.

Poor glycemic control and unstable blood sugar levels are often caused by having excess fat, so embarking on a fat loss journey can lead to better blood sugar levels. If your diet got you into this mess, then it can get you out. The choice and power to change are yours.

ACTION LIST

To kick off better glycemic control, I encourage you to pick one to three items you can implement today. Stick with them for at least three to four weeks, or until they become habitual, and then add another one to three habits to your daily routine.

As in other chapters, you may find that you can incorporate more than three. That's fine if it's sustainable, but don't overwhelm yourself. Restoring better glycemic control takes time, so make sure you can perform each task effortlessly and efficiently before moving on to another.

Also, you'll notice that each task except the last has a primary goal with three to four smaller stepping-stone goals beneath it. That's intentional, as establishing new habits often requires baby steps in the right direction. I urge you to start with the first stepping-stone and then work your way down before checking off the primary goal box.

- ☐ **Reduce your intake of digestible carbohydrates. (Note: this may not be necessary depending on your personal needs and dietary preferences.)**
  - ☐ Replace "avoid" foods with "no restriction" foods at 1 meal.
  - ☐ Replace "avoid" foods with "no restriction" foods at 2 meals.
  - ☐ Replace "avoid" foods with "no restriction" foods at every meal.

- ☐ **Confine your food and caloric beverage intake to a time-restricted window.**
  - ☐ Consume all your calories within 12 to 14 hours.
  - ☐ Consume all your calories within 10 to 12 hours.
  - ☐ Consume all your calories within 6 to 10 hours.

- ☐ **Eat sources of protein and fibrous vegetables before sources of digestible carbohydrate.**
  - ☐ At 1 meal.
  - ☐ At 2 meals.
  - ☐ At every meal.

- ☐ **Consume at least 5 grams of cinnamon per day, preferably spread across carbohydrate-containing meals.**
  - ☐ At 1 meal.
  - ☐ At 2 meals.
  - ☐ At every meal.

- ☐ **Drink 1 to 2 tablespoons of vinegar (diluted in water or used as a dressing over salad) before eating your meals.**
  - ☐ At 1 meal.
  - ☐ At 2 meals.
  - ☐ At every meal.

- ☐ **Obtain a healthy body composition by losing fat mass and building muscle mass. (Note: this may not be applicable to you if you're already at a healthy body composition.)**
  - ☐ Follow the recommendations put forth in Chapter 3.

CHAPTER 6

BOOSTING YOUR BRAIN FOR ENERGY PERFORMANCE

Stephanie had gone from climbing mountains to barely walking two blocks. "My energy levels are so low, all I do is mope around my apartment, and my brain function has been affected severely," she told me the first time we met. "My doctor told me that my cognitive decline is accelerating and I'm beginning to show signs of early-onset dementia."

In her early 50s, Stephanie felt miserable and lacked any motivation. "Socializing is an extreme effort, and I've started avoiding most situations because they become too overwhelming too quickly."

Stephanie felt like her brain had broken right along with her energy levels. She suffered from memory issues and brain fog—these symptoms, combined with her extreme fatigue, had exacerbated her anxiety and depression. "My life is intolerable. I'm existing in chronic pain, unhappiness, and exhaustion."

UNLOCKING THE MYSTERIES OF YOUR BRAIN

Most people I work with never suffer from just fatigue—it's usually multiple health conditions that leave them feeling worn out, desperate, and hopeless. It's been decades since I experienced the devastating impacts of mono, but I can still remember that feeling of despair and fear—fear because not only does getting to the underlying cause take time but there's never a silver pill or one Holy Grail switch that turns your life around.

And when your brain health is affected, it can feel more terrifying because you don't recognize yourself. You can't think clearly. Sometimes the most mundane daily tasks leave your brain fuzzy and confused. Your moods can quickly shift from irritable to anxious to depressed.

Your brain is the central hub of your life. It determines virtually all bodily commands and behaviors, from breathing to what you think to what you feel. If your brain isn't working at capacity, not only does it have grave consequences for your health but it also reduces your energy levels.

People struggling with energy and fatigue problems, especially in the more severe stages of chronic fatigue, often experience brain-related symptoms, including:

- Brain-related fatigue (feeling fatigued, exhausted, or sleepy, almost as if your brain turns off after a mentally demanding task such as working at your job, reading a book, studying, or driving a car)

- Brain fog (a type of cognitive dysfunction that involves memory problems, lack of ability to concentrate, lack of mental clarity, clouded thoughts, slow thought processes, and poor focus)

- Loss of resilience (to stress, fragility, and even relatively minor psychological stress or physical activity)

- Depression or anxiety

- Fibromyalgia or migraines

- Psychological conditions or psychiatric conditions

People often think of these conditions as separate and unrelated; however, they're intertwined.

Even if you have mild to moderate fatigue, it's likely that you also suffer from brain-related symptoms. Why? Because these health conditions and fatigue are connected at the cellular level in the brain.

UNDERSTANDING THE BRAIN HEALTH–MITOCHONDRIA LINK

Your brain is a complex organ, and two primary components of it that keep your body properly functioning are *neurons* and *neurotransmitters*. Neurons are information messengers, or the buildings in your brain's city. Neurons are responsible for generating signals and communicating within the brain and nervous system what is happening—or needs to happen—in the body.

Neurotransmitters are the chemical messengers carrying the signals and information from the neurons throughout the brain and nervous system. If neuronal buildings generate messages to be communicated, neurotransmitters are the people who carry messages from building to building.

You need both neurons and neurotransmitters—the signal and the unimpeded transmission—for optimal brain health, overall wellness, and strong energy levels. If your neurons get damaged or become dysfunctional, or if your neurotransmitters become disrupted and imbalanced, then your brain can't send or deliver the right signals for energy production.

There's a strong connection between chronic fatigue and widespread changes in brain structure and function. If you are battling with chronically low energy levels, then there is a good chance that poor brain health is at least partly responsible.

A systematic review of 55 studies involving chronically fatigued patients found widespread changes in brain structure and function compared to those without chronic fatigue, including:[1]

- Disrupted autonomic nervous system activity
- White matter volume loss and brain shrinkage
- Functional connectivity deficits between brain regions
- Impaired cognition and memory
- Reduced cerebral blood flow and nutrient delivery
- Predisposition to depression and anxiety

One of the biggest reasons for worsening brain health and mood disturbances is mitochondrial dysfunction. The brain is rich in mitochondria that are vital for proper neuronal firing and neurotransmission,[2] and the brain is a highly energy-dependent organ. As we discussed in Chapter 5, while making up only 2 percent of the body's weight, the brain uses 20 percent of the body's oxygen at rest.[3] We know that mitochondrial dysfunction is the keystone of chronic fatigue, and it may also be the keystone of neuroinflammation, cognitive decline, and neurodegeneration[4]—all of which can lead to fatigue.

Many of our brain-related health and energy issues can be traced back to *neuroinflammation* and a *leaky blood-brain barrier.*

You have more than 370 miles (600 kilometers) of blood vessels that deliver oxygen and nutrients to, and remove metabolic wastes from, your brain. To prevent unwanted molecules from getting into the brain, this vast expanse of blood vessels is coated with a *blood-brain barrier* (BBB) that serves as the gatekeeper to your brain,[5] much as the gut barrier serves as the gatekeeper to your body.

The blood-brain barrier plays an integral role in protecting your brain from all the things that shouldn't be allowed to enter, including toxins, pathogens, errant immune cells, foreign particles in the bloodstream, and so on. At the same time, the blood-brain barrier needs to let in materials such as glucose, carbohydrates, proteins, amino acids, ketones, vitamins and minerals, immune cells and cytokines, and hormones. The problem is that over time, due to things like toxins in the environment, chronic stress, or a poor diet, the blood-brain barrier can become dysfunctional or "leaky," allowing in particles that shouldn't be getting through. It's been shown that individuals with chronic fatigue have signatures of BBB dysfunction,[6] which could explain the predisposition to brain fog, cognitive decline, and mood disturbances.

When the BBB is leaky, our brain is hit with a one-two punch: (1) neurotoxic molecules enter the brain, causing neuroinflammation and neuronal injury, while (2) clearance of metabolic and toxic waste products becomes impaired, exacerbating harm to the brain.[7] It has been unequivocally established that BBB disruption is both necessary and sufficient to cause neurodegeneration and cognitive impairment.[8,9]

Neuroinflammation causes neurons to fire more slowly, or potentially to fire too much, which can slow down and disrupt brain cell communication and cognitive performance. Your brain cells become either sluggish or exhausted from firing excessively.

This causes mitochondrial dysfunction, and it alters other critical energy-related controls in the body.

Brain Signals Misread

Your brain and body constantly communicate with each other on a subconscious level. You don't have to consciously remind your lungs to breathe oxygen in and carbon dioxide out. Many of our subconscious biological and chemical processes are evolutionary designs to keep our body healthy, safe, and properly functioning.

The signals between our brain and body have a lot to do with our energy levels. Take "sickness behavior," which we looked at in Chapter 3. Sickness behavior occurs when your body must fight off a virus or bacteria or has suffered a trauma, or you have inflammatory cytokines flowing. Your brain picks up on these signals and "chooses" to cause fatigue by reducing neurotransmitters and hormones that would typically motivate you to feel awake, alert, and active. Your brain—as the central controller—recognizes the body needs rest and recovery, so it slows you down.

This is an incredible evolutionary adaptation that allowed the human body to overcome illness and injury. Yet we face an evolutionary mismatch in the modern day, where *chronic neuroinflammation* tricks the brain into making us feel sick and tired all the time.

If you're chronically inflamed from a poor diet, stress, or exposure to toxins—or some combination of these factors—your brain could be, and most likely is, intentionally sending your body into a fatigue state as it attempts to heal.

Another example of your brain "choosing" to make you feel tired and exhausted is something often related to sports performance: *central nervous system fatigue (central fatigue)*.

Central fatigue is a state of altered neurotransmitter signaling—particularly of the neurotransmitters noradrenaline, serotonin, and dopamine—that impedes muscle function independent from the state of the muscles themselves.[10,11,12,13] So even if your muscles could keep going, your brain will say no because the neurotransmitter signaling is off.

It's like your body is a car and your brain is the driver. If your car is out of oil, out of gas, or otherwise damaged, its ability to drive will be impaired regardless of how hard you push the gas pedal. Similarly, if your muscles are out of energy or injured, your physical performance will suffer regardless of the brain's commands. The reverse is also true. Even if your car (muscles) is in perfect shape, you won't go anywhere if the driver (brain) has their foot on the brakes.

As with sickness behavior, this is an evolutionary mechanism designed to protect us. Since our brain and body constantly communicate, if our brain perceives continued physical activity as a threat to our survival, it'll take action to prevent it.[14,15] As a result, our brains are on high alert for threats like dehydration, overheating, and insufficient nutrition and will reduce motor commands and increase perceived effort in the hopes of exhausting our body and causing it to stop moving.

With central and chronic fatigue, the brain misreads signals from the body and inappropriately slams on the energy brakes.

Individuals with chronic fatigue are unable to fully activate (contract) their muscles despite the absence of any abnormalities preventing total use, but they are able to increase muscle contraction by directly stimulating the muscle, indicating that the issue is with the brain signal rather than the muscle.[16]

When electrodes were used to directly measure the strength of the brain signal coming into the muscles of women with chronic fatigue as they physically exerted themselves, their muscles could contract as forcefully as those of healthy, non-fatigued adults when locally stimulated with electricity, but this was only 40 percent as powerful as if the muscles had been stimulated by their own accord (from the brain). Confirming the role of central fatigue, the electrical signal from the brain reaching the muscle tissue was equivalently reduced as well.[17]

Mood and Perception Changes

Do you feel more energized when you feel happy or when you feel sad? What about when you are focused and mentally sharp compared to having brain fog and difficulty concentrating?

Our perceptions about the world around us and our overall mental state play subtle but paramount roles in determining our daily energy levels. If we have poor brain health, it will impact our perceptions about the world, ourselves, and our feelings and desires around physically moving our body and acting.

Our mood plays a tremendous role in determining our energy levels. Having an unhealthy brain can predispose us to mood disorders like anxiety and depression, which can take a huge toll on our vitality and livelihood.

Greater fatigue has been linked to both worsening depression and higher anxiety, with fatigue increasing the economic burden of depression by 45 percent.[18] Yet one of the effects of resolving people's depression is a reduction in fatigue severity,[19] clearly showing that depression can lead to fatigue.

Neurotransmitter Deficits

For your body to have the energy it needs, the neurons in your brain must signal that it's time for abundant energy, to be awake and alert, and to feel happy. And once those neurons fire, you need enough neurotransmitters to transmit those signals.

But if you don't have enough neurotransmitters, or if they cannot properly bind to the neurons to communicate with them, then you may not think clearly, remember at capacity, be fully emotionally stable, or have the energy you need to go about your day.

Yet for many people, this is everyday life—and they have no idea why they can't focus, why their memory is fading, why their anxiety or depression is flaring, or why they feel tired all the time.

There are numerous neurotransmitters in the body, but the five most important for energy levels include:

- Acetylcholine

- Dopamine

- Serotonin

- Orexin

- GABA

Acetylcholine

When it comes to fatigue, acetylcholine is the neurotransmitter that our brain uses to tell our body to move. Studies have linked chronic fatigue to disturbed acetylcholine signaling, particularly an overreactive acetylcholinergic system that ultimately reduces the body's ability to appropriately respond to its signal.[20,21]

Acetylcholine is one of the most prevalent neurotransmitters in the body, involved in regulating muscle contractions of the heart, blood vessels, and skeletal muscle, as well as the ability to learn and remember. Disturbances in acetylcholine signaling can have widespread consequences for cognitive function, cardiovascular health, and physical function.[22]

For example, young adults whose acetylcholine signaling is inhibited by drugs demonstrate similar impairments in long-term and working memory as elderly adults suffering from cognitive decline.[23] Moreover, reductions in acetylcholine signaling set up the brain to be less plastic and more vulnerable from other insults like oxidative stress, inflammation, and injury.[24]

Dopamine

Dopamine is a tiny molecule with a big job: motivation and reward. Whenever you do something pleasurable, like eat cake, orgasm, or accomplish a goal, dopamine is released to help reinforce that behavior. It makes us feel good and motivates us to continue engaging in behaviors that bring us pleasure.

Addiction is probably the best-known example of dopamine involvement.[25] Whether it's a drug, food, or behavior, the dopamine burst we experience leads us to crave more of that experience. With regular exposure, we form habits or routines whereby the experience is expected to give us that pleasurable dopamine reward.

Yet there's a downside as well: regular exposure leads to tolerance. Tolerance means that we need more of the experience to get the same effect we once enjoyed in the beginning. This is why drug use tends to escalate with time. Tolerance also means that ceasing to use a drug or engage in a behavior causes a dopamine withdrawal, leading to agitation, irritability, difficulty concentrating, and excessive preoccupation of our thoughts with the pleasurable experience.

The reason we want to ensure that our dopamine system is functioning optimally is that low levels of dopamine can lead to apathy, a lack of motivation, an inability to complete or follow through with tasks, mood swings, and addictive tendencies.

If you're struggling with a maladaptive habit that you can't seem to kick, optimizing your dopamine system can help make establishing healthier habits easier, including those we've discussed for building up energy and overcoming fatigue. Plus, structural and functional neuroimaging studies have strongly supported the role of dopamine dysregulation in chronic fatigue patients.[26] In fact, giving chronically fatigued adults a dopamine-mimicking drug leads to significant increases in dopamine signaling and reductions in their fatigue.[27]

Serotonin

Serotonin is possibly the most diverse neurotransmitter in our body, regulating how we both think and behave, as well as numerous physiological processes involved in digestion and bowel motility, breathing, cardiovascular function, and sexual function.[28] Serotonin also modulates all behavioral and psychological processes, including mood, perception, reward, anger, aggression, appetite, memory, and attention.[29]

This ties into psychedelics. No matter what psychedelic you talk about—magic mushrooms, ayahuasca, LSD—all cause altered states of consciousness and hallucinations through potently binding with and activating serotonin receptors within the brain.[30]

On the flip side, many mood disorders are related to too little serotonin activity, a common example being depression.[31,32] While low levels of serotonin don't outright cause depression, they do alter the way in which we perceive and process information, predisposing us to negative thought patterns, apathy, and an inability to enjoy pleasurable things.[33]

If you aren't optimizing your serotonin levels, then you can expect to be moody, lose interest in things that once brought you pleasure, and worry needlessly. Plus, several studies have documented reductions in serotonin levels in chronically fatigued adults.[34,35,36]

Orexin

Orexin is one of the newest and least-known kids on the block, with its discovery occurring in 1998.[37] Prior to this, we didn't have a good understanding of what regulated sleep and wakefulness. But now we know that orexin is one of the most important players in our sleep-wake cycle.

Studies have shown that an orexin deficiency is the cause of narcolepsy, likely as the result of an autoimmune attack on orexin-producing neurons.[38] We have discovered that drugs inhibiting orexin signaling are an effective treatment for insomnia,[39] and that orexin signaling causes arousal and wakefulness.

In the decades since its discovery, orexin has been shown to play a significant role in regulating emotions, energy balance, and addictive tendencies.[40,41] Low levels of orexin are associated with lower levels of physical activity and obesity,[42] and orexin injections cause spontaneous increases in physical activity.[43] If you have low orexin levels, then it will reduce your desire to be active, reduce your energy expenditure, and increase your propensity for weight gain.

GABA

GABA (gamma aminobutyric acid) is the most potent inhibitory neurotransmitter in the brain and regulates many of the sedative actions required for relaxation.[44,45] It is also critical for the regulation of neuronal communication, cognition, emotion, and memory.[46,47,48]

Studies have suggested that higher GABA levels help reduce distraction in the brain,[49] which makes it possible to react and make decisions more quickly, and supplementing with GABA has been shown to improve attention and task switching in healthy young adults.[50,51]

Other research has documented a relationship between lower levels of GABA in the brain and a variety of cognitive deficits in humans including:

- Worse memory[52]
- Self-reported cognitive failures (e.g., inability to attend to relevant details while being distracted by irrelevant details)[53]
- Lower visuospatial IQ[54]
- Less empathy[55]

- Reduced resilience to stress and greater susceptibility to depression and anxiety[56]

- Susceptibility to addiction[57]

If you aren't supporting your GABA system, then you can expect to have difficulty concentrating, feelings of anxiety, a lower resilience to stress, and trouble sleeping, all of which can contribute to fatigue.

STRATEGIES FOR BETTER BRAIN HEALTH

Poor brain health can result from any of several factors, including neurodegeneration, neuroinflammation, oxidative stress, impaired synaptic connections, and neurotransmitter deficits. These issues can stem from stressors such as circadian dysregulation and sleep disruption, carrying too much fat mass, gut dysbiosis and systemic inflammation, and even poor glycemic control—all factors that can interfere with proper neuronal communication.

When it comes to improving brain health, we've already discussed multiple strategies, including:

- Fixing your circadian rhythm and getting deeper, more rejuvenating sleep

- Maintaining a healthy body composition and reducing excess fat mass

- Fostering a healthy microbiome and repairing your gut

- Stabilizing your blood sugar levels, eliminating big spikes and swings

Additionally, there are brain-specific nutritional strategies that you can use to directly boost your brain's performance, reduce cellular dysfunction, and improve your neurotransmitter levels and functioning. You'll notice that these recommendations are designed to improve your brain health and its ability to properly work, which will indirectly improve your energy levels.

Whole Foods, Mostly Plants

A healthy brain doesn't require any single diet. In fact, most research linking diet to brain health and better outcomes, including reducing risks of cognitive decline and mood disorders, recommends many of the tenets we've already mentioned, most particularly:

Eat a diet abundant in nutrient-dense,
whole foods, mostly plants.

If you're looking for a slightly more specific approach, then consider the *MIND diet*, developed by Dr. Martha Morris and her colleagues from Rush University Medical Center and based on the most compelling evidence in the diet-dementia field. The MIND diet is a blend of the Mediterranean diet and DASH diet, which is rich in fruits, vegetables, whole grains, and low-fat dairy foods and promoted by the National Heart, Lung, and Blood Institute to prevent and control high blood pressure.

The MIND diet promotes the consumption of 10 brain-healthy food groups:

- Green leafy vegetables—at least six servings per day
- Other fibrous vegetables—at least one serving per day
- Berries—at least two servings per week
- Nuts—at least one serving per day
- Beans—at least three servings per week
- Whole grains—at least three servings per day
- Seafood—at least once per week
- Poultry—at least twice per week
- Olive oil—primary added oil (if any)
- Wine—one glass per day (no more, no less)

Studies investigating the relationship between the MIND diet and cognitive function with aging have found that those with the highest adherence to this diet have a cognitive function equivalent to being roughly 7.5 years younger than those with the lowest score.[58] Adherence to the MIND diet has also been associated with 53 percent reduction in the odds of developing Alzheimer's disease over five years of follow-up.[59]

When I reviewed Stephanie's diet, I knew she wasn't eating enough and was possibly malnourished. She had almost no appetite, and most days she existed on chicken broth with some chopped vegetables like carrots and celery, baked or grilled chicken tossed with a salad, sometimes a baked potato, maybe an apple or banana, the occasional granola bar, and some eggs.

When we don't eat enough food or a variety of foods, we don't get the essential nutrients our bodies need to flourish. Also, undernourishment can send our bodies into a stress response in which we conserve energy since we lack fuel.

Stephanie needed a nutrition overhaul, but I didn't want to override her body's natural responses by having her eat when she really wasn't hungry. My plan was to have her eat three meals per day, with a snack. The meals could be on the small side (at least to start), and she had to eat most of her foods from the MIND diet list. Because Stephanie was fatigued and struggled with mental capacity, I wanted to keep the recipes simple and limit how much time she had to spend in the kitchen. This meant going with easy-to-prepare meals and ingredients. For instance, Stephanie would have sunny-side-up eggs over bok choy and kale with a cup of blueberries or strawberries for breakfast. To get grains into her diet, Stephanie would make a big batch of oatmeal that she could eat for a few days, which she topped with berries and/or walnuts or sunflower seeds.

Typically lunch was a big salad with different leafy greens such as spinach, kale, watercress, chard, arugula, or lettuce; an animal protein like fish or chicken; and fibrous vegetables like green beans, asparagus, broccoli, celery, cauliflower, garlic, and tomatoes. A few times per week, I had her toss in some beans—Stephanie's favorites were black beans and chickpeas. Her dressings were olive oil based.

For dinner, I wanted Stephanie to up her seafood intake, anything from a ginger shrimp stir-fry to snapper filets to Asian-style wild salmon served with mixed vegetables or salad.

Consume More Seafood (or Supplement with DHA and EPA)

All the food groups listed in the MIND diet play a critical role in brain health by supplying essential vitamins and minerals, fats and proteins, and phytochemicals (beneficial but nonessential nutrients originating in plants) that help your brain function better, but one that deserves special attention is the omega-3 fatty acid *docosahexaenoic acid*, or DHA.

The brain is the most lipid-dense organ in the body, second only to body fat, being 40 to 80 percent fat by weight depending on which part of the brain you're looking at.[60] Of that fat content, DHA is one of the most important molecules, increasing rapidly during early life and leveling off at approximately 14 percent of total brain mass or 20 to 30 percent of total brain fat content during adulthood.[61,62]

There are brain benefits from having sufficient DHA in our noggin, including the maintenance of neuronal membrane fluidity, potentiation of cell signaling, and use in the synthesis of anti-inflammatory docosanoid molecules.[63] Collectively these functions work to ensure our neurons aren't inflamed and can communicate with ease. These functions simply can't be maintained with other types of fats, leading to a widely accepted belief that an abundant intake of DHA in the diet was necessary for the evolution of the large human brain.[64]

Today most of us are doing dietary disservice to our brain by not getting enough DHA. The only populations that maintain an evolutionarily appropriate intake of DHA are Japan, Scandinavian countries, and areas of indigenous societies not yet influenced by the Western diet,[65] likely due to their high intake of fish and other seafood—the best natural sources of DHA.

The consequences of inadequate DHA intake may include increased risk for cognitive decline or dementia[66] and mental health conditions such as schizophrenia, bipolar disorder, anxiety, and depression.[67,68] In addition, individuals with Alzheimer's disease have shown lower brain concentrations of DHA.[69]

Importantly, DHA is not a magic pill for improving brain health but rather an essential nutrient that needs to be supplied regularly for its benefits to be realized. While there may be a memory benefit of DHA supplementation in those with cognitive impairment,[70] the greatest benefits of preventing neurodegeneration are seen when intake is adequate throughout one's lifespan.[71,72] It's also important to note that DHA, along with EPA—another "fish oil" omega-3—have potent anti-inflammatory effects both in the brain and throughout the body.[73,74]

In those with chronic fatigue, low omega-3 status is common.[75] The extent to which one is low in EPA and DHA also correlates with greater fatigue severity,[76] meaning that ensuring adequate DHA intake will not just help optimize brain health but also help optimize energy levels.

You don't need a lot of DHA; often 500 to 1000 mg per day is sufficient. This can be easily obtained by eating a couple of ounces of fatty fish or taking a supplement. But fish is the preferred choice for greater incorporation of EPA and DHA into blood lipids. For example, salmon is twice as efficient as supplements at increasing EPA status and ninefold more efficient at increasing DHA status.[77]

Nonetheless, not everyone likes eating seafood, so the next best option is supplements. If you want to go this road, there are several options on the market, including:

- Fish oil
- Krill oil
- Algae oil

Now, if you are vegan, fish and krill oils are out, so going with algae oil is your best bet. It won't supply as much EPA, but it does supply ample amounts of DHA.

In one study comparing algae oil supplements to salmon, both equivalently increased plasma DHA concentrations, although salmon was superior at simultaneously increasing plasma EPA concentrations.[78] Now, it is important to keep in mind that fish supplies vastly more nutrients than algae oil, which supplies only DHA, but when the goal is getting in your omega-3s, algae oil definitely serves its purpose.

As for fish oil and krill oil, each supplies EPA and DHA in a couple of different forms. Fish oil can come as an ethyl ester or a triglyceride, while krill oil comes as a combination of phospholipid and triglyceride. By far, most fish oil supplements on the market are triglyceride based, which makes sense, considering that 95 percent of all dietary fat and most of the storage fat on the body are triglycerides.

And that's okay, because standard triglyceride fish oil is likely to be the most affordable option. In a study comparing all three, four weeks of supplementing with EPA and DHA from a triglyceride-based fish oil was similar at raising EPA and DHA status compared to supplementing with equivalent amounts of EPA and DHA from both the ethyl ester fish oil and phospholipid krill oil.[79]

Lastly, the reason I haven't mentioned any vegan-friendly sources of EPA or DHA other than algae oil is that they don't exist. Plants do not contain EPA or DHA, but rather their parent fatty acid that our body must turn into EPA and DHA: alpha-linolenic acid (ALA). So when you see plants like flaxseed or chia seeds being advertised as having omega-3 fatty acids, they are supplying exclusively alpha-linolenic acid, not EPA or DHA.

Not only does alpha-linolenic acid lack the anti-inflammatory effects of EPA and DHA[80] but its conversion into EPA and DHA is inefficient. Studies show that less than 10 percent of alpha-linolenic acid is converted to EPA and less than 1 percent to DHA.[81] In addition, the enzymes required to make this conversion are shared between omega-3 and omega-6 fatty acids, so it's further reduced when the diet is high in omega-6 fatty acids, as is the case with the majority of the U.S. population, whose current ratio of omega-6 to omega-3 fatty acids is about 10 to 1.[82]

EPA and DHA Content of Common Seafoods			
Food Source (100 Grams or 3.5 Ounces)	EPA (grams)	DHA (grams)	Amount of Food Source Needed to Obtain 1 gram of EPA + DHA
Herring, Pacific	1.24	0.88	1.7 ounces
Salmon, Chinook	1.01	0.94	1.8 ounces
Mackerel, Pacific	0.65	1.20	1.9 ounces
Oysters, Pacific	0.88	0.50	2.5 ounces
Salmon, coho	0.54	0.83	2.5 ounces
Trout, rainbow	0.47	0.52	3.5 ounces
Salmon, sockeye	0.42	0.66	3.5 ounces
Tuna, canned White	0.23	0.63	4.0 ounces
Bass, freshwater	0.30	0.46	4.6 ounces
Salmon, pink	0.22	0.40	5.6 ounces
Lobster	0.34	0.14	7.0 ounces
Crab, Alaskan king	0.29	0.12	8.5 ounces
Lingcod	0.13	0.13	13.5 ounces
Tuna, canned light	0.05	0.22	13.5 ounces
Cod, Pacific	0.04	0.12	22.0 ounces

Now, the half-life of DHA in the human brain is roughly 2.5 years,[83] meaning that the DHA incorporated into our neurons stays there for quite some time. This provides ample time for this polyunsaturated fatty acid to become oxidized and dysfunctional, which has widespread consequences for brain health.

Both too little DHA and its oxidation are related to increased levels of neuroinflammation, neuronal dysfunction, and cell death, all of which are believed to contribute to the brain aging process.[84]

I'm a big believer in first trying to get what you need from fresh foods, but I also know that sometimes targeted supplements really are the best choice. When it came to Stephanie, I wanted her to introduce more seafood into her diet, but I also told her that if she was struggling to eat because she lacked an appetite, then she should try supplementing. There was no shame in that, and that was what she opted to do. To Stephanie's credit, she did increase her fish intake to twice per week, and she added a fish oil supplement that she took daily.

Eat Your Leafy Greens

To help protect your brain against neuroinflammation, neuronal dysfunction, cell death, and DHA oxidation, your brain harnesses two potent antioxidants: *lutein* and *zeaxanthin*.

Lutein is a carotenoid abundant in green leafy vegetables. It makes up a significant portion of our antioxidant defenses.[85] In particular, lutein has been shown to protect against DHA oxidation within the brain,[86] and brain concentrations of lutein are correlated with better cognitive function with aging.[87]

Supplements can play a huge role in boosting your brain health. Make sure to check out Chapter 8 to learn about the most effective supplements to optimize your brain function, mood, long-term brain health, and neurotransmitter balance.

BRAIN LUTEIN CONCENTRATION

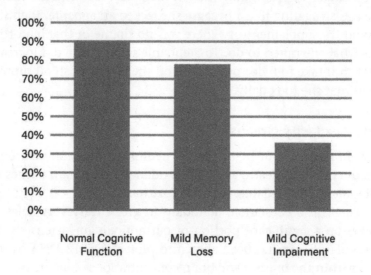

A systematic review of several studies investigating the impact of lutein supplementation on cognitive performance in otherwise healthy adults without cognitive impairment found that daily doses of 10 mg of lutein consistently improved episodic memory and inhibition, with potential additional benefits for improving attention.[88] Other studies have reported that lutein supplementation increases neurotrophic factors (molecules that support the growth and survival of neurons) and antioxidant capacity.[89]

The humble egg is a terrific source of lutein in a far more bioavailable form than that found in leafy green vegetables like spinach. In one study healthy adults who ate 6 mg of lutein through eggs every day for 10 days were found to have 68 percent more lutein in their bodies, significantly more than when the lutein was provided from spinach or two different forms of a lutein supplement.[90] In another study, having vegetarians eat just six eggs per week was enough to boost their lutein status by 20 percent.[91]

Lutein Content of Common Foods		
Food	Measurement	Lutein content (mg)
Spinach, raw	1 cup (30 grams)	3.7
Green peas	1 cup (145 grams)	3.6
Zucchini, boiled	1 cup (180 grams)	2.1
Broccoli, boiled	1 cup (156 grams)	2.0
Marigold-fed egg	1 large (50 grams)	1.6
Kale, raw	1 cup (21 grams)	1.3
Corn kernels	1 cup (145 grams)	1.1
Asparagus, boiled	1/2 cup (90 grams)	0.7
Celery, boiled	1 cup (150 grams)	0.5
Carrots, raw	1 cup (128 grams)	0.3
Conventional egg	1 large (50 grams)	0.25

Now, none of this means to ditch the spinach for eggs; it only means that eggs provide more bioavailable lutein. Your best bet: eat both. And don't throw out the yolks, since that is where the lutein is found.

Boost Key Nutrients for Neurotransmission

By following the nutritional strategies in this book, most people should get the essential nutrients they need to support their neurotransmitters. But sometimes we must intentionally increase our consumption of certain foods, and sometimes supplements, to ensure we're getting the right amounts. The MIND diet includes most of the foods we will want to eat and use to build a brain-healthy nutritional plan. But understanding *why* certain foods are critical, especially for our neurotransmitters, can help make adopting and embracing new nutritional strategies more successful.

Protein

First up is our good friend protein. It's essential not only for a healthy body composition but also for optimal brain health and neurotransmission. When eating a meal, we want it to contain protein regardless of our other choices. The absolute worst food choice we can make is to eat a pure carbohydrate meal and very little protein, which would lower orexin and cause sleepiness or fatigue. Protein supplies the dopamine precursor *tyrosine* and the serotonin precursor *tryptophan*. Without sufficient protein, we won't have enough building blocks to make dopamine or serotonin, which will lead us to feeling apathy and fatigue.

Our body requires several nutrients that we get from protein to create dopamine, including the amino acid tyrosine, vitamin B_6, folate, and iron. Basically, tyrosine is converted into the molecule L-DOPA with the help of folate and iron, which is then converted into dopamine with the help of vitamin B_6. Animal studies have shown that being deficient in any of these nutrients leads to disruptions in dopamine metabolism,[92,93,94,95] so it makes sense to ensure that your diet supplies ample amounts of each.

Vitamin B_6

Regularly eating lean meats, poultry, and seafood makes it easy for us to get the vitamin B_6 we need. You can also meet daily requirements from plants by regularly consuming nuts, seeds, potatoes, sweet potatoes, shiitake mushrooms, and cabbage.

Best Foods for Supplying Vitamin B$_6$ (per 100 Grams or 3.5 Ounces)			
	Percent of Daily Requirement Supplied	Animal Products	Plant Foods
"Green" range	>50 percent	Liver (all types) Tuna	Pistachios
"Orange" range	25 to 50 percent	Lean red meat Lean pork Fish and seafood Poultry	Sunflower seeds Hazelnuts Walnuts Hearts of palm
"Yellow" range	10 to 25 percent	Eggs	Most nuts and seeds Potatoes Shiitake mushrooms Brussels sprouts Sweet potatoes Sweet peppers Cabbage

Iron

Iron, the third nutrient for optimizing dopamine metabolism, is abundant in animal-based foods, but it requires a more conscious effort to obtain it from plants because plant-based forms of iron have a lower bioavailability than animal-based forms.

Best Foods for Supplying Iron (per 100 Grams or 3.5 Ounces)			
	Percent of Daily Requirement Supplied	Animal Products	Plant Foods
"Green" range	>50 percent (men) >25 percent (women)	Lean red meat Oysters Cuttlefish Octopus	Potatoes
"Orange" range	25 to 50 percent (men) 10 to 25 percent (women)	Sardines Dark poultry meat	Amaranth Teff Most beans Spinach
"Yellow" range	10 to 25 percent (men) 5 to 10 percent (women)	Most fish White meat Eggs Cheese	Most whole grains Kale Asparagus Mushrooms Peas

There are two forms of iron in the diet: heme and nonheme. Heme iron is supplied only by animal foods and has a bioavailability of 15 to 35 percent, while nonheme iron is the form of iron in plants and has a much lower bioavailability of less than 10 percent.[96,97] If you don't eat meat, then iron supplementation may be prudent to ensure you get the iron you need for dopamine production.

Folate

We need to get adequate folate, particularly in the form of methylfolate, which is the form required for dopamine synthesis.[98] It is readily obtainable from fibrous vegetables and beans, where roughly 45 to 65 percent of the folate is in methylfolate form.[99]

Best Foods for Supplying Folate (per 100 Grams or 3.5 Ounces)			
	Percent of Daily Requirement Supplied	Animal Products	Plant Foods
"Green" range	>50 percent	Liver	—
"Orange" range	25 to 50 percent	—	Most leafy green and fibrous vegetables Most beans
"Yellow" range	10 to 25 percent	Fish roe Mussels Crab	Most nuts and seeds

The only way we can make methylfolate within our body is through the MTHFR enzyme (methylenetetrahydrofolate reductase). Yet many people have polymorphisms that impair its functionality. Thus if you opt to supplement with folate, then please choose the methylfolate form, particularly if you have any polymorphisms in MTHFR. It's the most biologically active form and circumvents any issues with genetics.

Tryptophan

In addition to vitamin B_6, folate, and iron, your body also needs *amino acid tryptophan* to synthesize serotonin. Tryptophan needs to cross the blood-brain barrier to be used for serotonin production within the brain, but it competes with several other amino acids for transport across this barrier.

When we eat carbohydrates, the insulin response will preferentially shuttle many of these other amino acids into muscle tissue, leaving tryptophan with less competition for getting across the blood-brain barrier.[100] Mood disturbances like depression, being quick to anger, irritability, a big appetite, a poor memory, and/or a short attention span can be signs that your body isn't producing enough serotonin. As such, if you tend to run on the lower end of serotonin production, you may benefit from eating a higher-carbohydrate diet that you would get from grains, legumes, starchy vegetables, and fruit (alongside adequate protein, of course).

Choline

Choline is an essential nutrient within the brain required for the synthesis of acetylcholine (the primary neurotransmitter involved in executive functions) and phosphatidylcholine (one of the most abundant and important structural components of cell membranes).

Best Foods for Supplying Choline (per 100 Grams or 3.5 Ounces)			
	Percent of Daily Requirement Supplied	Animal Products	Plant Foods
"Green" range	>50 percent	Liver (all types) Whole eggs Caviar and fish roe	Sunflower lecithin
"Orange" range	25 to 50 percent	Lean red meat Lean pork Oysters Salmon	—
"Yellow" range	10 to 25 percent	White fish Most mollusks Poultry	Beans and legumes Nuts and seeds Cauliflower Mushrooms Collard greens Broccoli Brussels sprouts

It's well established that choline within the brain plays a critical role in neuronal plasticity, membrane stability, signaling events, and neurotransmission, all of which are important for communication within the brain and nervous system.[101]

An omnivorous diet should provide sufficient choline, as most meat is a decent source of it. Even if you don't eat meat, just three eggs per day will satisfy your needs, and sunflower lecithin represents a solid vegan option.

Stay Hydrated

Brain cells need a fresh supply of clean, pure water every day to function well. It's so critical for all our cells, which is why our bodies can exist without food for several weeks but can only function for three to four days at most without water. It takes just hours for dehydration to impair physical energy levels, mood, and brain function.

Proper hydration causes increased blood pressure and arterial vessel expansion (vasodilation), which promotes increased blood flow to the brain, which, in turn, enhances oxygen and glucose delivery to brain cells and improves mood, energy levels, and cognitive performance.

When it comes to how much water you should drink, there is no one-size-fits-all amount. It's not "drink your body weight in ounces each day" either. How much water you need depends on your daily activity levels and the climate you live in. If you are someone who spends hours outdoors each day, does lots of intense exercise, and uses a sauna daily, then your water needs will be drastically more than someone who has a sedentary desk job and who spends most of their time in a climate-controlled room.

The best way to gauge how much water you need to drink is to check the color of your urine. The lighter the color, the more hydrated you are, while the darker the color, the more water you need to drink.

A word of caution: some substances, like beets, carrots, black-berries, and paprika, and large doses of some B vitamins (such as riboflavin) can alter your urine color.

My final tip: don't just run to the faucet for tap water. If you live in the U.S., your public tap water supply likely contains chemicals that may harm your gut health. You want pure, clean water, so check your area.

This was one area Stephanie admitted she could improve. Like many people, she relied on coffee to keep her going in the morning and afternoon, so I encouraged her to slowly cut back on the caffeine—even tea—and up her water intake. She said she didn't like the taste of water on its own, but I encouraged her to buy a home water filter that she could connect to her faucet and to add a spritz of lemon or lime or a few slices of cucumber.

MAKING THE CHANGES STICK

Poor brain function, brain fog, and brain-related fatigue make daily life hard. Healing your brain, balancing your neurotransmitters, and optimizing your brain function will not only improve your mental capacity but will shift your energy. For Stephanie it truly was a journey. Switching to the MIND diet started moving her in the right direction within a month, but it wasn't a miraculous recovery.

Restoring vitality and energy is often a gradual reawakening, which was hard for Stephanie to embrace. But I emphasized to her that she would enjoy better results by loosening the reins on needing to see immediate transformation and instead tracking how she felt monthly. For five days, Stephanie would track her foods, moods, sleep patterns, memory, and overall energy; then a month later, she would track it again.

While it took Stephanie almost a year before she returned to rock climbing, the steady progress each month helped motivate her to continue the work. "For the first time in so long, I feel like I'm moving in the right direction," Stephanie told me about two months into our work together. "I know I'm not fully back, but I feel better, and I feel like I will make it someday."

As each month passed and she saw more results, we kept adding nutritional strategies, such as rewiring her circadian rhythm and repairing her gut.

Stephanie's journey reflects that we don't control the pace of our healing—whether it involves restoring our brain health or energy. But we can support our brains and our bodies on this journey by nourishing ourselves with the foods we need to return to our optimal capacity.

ACTION LIST

The following checklist is here for you to pick from to start on your energy healing journey for brain health. As with previous chapters, I encourage you to pick no more than three items to implement. Give it at least two to four weeks, or until those actions become habitual, and then pick up to three more challenges.

- ☐ **Get your daily dose of DHA and EPA.**
  - ☐ Eat fish or seafood 1 time per week.
  - ☐ Eat fish or seafood 2 to 3 times per week.
  - ☐ Eat fish or seafood 4 to 6 times per week.

- ☐ **Get your daily dose of lutein and zeaxanthin.**
  - ☐ Eat 1 to 2 servings (1 cup raw or 1/2 cup cooked) of leafy green vegetables per day.
  - ☐ Eat 3 to 4 servings of leafy green vegetables per day.
  - ☐ Eat 5-plus servings of leafy green vegetables per day.

- [ ] **Incorporate berries into your diet.**
  - [ ] Eat 1 cup of berries 1 to 2 times per week.
  - [ ] Eat 1 cup of berries 3 to 4 times per week.
  - [ ] Eat at least 1 cup of berries daily.

- [ ] **Incorporate nuts into your diet.**
  - [ ] Eat a handful (1 ounce) of nuts 1 to 2 times per week.
  - [ ] Eat a handful of nuts 3 to 4 times per week.
  - [ ] Eat a handful of nuts daily.

- [ ] **Incorporate beans and legumes into your diet.**
  - [ ] Eat 1 cup of beans 1 to 2 times per week.
  - [ ] Eat 1 cup of beans 3 to 4 times per week.
  - [ ] Eat 1 cup of beans every day.

- [ ] **Consume adequate choline to support acetylcholine signaling.**
  - [ ] Eat 1 serving of the "yellow" choline foods per day.
  - [ ] Eat 1 serving of the "orange" or two servings of the "yellow" choline foods per day.
  - [ ] Eat 1 to 2 servings of the "green," 2 to 3 servings of the "orange," or 4 to 5 servings of the "yellow" choline foods daily.

- [ ] **Consume adequate vitamin B_6 to support GABA, dopamine, and serotonin signaling.**
  - [ ] Eat 1 serving of the "yellow" B_6 foods per day.
  - [ ] Eat 1 serving of the "orange" or 2 servings of the "yellow" B_6 foods per day.

☐ Eat 1 to 2 servings of the "green," 2 to 3 servings of the "orange," or 4 to 5 servings of the "yellow" B_6 foods daily.

☐ **Consume adequate folate to support dopamine and serotonin signaling.**

    ☐ Eat 1 serving of the "yellow" folate foods per day.

    ☐ Eat 1 serving of the "orange" or 2 servings of the "yellow" folate foods per day.

    ☐ Eat 1 to 2 servings of the "green," 2 to 3 servings of the "orange," or 4 to 5 servings of the "yellow" folate foods daily.

☐ **Consume adequate iron to support dopamine and serotonin signaling.**

    ☐ Eat 1 serving of the "yellow" iron foods per day.

    ☐ Eat 1 serving of the "orange" or 2 servings of the "yellow" iron foods per day.

    ☐ Eat 1 to 2 servings of the "green," 2 to 3 servings of the "orange," or 4 to 5 servings of the "yellow" iron foods daily.

☐ **Ensure that your diet is providing you with adequate daily protein to support neurotransmitter synthesis (refer to Chapter 3 for adequacy information).**

    ☐ Calculate your ideal protein intake and eat it 1 to 2 days per week.

    ☐ Eat sufficient protein 3 to 4 days per week.

    ☐ Eat sufficient protein 5 to 6 days per week.

    ☐ Eat sufficient protein every day.

☐ **Drink enough water throughout the day to have most of your urine be lemonade-colored.**

PART II

SUPERCHARGE YOUR MITOCHONDRIA

CHAPTER 7

ENERGY SUPERFOODS

Food is fuel, and some food choices are "super" fuel in their health-promoting and mitochondria-boosting properties.

You now have numerous nutritional strategies for beating fatigue, supercharging your mitochondria, and improving several areas of your health and well-being. If you find yourself pulled to address one particular stressor—say, your gut health—then start there, incorporating those recommendations and foods first. If you're unsure where to start, or you want broader suggestions for what to eat that will improve the health, strength, and number of your mitochondria, then this chapter on superfoods is for you.

Some of these superfoods will directly impact your mitochondria and energy levels, while others may benefit critical systems and functions that indirectly enhance your energy levels.

To make this chapter easy to navigate, these superfoods are divided into their general food groups, so the next time you're looking for the best fruit, veggie, or nut to eat, you'll pick one that enhances rather than depletes your energy. I've included suggested serving or supplement sizes as appropriate when supported by the evidence.

FRUITS

Pomegranates

Pomegranate is a rich source of ellagitannins, potent antioxidants that can be further broken into other antioxidant compounds like ellagic acid and urolithins.[1,2] These substances have been heavily investigated for their cardiovascular, anticancer, and mitochondrial benefits.

Regular intake of pomegranate juice has been shown to reduce blood lipid oxidation and the accumulation of plaque in arteries over the course of 1 to 3 years,[3] particularly in people who have higher levels of oxidative stress.[4,5]

The most important benefit of pomegranates is their ability to stimulate mitochondrial function and mitophagy, which is done primarily through a compound called urolithin A.[6] Mitophagy (mitochondria + autophagy) is a quality-control pathway that preserves mitochondrial health by targeting damaged mitochondria for autophagic degradation, making anything that facilitates mitophagy vital for optimal health and disease prevention.

In recreational endurance athletes, supplementing with 750 mg of pomegranate extract for just two weeks increased the total time the athletes could cycle before complete exhaustion by 14 percent and increased the amount of time they could rely on their mitochondria to supply most of their energy by 10 percent.[7]

Recommended Dose: Supplement with 750 to 1500 mg of pomegranate extract or eat ½ to 1 pomegranate daily

Blueberries

If you want to boost your brain power, memory, learning ability, and executive functioning skills, then look to the blueberry. Numerous studies have reported that consuming the equivalent of 1 to 2 cups of blueberries per day improves learning ability, memory, and executive cognitive function in healthy older adults,[8,9,10] older adults with cognitive impairment,[11,12] and young, healthy adults.[13]

Additionally, an ever-growing body of evidence suggests that blueberries and their constituent phytochemicals are protective against the development of cancer, obesity, cardiovascular diseases, diabetes, bone loss, poor immune function, fatty liver, vision loss, and chronic inflammation.[14]

Recommended Dose: Eat 1 to 2 cups of blueberries per day.

Acai Berries

Acai berries are an antioxidant- and phytochemical-rich fruit native to the Amazon rainforest. Regular consumption of acai may help battle cardiovascular disease through reducing blood lipid oxidation,[15,16,17] fight cognitive decline with aging,[18,19,20,21] protect against cancer and reduce its ability to spread and proliferate,[22] and protect against liver damage and inflammation.[23]

Consuming acai can help reduce biomarkers of muscle damage following strenuous exercise. It increases serum antioxidant status and lowers blood lipids,[24] as well as improving physical performance and reducing perceived exertion.[25] Furthermore, consumption of acai berries has been reported to reduce markers of inflammation and oxidative stress while improving blood vessel function, particularly in overweight and obese adults.[26,27]

Recommended Dose: Eat 1 to 2 cups of acai berries per day

Bilberries

Bilberries are a dark-purple berry originating in Europe that possesses a diverse array of anthocyanin phytochemicals similar to blueberries,[28,29] which have potent antioxidant and anti-inflammatory effects.[30,31]

Studies have reported reductions in inflammation with the addition of 330 mL of bilberry juice in adults at an elevated heart disease risk,[32] and with 300 mg of bilberry anthocyanins in otherwise healthy adults.[33] Additionally, in adults with type 2 diabetes, eating the equivalent of 50 grams of fresh bilberries before drinking a sugary beverage lowered their glycemic and insulin responses by 18 percent each.[34]

Recommended Dose: Eat 1 to 2 cups of bilberries per day

Maqui Berries

Maqui berries are an exotic, dark-purple fruit native to South America. They are a rich source of anthocyanins that possess strong antioxidant abilities,[35,36] and ultimately provide up to three times more antioxidants than blackberries, blueberries, strawberries, or raspberries.[37,38]

Studies have shown that maqui berries could be a powerful ally against inflammatory diseases.[39] Particularly, they have been shown to reduce blood vessel inflammation,[40] and in one study of smokers, 2 grams of maqui berry extract per day reduced markers of lung inflammation after two weeks.[41]

In a three-month clinical study in people with prediabetes, 180 mg of maqui berry extract once daily reduced average blood sugar levels by 5 percent, which was enough to bring their blood glucose levels back into normal range.[42] It also reduced their LDL and increased their HDL (i.e., improved their blood lipid profile).

Other research has found that 30 to 60 mg of a concentrated maqui berry extract each day increased tear production by roughly 50 percent,[43] with follow-up research demonstrating similar effects after just a month, along with reduced eye fatigue.[44]

Recommended Dose: Supplement with 100 to 2000 mg of maqui berry extract daily

Cranberries

Cranberries are pinkish-red berries that are rich in A-type pro-anthocyanidins (PACs), in contrast to the B-type PACs present in most other fruits. Studies in animals and humans have shown that adding cranberries to the diet reduces markers of oxidative stress and inflammation and thereby protects against mitochondrial dysfunction.[45]

Numerous randomized, controlled trials in adults with metabolic dysfunction have also shown that drinking 1 to 2 cups of cranberry juice or taking 1500 mg of cranberry extract improves blood lipids, blood pressure, vascular function, and insulin sensitivity.[46]

Recommended Dose: Eat 1 to 2 cups of cranberries per day

Camu Camu

Camu camu is an Amazonian berry renowned for its high levels of vitamin C and phytochemicals,[47,48] which have been consistently associated with health benefits.[49,50,51,52]

In animals, camu camu has been shown to reduce inflammation,[53] reduce fat gain and mitigate metabolic dysfunction,[54] and protect the liver from injury.[55]

In humans, drinking 70 mL (⅓ cup) of camu camu juice per day for just one week has been shown to reduce markers of oxidative stress and inflammation in healthy adults, versus no benefits with an equivalent amount of supplemental vitamin C.[56] Camu camu has also been shown to blunt the glycemic response to eating,[57] and improve blood vessel function.[58]

Recommended Dose: Drink ¼ to ½ cup per day (or 500 to 3000 mg powder)

Amla

Amla is an Ayurvedic herb used traditionally for enhancing vitality and promoting longevity, with studies in animals and isolated cells showing that it enhances mitochondrial energy production, stimulates mitochondrial biogenesis, increases antioxidant enzyme production, and protects cells and mitochondria from oxidative damage.[59,60]

Researchers have been investigating its potential as a neuroprotective,[61] anticancer,[62] and general health agent.[63] However, the most promising avenue of benefit is toward metabolic health.

Amla has been shown to have improved metabolic health in adults with and without type 2 diabetes, with the greatest benefits coming from the higher dose. Amla has also been shown to be more effective than a placebo at improving glycemic control and blood lipids, and just as effective as antidiabetic medication at lowering blood glucose in those with diabetes.[64]

In a study of adults with diabetes, 1000 mg per day of amla was as effective as a statin at improving endothelial function, reducing oxidative stress, increasing antioxidant enzyme activity, and reducing inflammation, while 500 mg/d of amla had beneficial effects, albeit less pronounced.[65] These findings were confirmed in a study focused on metabolic syndrome.[66] Furthermore, taking 500 mg/d of amla for four weeks has been shown to improve vascular fluidity, reduce an index for vascular age, and reduce markers of oxidative stress.[67]

Recommended Dose: Supplement with 500 to 3000 mg of amla daily

MICROALGAE

Spirulina

For centuries, natives living around Lake Chad in Africa have consumed spirulina, and it was an important trading commodity between the Aztecs of Central America and Spanish conquistadors.[68] Today you can find it lining the shelves of many health food stores.

Spirulina is one of the most powerful superfoods in existence, possessing amazing, evidence-backed benefits for metabolic health and energy production.

Several studies have shown that spirulina protects the heart, liver, and intestinal cells from oxidative stress and mitochondrial damage, stimulates mitochondrial biogenesis, and attenuates metabolic dysfunction.[69,70,71] These benefits are largely due to a little molecule it contains called C-Phycocyanin, the potent phytochemical that mimics the structure of bilirubin and has similar physiological effects.[72,73,74,75]

Bilirubin is a potent antioxidant and anti-inflammatory molecule that's been implicated in the prevention of metabolic syndrome and diabetes, cardiovascular diseases, and kidney disease.[76,77,78,79]

On top of improving metabolic health, an abundance of evidence shows spirulina improves endurance exercise performance and reduces fatigue in people who exercise.[80,81,82]

Recommended Dose: Take at least 2 grams per day, ideally 6 to 8 grams

Chlorella

Chlorella is roughly 2.5 billion years old, one of the first single-celled organisms to inhabit the planet. In order to survive and replicate over that inconceivable span of time and to protect against famine, drought, radiation, and poisoning, this little algae developed an impressive array of carotenoids, antioxidants, and enzymes to create energy, minimize oxidative stress, and neutralize toxicants, all housed within a fibrous armor shell. When we eat chlorella, it passes on many of these defenses to us,[83] and it does so with relatively small doses.

Supplementing with chlorella has been shown to increase antioxidant status in patients with chronic obstructive pulmonary disease (COPD)[84] while also cutting levels of oxidative stress in smokers by 20 percent.[85]

A meta-analysis of 19 randomized, controlled trials reported that supplementing with an average of just 4 grams per day of chlorella significantly reduced LDL-C, blood pressure, and fasting blood glucose after an average of two months.[86]

And this plays out in people struggling with chronic fatigue too. In adults with fibromyalgia, supplementing with 10 grams of chlorella plus a liquid chlorella extract daily for two months has been shown to have significantly reduced the number of tender muscle points by 8 percent and pain intensity by 22 percent.[87]

The participants also reported improvements in most of their fibromyalgia symptoms, like general well-being and the ability to be active.

Recommended Dose: Take 500 to 3000 mg of chlorella per day

GARNISHES

Broccoli Sprouts

Broccoli sprouts are the richest source of sulforaphane in the world, a molecule that strongly upregulates the master regulator of the antioxidant response element Nrf2 (nuclear factor erythroid 2-related factor 2).[88] Nrf2 not only protects cells from oxidative damage and other stressors but also induces phase II of the liver's detoxification pathways and thereby helps the body neutralize toxicants and prepare them for excretion.

Studies have shown that individuals who regularly consume cruciferous vegetables (like broccoli sprouts) have enhanced detox-ification capabilities that could impact drug metabolism.[89] These benefits can be obtained with 24 to 48 grams of fresh broccoli sprouts, which provides roughly 20 to 40 mg of sulforaphane.[90]

Moreover, a systematic review of 17 clinical trials found that consuming upward of 100 grams of broccoli sprouts per day reduced fasting glucose, insulin resistance, blood lipids, oxidative stress, and inflammation in those with type 2 diabetes or car-diovascular disease.[91] Even in overweight but otherwise healthy adults, consuming 40 grams of broccoli sprouts has been shown to cut inflammatory biomarkers like C-reactive protein and interleukin-6 by half.[92]

Recommended Dose: Eat 25 to 100 grams (1 to 4 ounces) of fresh broccoli sprouts daily

Garlic

Garlic (*Allium sativum*) is a bulbous plant related to onions, shallots, leeks, and chives that has been consumed for thousands of years as both food and medicine among the Babylonians, Egyptians, Phoenicians, Vikings, Chinese, Greeks, and Romans.[93]

Numerous controlled trials have supported the use of garlic as a health tonic. Meta-analyses of these studies have found that supplementing with 600 to 2400 mg of garlic extract (2 to 4 cloves) per day reduces markers of oxidative stress,[94] markers of inflammation,[95,96] blood lipids and fasting glucose in adults with type 2 diabetes,[97] blood lipids in those with elevated levels,[98] and blood pressure in those with hypertension.[99] It may also improve liver function.[100]

Recommended Dose: Take 600 to 2400 mg of garlic extract or eat 2 to 4 cloves per day

Ginger

Ginger is a culinary and medicinal herb in many cultures, often used as a tonic for the digestive system, including symptoms such as bloating and nausea.[101,102]

In fact, just 1 to 2 grams of ginger is as effective as vitamin B_6 and certain medications for treating nausea during pregnancy[103] and can help alleviate nausea and vomiting in those undergoing chemotherapy for cancer.[104]

Several meta-analyses have also reported that ginger consumption alleviates menstrual cramp pain,[105] lowers markers of inflammation and oxidative stress,[106] reduces blood pressure (with doses above 3 grams daily),[107] reduces blood lipids,[108] and facilitates weight loss among overweight and obese adults.[109]

Recommended Dose: Consume at least 3 grams of ginger daily (about 1.5 tea bags if you drink ginger tea or about ½ teaspoon ground ginger)

Cacao

Cacao has been used by humans for more than 3,000 years as a nutritional and medicinal food, drawing fame throughout the world thanks to its heavy use by the Olmec, Maya, and Aztec cultures of Central America.[110,111]

While many people may only think of cacao as being used in a dessert or candy, it actually has more phytochemicals and a higher antioxidant capacity than most other flavonoid-rich foods, including both green tea and red wine.[112] Of course, the source and processing methods of cacao beans will influence this, and your best bet is to find a non-alkalized (raw) cacao powder.

Meta-analyses suggest that cacao consumption benefits vascular health (lower arterial stiffness and increased endothelial function),[113,114] reduces biomarkers of oxidative stress,[115] modestly lowers blood pressure,[116] and improves several other cardiometabolic risk factors like inflammation, insulin sensitivity, and blood lipids.[117]

Just remember: you want non-alkalized cocoa powder, as the alkalizing ("Dutch") process destroys the flavanols (which is why this type of cocoa isn't as bitter). If you opt for chocolate, then get the darkest you can tolerate, and avoid milk chocolate.

Recommended Dose: At least 50 grams (about 2 ounces) dark chocolate or 40 grams pure cocoa powder

NUTS, SEEDS, AND FATTY FRUITS

Almonds

Almonds are a type of drupe (also called stone fruits), like peaches and apricots, only the part we eat is the seed of the tree. Nonetheless, almonds are nuts from a culinary and nutritional standpoint, and they are rich in vitamin E, fiber, and phytochemicals that all converge to provide a nutrient-dense source of fat in our diet.[118]

Meta-analyses of randomized, controlled trials have shown that eating at least 1 ounce (a handful) of almonds per day can lower blood lipids implicated in cardiovascular disease[119] and reduce body weight and fat mass.[120] A variety of clinical trials have also suggested that regular almond consumption lowers markers of oxidative stress and inflammation.[121]

Another cool thing about almonds is that they contain a resilient plant cell wall that encloses the fat particles, rendering the fat unavailable for digestion and absorption.[122] Thus, less chewing means more intact cell walls that interfere with the digestive process,[123] which means fewer calories available for the body to use while allowing more fiber to reach the microbiome. Eating just 2 ounces of almonds per day has been shown to increase microbial diversity in otherwise healthy adults.[124]

Recommended Dose: 1 ounce per day minimum

Avocado

Avocados are a fatty fruit rich in healthy monounsaturated fatty acids, fiber, and phytochemicals, particularly the carotenoid lutein. Eating just one avocado per day has been shown to increase macular pigment density (the primary location of lutein in the body that correlates with brain concentrations).[125]

Meta-analyses have reported that substituting avocados for other food in the diet results in moderate-to-large reductions of LDL cholesterol and triglycerides,[126,127] which are key cardiovascular disease risk factors.

Other clinical trials in which participants are instructed to eat more avocados have reported improved autonomic (rest-and-recover) nervous system activity following exercise,[128] increased serum antioxidant status and lower levels of oxidized LDL particles,[129] and an improved metabolic response to eating when the avocado replaces carbohydrate in the meal.[130]

Recommended Dose: Eat ½ to 1 large avocado per day

FIBROUS VEGETABLES

Tomatoes

Tomatoes are a fruit best known for their high concentration of the red color pigment lycopene, which is named after the tomato plant (*Solanum lycopersicum*). This carotenoid is considered one of the most efficient singlet oxygen quenchers,[131] which are primary sources of oxidative stress in the body, especially the skin.[132]

In one study, researchers found that eating 55 grams of tomato paste (16 mg lycopene) reduced mitochondrial damage and increased collagen deposition in the skin.[133]

Of course, if tomatoes aren't your thing, you can still reap a benefit from pure lycopene supplements,[134,135] albeit a little less than the benefit from an equivalent amount of lycopene supplied from whole tomatoes.[136] That makes sense given that tomatoes contain not just lycopene but other carotenoids that have biological effects in the body.[137]

Aside from making your skin shine, tomato consumption has been linked to lower risks of dying from any cause or heart disease,[138] modest improvements in blood lipids,[139] and lower risk of developing prostate cancer.[140,141]

Recommended Dose: 40 grams tomato paste or 1 to 2 whole large tomatoes per day

Beets

Beets are a food best known for their high concentration of dietary nitrates, which are molecules that are transformed into nitric oxide within the body.[142] Nitric oxide is a signaling molecule within the cardiovascular system that plays a central role in relaxing blood vessels, promoting vasodilation, and reducing blood pressure.[143]

Studies have shown that consuming nitrates from foods like beets increases nitric oxide concentrations in the body and consequently improves blood pressure, endothelial function, arterial stiffness, platelet function, and exercise performance.[144]

For example, an average-sized beet (about 80 grams) provides about 200 mg of nitrates,[145] and a meta-analysis of 47 randomized, placebo-controlled trials reported that supplementing with 250 to 1200 mg of nitrates from beetroot and other sources improved several assessments of endurance exercise performance, particularly the amount of time that healthy adults could exercise before exhausting themselves.[146]

Recommended Dose: Supplement with 250 to 1200 mg of nitrates daily or eat 1 to 6 beets

Mushrooms

Mushrooms have been an important part of the human diet and used medicinally to treat countless ailments for thousands of years. Although medicinal mushrooms are considered distinct from dietary ones, the division is becoming increasingly blurred as we learn more about the potent health-promoting properties of mushrooms.

Mushroom species such as cremini, shiitake, and oyster are a rich source of essential minerals like potassium, copper, and zinc, and are also full of prebiotic fiber and bioactive polysaccharides with antiviral, antibacterial, and antibiotic properties that protect against cancer and metabolic dysfunction.[147,148,149]

The most common culinary mushroom is the cremini or button mushroom, which is an immature portabella mushroom. The polysaccharides contained within this mushroom have been shown to lower the inflammatory response to microbial endotoxins commonly absorbed from the gut,[150] and eating just 100 grams of this mushroom per day for a week increases mucosal immunity via enhanced immunoglobulin A secretion.[151]

Moreover, in animals, regular consumption of the cremini or button mushroom has been shown to improve microbiome diversity and protect against pathogenic infections,[152] as well as improve innate immune function.[153]

Clinical trials with oyster mushrooms, mainstays in Asian cuisine, have shown enhanced immune function among healthy adults,[154,155,156] while those with shiitake have shown it to have immune-boosting effects alongside protecting against dental cavities.[157,158]

Recommended Dose: Eat regularly (ideally at least 3 times per week)

ANIMAL-BASED PROTEINS

Eggs

High-quality pastured eggs are a rich source of protein and many nutrients, particularly choline, DHA, and lutein. Obtaining pastured eggs is important because the chickens' diet significantly impacts the nutritional quality of their eggs.

Pastured hens lay eggs with significantly more omega-3 fatty acids, including a notable increase in DHA[159] (an amount comparable to seafood), less omega-6 fatty acids, and an improved omega-3 to omega-6 ratio than their conventional or organic counterparts.[160,161] Additionally, eggs from pastured hens contain significantly more vitamin E and bioactive compounds, including lutein and zeaxanthin.[162,163]

With choline, a single large egg provides about 170 mg, or about 30 to 40 percent of the adequate intake for men (550 mg) and women (425 mg). In other words, eating 3 to 4 eggs per day could get you all the choline you need to support neurotransmission, brain health, and liver function.

Recommended Dose: Eat 1 to 4 pastured eggs per day

Beef Liver

Beef liver is one of the most nutrient-dense foods on the planet, although the taste does admittedly leave much to be desired. Still, just 3.5 ounces (100 grams) meets your daily requirements for most B vitamins, vitamin A, and copper, while providing over half your requirements for choline, zinc, iron, selenium, and folate.

Beef liver is basically nature's multivitamin, although you don't want to eat too much due to the risk of vitamin A and copper toxicity. It's best to limit yourself to eating no more than a pound per week.

Also, there's a common belief that the liver is full of toxicants due to its detoxification job in the body, but this is a myth. The liver doesn't store toxicants; it processes them and prepares them for excretion from the body.

Recommended Dose: Consume 4 to 8 ounces of beef liver 2 to 4 times per week (8 to 16 ounces in total per week)

Salmon Roe

Salmon roe consists of red-orange unfertilized salmon eggs, like caviar (salt-cured fish eggs from the sturgeon family). They are rich in many nutrients, including vitamin A, choline, iron, magnesium, calcium, selenium, and omega-3 fatty acids (EPA and DHA); one of nature's richest sources of phospholipids; and can be considered a nutrient powerhouse when added to the diet.

Recommended Dose: To taste

Oysters

Oysters are possibly the best source of zinc in existence, an essential mineral required for proper immune function, wound healing, and metabolism. Just one medium oyster provides you with all the zinc you need for a day, along with a generous serving of iron, selenium, and omega-3 fatty acids (EPA and DHA).

A randomized clinical trial involving 94 healthy adults found that eating 40 grams of boiled oysters (15 mg of zinc) daily for 12 weeks significantly improved sleep efficiency, shortened the time it took to fall asleep, and reduced nightly restlessness compared to a placebo.[164]

Recommended Dose: 1 to 3 oysters per day if you enjoy them

WHOLE GRAINS

Oats

If you eat only one grain, choose oats. They are an excellent source of complex carbohydrates, a special type of fiber called beta-glucan, and numerous minerals such as manganese, magnesium, iron, selenium, zinc, and copper.

The beta-glucan fiber of oats has been consistently linked to improved cardiovascular health through its ability to help lower blood lipids.[165] Moreover, including oats in a diet has been shown to reduce fasting insulin and improve glycemic control,[166,167] but likely only when the oats are minimally processed, such as with steel cut and thick rolled oatmeal.[168]

Another unique benefit of oats is their avenanthramide content, an oat-specific phytochemical that increases antioxidant status after consumption[169] and can also reduce exercise-induced inflammation in younger and older adults.[170,171,172]

Recommended Dose: 1 to 2 servings (about 40 to 80 grams dry oats) per day

LEGUMES

Black Beans

Black beans are a rich source of fiber, protein, phytochemicals, and multiple vitamins and minerals, like calcium, magnesium, potassium, zinc, and folate. Consuming black beans has been shown to improve antioxidant capacity and lower the insulin response to eating more than either an equivalent amount of supplemental fiber or antioxidants alone, suggesting a synergistic effect of the whole black bean.[173]

Other research has shown that black beans can lower the glycemic response of eating,[174] meaning they can minimize those post-meal surges and drops in blood glucose that often lead to fatigue. They also improve cardiovascular health after eating (improved vascular tone) compared to other beans.[175]

Recommended Dose: Eat regularly

Soy

Soybeans and many (but not all) of the products made from them are a rich plant-based source of high-quality protein and generous amounts of fiber. Soybeans are part of the traditional diets of many Asian societies, where they undergo minimal processing to become wholesome foods such as natto, tofu, tempeh, miso, soy sauce, and soy milk.

Many soy products are rich in isoflavones, a type of phytochemical whose consumption has been associated with lower blood lipids,[176] lower blood pressure,[177,178] and improved endothelial function[179]—which could possibly explain the association between soy consumption and reduced risks of developing cardiovascular disease.[180] If you include soy in your diet, we strongly advise consuming only organic soy foods, ideally traditionally fermented soy products like tempeh and natto.

Recommended Dose: Eat soy foods at least several times per week (ideally organic and fermented soy products)

CHAPTER 8

ENERGY SUPER SUPPLEMENTS

The nutritional strategies that we've covered so far create a strong foundation for optimizing your energy levels and mitochondrial function. By using your diet to address the most common cell danger response triggers, you can experience renewed vitality and livelihood.

However, implementing dietary changes takes time. Many strategies involve the altering of eating times and schedules, types of foods, and preparation and cooking techniques. These adjustments are incredibly important, but they can be an involved process that takes weeks before you experience positive changes.

Comparatively, some supplements have been shown to improve people's energy levels in as little time as *one week*.

Supplements are called *supplements* because they're meant to supplement the diet, and to provide nutrients and other compounds that can't be obtained through foods. Truly, at drug-level potency, they have qualities that you will not find in food. For many people suffering debilitating and persistent fatigue, sometimes taking a supplement or two gives just enough relief to start experiencing better energy levels. Feeling slightly better then becomes a motivating factor that inspires them to keep making, and sticking with, the dietary revolutions.

Supplements can play such a powerful role in restoring and enhancing energy levels that my team at *The Energy Blueprint* created a line of ultra-premium supplements. For many people, experimenting with supplements one at a time can be overwhelming and expensive, so our products were created using multiple clinically effective doses of key ingredients, backed by scientific evidence.

While we encourage anyone to try the "20-in-1" approach using our supplements (or other high-quality products), our aim in this chapter is to explain some of the most powerful and effective supplements individually. We share the science behind how these supplements and compounds work, the suggested doses based on the scientific evidence, and some of the most common benefits that people often experience when adding supplements to their diets. We use many of the supplements described in this chapter in *The Energy Blueprint* products too.

These supplements and compounds can help rejuvenate your mitochondria, get deeper and more regenerative sleep, strengthen the integrity of your gut, improve your glycemic control, and bolster your brain function and moods—each of which will help bring you one step closer to overcoming fatigue and reclaiming your lost energy.

This information can also help you have more informed conversations with health and wellness professionals. If you are uncomfortable identifying and determining the right supplements to take by yourself, that's okay. Please seek out health care practitioners like functional, integrative, or naturopathic providers who recommend targeted supplements and compounds for their patients.

Of course, taking supplements—whether you're experimenting with them one at a time or as compounds that include multiple ones—is *not required* for achieving optimal health, mitochondrial function, and top energy levels.

But for some people, supplements can be game changers.

The key lesson with supplements—and with any strategy—is to always *listen to your body*. We've included suggested doses for each supplement along with the typical improvements that many people will experience, but feel free to start with lower doses and gradually work your way up. None of the supplements we talk about have notable adverse effects when used at the recommended doses. Still, bodies are unique, so do your best to notice how yours feels after you start taking a supplement.

Remember, our aim is to increase your energy and make your body feel amazing. If any supplement (or strategy) ever causes a *negative* reaction, get rid of it.

And if something isn't working, don't let that discourage you. Instead, try shifting your perspective. Remind yourself that you're one supplement (or strategy) closer to finding the one(s) that will help you regain your energy.

MITOCHONDRIAL SUPPORT AND ENERGY ENHANCEMENT

First up on our list are supplements that get to the heart of your energy problems by directly bolstering mitochondrial function and helping build their resilience to harm. Given the ubiquitous nature of mitochondria throughout your body, the benefits of bolstering mitochondrial energy production are vast, ranging from the obvious benefit of lessened fatigue to the more subtle: improved metabolic health and cognitive function.

Importantly, none of these compounds are stimulants like caffeine, which serve only to provide a temporary energy jolt through causing a stress response within the body. Worse yet, regular use of stimulants causes habituation: they no longer enhance energy levels but instead just maintain a new baseline. And regular intake must continue lest you suffer withdrawal and lower energy levels until the habituation fades.

Instead, these supplements build your "cellular engine"—your mitochondria—over time, so they become stronger and capable of producing more energy. They essentially raise your baseline energy levels by building up your mitochondria and your body's capacity to produce more energy on its own.

Fortunately you can experiment with a number of supplements and compounds to boost your mitochondria. To start, I recommend working with one of the top seven listed, as they are the best investigated. If you aren't getting the results you want from these, or if you simply want to see if your body responds better to other supplements, then try delving into any of the others outlined in this section.

The Top Seven

1. Comprehensive Vitamin and Mineral Formula

Multivitamins are like a safety net, which most people need. An analysis of 70 diet plans created for athletes and sedentary adults looking to improve their nutrient intake found 3 to 15 vitamin and mineral deficiencies.[1] Another study analyzing four popular diet plans (Atkins for Life, South Beach, Best Life, and DASH) found that a person would need to consume more than 18,000 calories per day to ensure an adequate intake of all essential micronutrients.[2]

Unsurprisingly, when we look at the average American, things are not any different. More than half of Americans do not meet the estimated average requirement for vitamins A, D, E, or K, calcium, magnesium, or potassium even after taking into account fortified foods.[3] In other studies, 33 to 58 percent of U.S. adults are deficient in at least one major vitamin like A, B_6, B_{12}, C, D, and E when looking at diet alone, but only 8 to 19 percent have at least one deficiency when a multivitamin is used.[4]

Given these numbers, almost everyone has *at least one* key nutritional deficiency, if not several. We won't cover every essential nutrient in detail, but it goes without saying that they are all important for your energy levels in one way or another.[5]

- B vitamins are necessary for turning food into cellular energy.
- Vitamin C reduces oxidative stress and is necessary for carnitine synthesis.
- Vitamin E prevents mitochondrial membrane oxidation.

- Vitamin A maintains healthy rates of mitochondrial respiration.

- Vitamin D has countless energy-relevant functions throughout the body.

- Iron is essential for the transport of oxygen throughout the body.

- Magnesium is required for cellular energy creation.

- Zinc is required for antioxidant enzyme activity that protects mitochondria.

And for those taking a multivitamin, there does appear to be a modest health benefit. A meta-analysis of 21 randomized, controlled trials lasting longer than one year found that they tended to reduce the risk of dying from any cause by 6 percent,[6] likely through preventing clinical and subclinical deficiencies.

More importantly, daily supplementation with a comprehensive vitamin and mineral formula has been shown to reduce fatigue by 35 percent and reduce sleep disturbances by 39 percent after two months in women with chronic fatigue.[7] Without doing expensive testing to look at what specific nutrients you may be low in, using a high-quality comprehensive vitamin and mineral formula is a powerful way to cover your nutritional bases and correct common nutritional deficiencies that frequently contribute to fatigue.

As an aside, not all studies find benefits in multivitamin use. It's a topic too complex and nuanced to address here, but it's worth mentioning that a primary reason for most negative findings is the use of inferior forms of many vitamins and minerals. As you'll read shortly, using certain forms of B vitamins can reduce their effectiveness or increase the risk of adverse effects, and these forms are often included in common multivitamins.

Vitamin E is another example. It consists of eight molecules, but most supplements only use one, alpha-tocopherol, which has limited benefits compared to the more bioactive tocotrienols.[8] Worse yet, they may use the synthetic DL-alpha-tocopherol that not only has lower bioavailability than natural alpha-tocopherol but may cause harm like liver damage and prostate cancer.[9,10]

Recommended Dose: Aim for a multivitamin that provides an array of biologically appropriate vitamins and minerals in their ideal forms. Seemingly small details like the form of each nutrient can ultimately determine whether you get energy and longevity benefits, making it critical to use an ultra-high-quality multivitamin and mineral formula rather than the typical stuff you find in your local drug or health food store.

Common Benefits: Ensures nutrient adequacy for your mitochondria and every other cell to function optimally

2. Methyl B Complex

Of all the essential vitamins and minerals, the B vitamins deserve special attention because without them, we wouldn't be able to turn the food we eat into cellular energy and our mitochondria couldn't function. The specific vitamins include:

- **Thiamine** (B_1)—required to harvest energy from glucose and for the synthesis of energy-carrying molecules within mitochondria

- **Riboflavin** (B_2)—the central unit for flavoproteins, which are necessary for mitochondrial energy production and antioxidant defenses

- **Niacin** (B_3)—the central unit for NAD+ and NADP, which are necessary alongside flavoproteins for mitochondrial energy production and antioxidant defenses

- **Pantothenic acid** (B_5)—the central unit of coenzyme A, which plays a vital role in energy production and the metabolism of many nutrients

- **Pyridoxal** (B_6)—required for amino acid metabolism, gene expression, and the breakdown of homocysteine

- **Biotin** (B_7)—the central component of several enzymes involved in energy production, amino acid metabolism, gene expression, and cell growth

- **Folate** (B_9)—required for methylation reactions, DNA synthesis, and the breakdown of homocysteine

- **Cobalamin** (B_{12})—necessary for the breakdown of certain amino acids and fatty acids, as well as for the breakdown of homocysteine and recycling of folate

Aside from energy production, three of the B vitamins are essential for another critically important job within the body: the breakdown of *homocysteine*, an excess of which has a diversity of harmful effects on our body, particularly when it comes to our cardiovascular system, brains, bones, and joints.[11] Individuals with chronic fatigue have significantly elevated levels of homocysteine in their cerebrospinal fluid that nourishes the brain and spinal cord, and the amount of homocysteine is related to one's fatigability—more homocysteine, more fatigue.[12] Higher homocysteine levels have also been identified as a significant cause of neurodegeneration and cognitive decline with aging.[13,14]

The breakdown of homocysteine involves three B vitamins: folate, vitamin B_{12}, and vitamin B_6. Folate is the most important and requires the most attention because we need a special form called *5-methyltetrahydrofolate*, or methylfolate for short, to break down homocysteine. As we covered in Chapter 6, the only way our body can create methylfolate is through the enzyme methylenetetrahydrofolate reductase (MTHFR). Yet many people have genetic polymorphisms (a type of mutation) that impair the ability of this enzyme to function.[15,16,17]

This means that you're going to have a hard time detoxifying homocysteine unless you directly consume methylfolate to bypass this bottleneck process. While eating a diet rich in fibrous vegetables and legumes can help, since roughly 45 to 65 percent of their folate is in methylfolate form,[18] many people need additional supplementation to keep homocysteine levels in check.

The amount of supplemental folate needed to maintain a healthy homocysteine range of 5 to 7 μmol/L is variable between individuals. The best thing to do is monitor your own homocysteine level and modify the dose of folate you take until homocysteine is in a healthy range. If you don't want to do regular blood work, then make sure you have a more than adequate intake of folate (at least 400 micrograms of methylfolate per day) and other methylated B vitamins.

Next up is vitamin B_{12}, which we need to use folate in the breakdown of homocysteine. You'll find several forms of B_{12} on the market, including methyl-, adenosyl-, hydroxy-, and cyano-B_{12}, but all get broken into their core B_{12} molecule during digestion and absorption.[19]

Still, some studies have suggested that retention rates with methyl- and hydroxy-B_{12} are greater than that of cyano-B_{12}, largely due to lower excretion.[20,21] Plus, there may be yet unidentified polymorphisms in B_{12} receptors and transporters that impact how someone responds to specific forms of B_{12} supplements. As such, it makes sense to supplement with methyl-, adenosyl-, or hydroxy- forms of B_{12}—the forms that we naturally obtain in our diet—rather than cyano-.

Recommended Dose: Aim for an adequate intake of all B vitamins.

- B_1: 1.2 mg
- B_2: 1.3 mg
- B_3: 16 mg
- B_5: 5 mg
- B_6: 1.3 mg
- Biotin: 30 mcg
- Folate: 400 mcg
- B_{12}: 2.4 mcg

Pay special attention to the form of folate (methylfolate), B_6 (pyridoxal-5-phosphate), and B_{12} (methyl-, adenosyl-, or hydroxy-B_{12}).

Common Benefit: Ensuring nutrient adequacy for optimal energy production within mitochondria and maintenance of healthy homocysteine levels

3. NTFactor Phospholipid Complex

One of the primary determinants of whether mitochondria switch from energy mode to danger mode is the integrity of their membranes. Damage to mitochondrial membranes signal danger and a need to shift resources away from energy production and to defense.

Lipid replacement therapy is based on the idea that you can take a supplement containing cell membrane phospholipids to repair damaged mitochondrial membranes that accumulate through life.[22] Accomplishing such a feat requires a compound that can survive degradation during digestion and avoid oxidation during transport throughout the body.

NTFactor is a phospholipid complex that supplies the primary cell membrane phospholipids along with antioxidants and fructooligosaccharides to protect the phospholipids from enzymatic degradation and oxidation.[23] This phospholipid complex is absorbed relatively intact and is readily transported throughout the body.

The result is a supply of bioactive phospholipids that naturally replace damaged mitochondrial membrane components, leading to a regeneration of dysfunctional mitochondria.

In a study of older adults with mild to moderate fatigue, 2 to 3 grams per day of NTFactor improved mitochondrial function by 24 percent after 12 weeks, restoring it to a level similar to *healthy 29-year-olds*.[24] This improvement in mitochondrial function was accompanied by a 33 percent reduction in self-reported levels of fatigue. In addition, numerous studies have shown that supplementing with 1.5 to 3 grams of NTFactor reduces fatigue by 24 to 43 percent among those with chronic fatigue syndrome or conditions associated with fatigue, like general aging, obesity, Lyme disease, and Gulf War illness.[25]

Recommended Dose: Take 1 to 4 grams of NTFactor daily

Common Benefits: Repairs mitochondrial membranes and bolsters energy production

4. Acetyl-L-Carnitine

Our mitochondria cannot make energy out of nothing, and our body uses intricate transport systems to get raw materials inside the mitochondria so they can make fuel. One of those transport systems is called the *carnitine shuttle system*, which is essential for bringing fatty acids inside mitochondria.

If you don't have enough carnitine, you won't burn fat and your mitochondria are going to have one hell of a time making energy. Even if everything else about your mitochondria is optimally functioning, a lack of carnitine will cause them to act as if they are damaged and dysfunctional.

While complete carnitine deficiencies cause a host of nasty effects like liver and brain damage, weakness, and lethargy,[26] even mild subclinical insufficiencies can cause problems. A systematic review of 25 studies investigating the relationship between mitochondrial function and fatigue reported that carnitine deficits were one of the most common biomarkers linked to fatigue status.[27]

Acetyl-L-carnitine (ALCAR) is a special form of carnitine that achieves two transformations: (1) it supplies the carnitine your mitochondria need to produce energy, and (2) it provides an acetyl constituent that your mitochondria use to remain youthful and healthy.

To illustrate these benefits, one study of chronically fatigued older adults found that taking 4 grams of ALCAR daily over six months led to profound benefits to their well-being, including a 15 percent increase in cognitive function, 24 percent increase in physical function, and close to a whopping 50 percent reduction in mental fatigue, physical fatigue, and overall fatigue severity.[28]

Through increasing mitochondrial acetylation and carnitine levels within the brain, ALCAR supplementation:

- Improves mitochondrial function within brain cells[29,30]

- Increases acetylcholine signaling and improves learning capacity[31,32]

- Increases brain energy availability[33]

- Protects against β-amyloid neurotoxicity and reduces oxidative stress[34,35]

Accordingly, ALCAR can be a powerful ally in the fight against neurodegeneration and cognitive decline with aging.[36] For example, a meta-analysis of 21 randomized, double-blind, placebo-controlled trials reported that 1.5 to 3 grams per day of ALCAR significantly improved cognitive function assessed by a variety of methods in older adults with mild cognitive impairment or early Alzheimer's disease.[37]

It can also be a powerful ally against mood disorders like depression, with one meta-analysis of 12 randomized controlled trials showing that ALCAR significantly reduced depressive symptoms with an efficacy like antidepressant medications but with fewer side effects.[38]

Recommended Dose: 1.5 to 4 grams per day, divided across 2 to 3 doses

Common Benefits: Optimizes mitochondrial energy production, increases energy levels, and protects against neurodegeneration and depression

5. Creatine Monohydrate

We rely on our mitochondria to supply virtually all our energy throughout the day, but sometimes they cannot support our energy demands. In situations where we require instantaneous energy bursts, our cells get their energy (ATP) from a molecule called *phosphocreatine.*

It's like gunpowder for your muscles, providing near-instantaneous regeneration of ATP. When we sprint, for example, it is the phosphocreatine that is responsible for exploding with energy (ATP) that our muscles can immediately use to sustain that sprint. The most prominent use of phosphocreatine is by our muscles, which use it to contract whenever we sprint, jump, lift heavy weights, or throw a punch. Creatine supplementation works, quite simply, by saturating our body with phosphocreatine and increasing the amount of readily available energy we have to use. This is why creatine is such a heavily researched ergogenic supplement for bolstering exercise performance, and studies clearly indicate that it can increase muscle strength, power output, and lean body mass in younger and older adults alike.[39,40,41,42,43]

The benefits go far beyond just improving muscle function; studies show that creatine protects muscle fibers from high levels of oxidative stress and preserves their ability to grow and differentiate.[44,45] One of the most important ways it does this is by increasing mitochondrial biogenesis, structural integrity, and function.[46]

On top of that, higher levels of creatine sensitize mitochondria to energy production signals, meaning that they will ramp up their energy production more effectively when faced with signals to do so.[47] In other words, creatine stimulates mitochondrial respiration.

And muscle contractions aren't the only cellular function reliant on phosphocreatine. Neurons require it to support their intense and fluctuating bursts of communication, with impairments in creatine metabolism linked to neurodegeneration.[48] Several studies have established that creatine supplementation increases brain creatine stores by 5 to 15 percent, depending on concentrations before supplementation and the size of the person supplementing.[49,50,51]

Through increasing the supply of readily available energy, acting as an antioxidant, and protecting against mitochondrial dysfunction, creatine is a powerful ally for supporting optimal brain health and physical energy levels.[52]

Recommended Dose: 3 to 5 grams per day

Common Benefits: Improves strength, physical function, and mitochondrial energy production

6. Taurine

Taurine is an omnipresent amino acid within the body, essential for the development and function of our cardiovascular, muscular, nervous, and ocular systems.[53] Taurine is such a powerful amino acid that deficiencies are implicated in numerous chronic disease states.[54,55]

There are many reasons why taurine plays a role in these conditions. It's required to regulate water balance, for cell signaling, to make bile and excrete toxicants, and, most importantly, for mitochondrial function and energy production.

The highest amounts of taurine are in tissues with huge energy requirements and a lot of mitochondria, such as the retina, nerves, kidney, heart, and skeletal muscles.[56] That's because taurine is essential for mitochondrial function.

If mitochondria don't have enough taurine, energy production decreases and oxidative stress increases.[57] To that effect, several clinical trials have shown that supplementing with 3 grams of taurine per day reduces biomarkers of oxidative stress and inflammation in those with metabolic dysfunction.[58,59,60] Additionally, a meta-analysis of 10 studies reported that 1 to 6 grams of taurine improved endurance exercise performance, particularly power output and the amount of time that people could run before exhaustion.[61]

Recommended Dose: 1 to 6 grams per day

Common Benefits: Supports mitochondrial function and enhances physical performance

7. Astaxanthin

Astaxanthin is a carotenoid produced by the microalgae *Haematococcus pluvialis* as protection for its cells against oxidative stress.[62] Of course, you've likely seen it in the many creatures that eat it—krill, shrimp, crab, and salmon are all rich sources of astaxanthin that pigments their flesh and shells with a red-orange hue.

While eating astaxanthin won't turn our skin red, it will bestow us with some incredibly potent antioxidant benefits, improved mitochondrial health, and increased energy levels, among many other benefits.

Astaxanthin is an incredibly efficient antioxidant. While other types of antioxidant molecules generally act either inside or outside the membrane, astaxanthin's structure allows it to do both, thereby helping stabilize mitochondrial membranes and protect them from oxidative damage.[63,64,65]

Ultimately, astaxanthin's polarity and antioxidant properties have afforded it a powerful ability to prevent mitochondrial dysfunction and help reverse the mitochondrial dysfunction associated with aging,[66,67] leading some researchers to call it a "mitochondria-targeted antioxidant."[68]

For example, just three weeks of supplementing with 5 mg of astaxanthin per day reduced oxidative stress and increased antioxidant status in individuals carrying around too much body fat to levels seen in those at a normal body weight.[69] In fatigued elderly adults, four months of supplementation with 12 mg of astaxanthin was found to increase maximal strength by 14 percent, muscle size by 3 percent, and force production by 12 percent compared to a placebo.[70]

Similar benefits have been observed in young adults too. Recreationally active college students who supplement with 4 mg of astaxanthin per day were found to increase their muscular endurance threefold compared to the placebo group.[71] Other studies have found that astaxanthin helps prevent the decrease in antioxidant defenses that occur from prolonged endurance exercise in elite-level soccer players and helps improve endurance exercise recovery in recreational athletes.[72,73]

Recommended Dose: 4 to 12 mg per day

Common Benefits: Lowers oxidative stress, improves mitochondrial integrity, increases energy levels, and enhances athletic performance

More Mitochondria- and Energy-Enhancing Supplements

Alpha-Lipoic Acid

Alpha-lipoic acid (ALA) is a mitochondrial molecule involved in energy metabolism and the antioxidant system. It is not only essential for mitochondria to create cellular energy but also serves to function as an antioxidant, replenish other antioxidants, and stimulate the production of antioxidant enzymes like glutathione.[74]

ALA has been heavily investigated as a mitochondrial rejuvenator that helps reverse age-related declines in mitochondrial energy production,[75] particularly within the brain.[76,77] Additional research has suggested that ALA benefits neurodegenerative disorders and age-related cognitive decline.[78,79] ALA accumulates in various brain regions as soon as an hour after ingestion,[80,81] and it has been shown to protect against neuronal cell death.[82] In patients with Alzheimer's disease, supplementing with 600 mg of ALA per day alongside fish oil prevented a decline in cognitive function over one year compared to both fish oil alone and a placebo.[83]

The mitochondrial benefits of ALA supplementation seem to extend to metabolic health as well.[84,85] Several studies have shown that supplementing with 800 to 2000 mg per day facilitates weight loss and reductions in waist circumference among both men and women using it for several months.[86,87,88]

Recommended Dose: 600 to 1800 mg per day, divided across 2 to 3 doses (or 100 to 600 mg if using R-ALA)

Common Benefits: Protects against mitochondrial dysfunction, oxidative stress, neurotoxicity, and weight gain

Butyrate

Butyrate is a short-chain fatty acid that is important for our health, particularly the gut and brain. While the primary source of butyrate is fermentation of prebiotic fibers by our intestinal microbes, eating a ton of prebiotic fiber isn't always feasible, depending on one's preferences and sensitivities. As such, supplementing with butyrate can provide great therapeutic value.

Tributyrin is a supplemental form of butyrate. Studies have shown that supplementing with tributyrin efficiently increases serum levels of butyrate,[89,90] making it a potential candidate for reaping many of the systemic effects that butyrate provides.

Animal research has shown that tributyrin protects the liver from endotoxin and alcohol injury,[91,92] reduces inflammation and insulin resistance associated with obesity,[93] enhances mitochondrial function,[94] and facilitates muscle growth and development.[95] With regard to the brain specifically, tributyrin has been shown to enhance non-REM sleep,[96] and may be able to protect the brain against neurodegeneration and neuroinflammation.[97]

The reason butyrate is critical for mitochondrial function is that it doesn't require any special machinery to be used for energy production—it just moves into our mitochondria and is transformed into cellular energy with ease, which can be a lifesaver when those mitochondria are dysfunctional and having a hard time making energy to begin with.

Recommended Dose: 500 to 3000 mg per day (ideally of tributyrin)

Common Benefits: Enhances mitochondrial energy production and protects against cardiometabolic diseases

Coenzyme Q10

Coenzyme Q10 (CoQ10) is an essential component of the electron transport chain through which mitochondria generate energy. It serves a dual purpose: as an antioxidant within the chain and as an energy-transferring molecule. As such, deficits in CoQ10 will not only lead to a cessation of energy production, but also an increase in oxidative damage. Individuals with chronic fatigue regularly show deficiencies in CoQ10 concentrations throughout the body,[98] as do those with conditions in which fatigue is a common symptom, like fibromyalgia;[99,100,101] those who have survived heart attacks or heart failure;[102,103] and people with multiple sclerosis.[104,105]

CoQ10 will enhance blood flow, protect blood vessels, lower oxidative stress, and boost vitality in anyone who suffers from fatigue, but especially in those people with the aforementioned conditions. Just several months of supplementing with 150 to 300 mg of CoQ10 decreases fatigue and improves autonomic nervous system activity (the part of the nervous system involved in rest and recovery) and biochemical parameters of mitochondrial energy production.[106,107,108,109]

Even in healthy adults, CoQ10 supplementation improves general fatigue and reduces oxidative stress.[110,111]

Recommended Dose: 150 to 300 mg per day

Common Benefits: Promotes mitochondrial energy production, reduces oxidative stress, and reduces fatigue

Curcumin

Curcumin is the yellow pigment and primary bioactive substance in turmeric, with powerful anti-inflammatory and antioxidant properties that protect and stabilize mitochondrial membranes and help the body build more mitochondria (mitochondrial biogenesis).[112,113]

These effects have led to vast investigation of its benefits for human health, with evidence suggesting curcumin supplementation can help slow cognitive decline with aging, improve cardiovascular health, reduce the risk of developing diabetes, and alleviate other inflammation-related conditions, including chronic fatigue.[114,115,116]

A systematic review of 11 studies reported that curcumin supplementation in athletes and active adults reduced inflammation and oxidative stress, decreased pain and muscle damage, and improved recovery and muscle performance.[117] These studies used 180 mg of Theracurmin, 500 mg of Meriva, 400 mg of Longvida, and 6 grams of regular curcumin combined with piperine.

Notably, there are many forms of curcumin on the market that have increased bioavailability compared to pure curcumin that you'd find in turmeric. Studies in humans have determined that the bioavailability of these various forms are: NovaSol (185-fold), CurcuWIN (136-fold), Longvida (100-fold), Cavacurmin (85-fold), Meriva (48-fold), BCM-95 (27-fold), Theracurmin (16-fold), Cur-Qfen (16-fold), MicroActive Curcumin (10-fold), and micronized curcumin (9-fold).[118]

Recommended Dose: 400 to 1000 mg per day of an enhanced curcumin form like NovaSol, Longvida, CurcuWIN, or Meriva

Common Benefits: Reduces inflammation and improves mitochondrial function

D-Ribose

D-Ribose is a naturally occurring sugar molecule that assists in the production of cellular energy by virtue of being a necessary component of ATP, DNA, and RNA.[119]

Evidence suggests that D-Ribose can help boost energy and physical function in situations where energy levels are reduced, such as in people who have suffered from heart disease or stroke[120,121,122] or people engaging in regular intense exercise.[123,124]

In adults with chronic fatigue, supplementing with 5 grams of D-Ribose three times per day (15 grams per day in total) led to 45 percent greater energy levels, 25 percent better sleep quality, 16 percent more mental clarity, 14 percent less pain, and 30 percent greater overall well-being.[125] Another study reported similar findings after using 10 grams per day, with all benefits disappearing within a week of stopping supplementation.[126]

Recommended Dose: 10 to 15 grams per day, divided across 2 to 3 doses, taken with meals. Please be aware that this is a unique kind of "sugar" molecule that can cause *low* blood sugar (hypoglycemia)

in some people, so start with 2 to 3 grams and work your way up to a larger clinical dose.

Common Benefits: Increases energy levels and physical function by supporting mitochondrial energy production

Forskolin

Forskolin is the primary bioactive in the *Coleus forskohlii* herb that has historically been used in Ayurvedic medicine. It works by increasing levels of cyclic adenosine monophosphate (cAMP),[127] which maintains mitochondrial health through regulating mitochondrial dynamics like biogenesis and energy production.[128]

This effect has ultimately translated into less fatigue and improved body composition in clinical trials of supplementation. For example, in overweight women 50 mg of forskolin per day was able to prevent an increase in fat mass experienced by the placebo group and reduce self-perceived fatigue.[129] In overweight men 50 mg of forskolin per day for 12 weeks cut the average body fat percentage from 35 percent down to 31 percent—about 10 lbs (4.5 kg) of fat loss.[130] And in a study with both overweight men and women, 50 mg of forskolin per day alongside a 12-week weight loss diet not only cut waist circumference by 2 inches but led to superior reductions in fasting insulin and insulin resistance compared to placebo.[131]

Recommended Dose: 50 mg per day

Common Benefits: Increases energy levels and physical function by supporting mitochondrial energy production

Green Tea EGCG

Green tea (*Camellia sinensis*) catechins include four phytochemical molecules, the most potent one being epigallocatechin-3-gallate (EGCG). Studies show it benefits almost every organ system in the body in doses you can obtain easily from simply drinking green tea.[132,133,134]

EGCG is neuroprotective,[135,136] cardioprotective,[137,138] anti-obesity,[139,140,141] anticarcinogenic,[142,143] and antidiabetic,[144] all due primarily to its ability to stimulate mitochondrial biogenesis, enhance energy production, and protect mitochondria from oxidative stress.[145,146]

Over the course of 12 weeks, daily supplementation with 280 mg of EGCG with 80 mg of resveratrol (a phytochemical found in grape skin) was found to significantly increase the use of fat as an energy source and mitochondrial function (oxidative metabolism) compared to a placebo.[147] Moreover, several meta-analyses of clinical trials concluded that 100 to 500 mg of EGCG reduces body weight and body fat,[148,149,150,151] particularly abdominal fat.[152]

A single cup (8 ounces or 250 ml) of brewed green tea typically contains about 50 to 100 mg of EGCG, with variation from one cup to another depending on many factors (species of tea, length of time steeping, time spent oxidizing, etc.). I prefer ceremonial matcha or EGCG supplementation as my own go-to.

Recommended Dose: 100 to 500 mg per day

Common Benefits: Reduces oxidative stress, improves mitochondrial function, and protects against cardiometabolic disease development

Gynostemma

Gynostemma pentaphyllum is a vine indigenous to and widely used in Korea, China, and Japan as traditional medicine and tea. It is a potent activator of numerous signaling pathways involved in mitochondrial health and biogenesis, including AMP-activated protein kinase (AMPK) and sirtuin 1.[153,154]

Several studies have reported metabolic and mental health benefits. In an 8-week study, chronically stressed adults supplementing with 400 mg per day of a gynostemma extract led to twice the reduction in anxiety compared to a placebo group—a 17 percent reduction.[155]

And in a 12-week study, overweight and obese adults supplementing with 450 mg of gynostemma (Actiponin extract)

experienced a 6 percent reduction in abdominal fat, half of which came from their more harmful visceral fat, compared to those taking a placebo.[156] And all without any apparent changes in food intake.

In another study of adults with diabetes, drinking tea made from 6 grams of gynostemma leaves daily over 12 weeks reduced fasting glucose by 24 percent and insulin resistance by 50 percent compared to a placebo.[157]

Recommended Dose: 400 to 500 mg per day of a gynostemna extract

Common Benefits: Increases mitochondrial biogenesis, facilitates fat loss, and improves mental health

N-Acetylcysteine

N-Acetylcysteine (NAC) is a molecule our body naturally creates from the amino acid cysteine as a precursor to one of our body's master antioxidants, glutathione. Supplemental NAC is an effective way to increase glutathione concentrations in our body and often the supplement of choice in conditions of glutathione deficiency.[158,159]

The depletion of glutathione ultimately causes Tylenol-induced liver failure, and NAC is the go-to of the medical profession to prevent this. NAC acts to replenish depleted glutathione reserves in the liver, thereby reversing the buildup of free radicals and maintaining mitochondrial energy production within the liver.[160]

Glutathione itself has numerous essential functions in the body, so much so that cellular concentrations match those of glucose, potassium, and cholesterol—some of the highest in the body. It is not only a potent antioxidant but a molecule required to recycle other antioxidants, detoxify and excrete toxins, and maintain mitochondrial function.[161]

Because it helps sustain optimal glutathione concentrations, NAC has been demonstrated to reduce mitochondrial oxidative damage and preserve cellular life in the face of genetic mitochondrial mutations that cause dysfunction or toxic conditions that directly damage mitochondria.[162,163,164,165] In fact, by serving as an antioxidant precursor rather than an antioxidant itself, NAC shows greater promise than other antioxidant compounds for supporting mitohormesis,[166] a process whereby the mitochondria adapt to stress by growing bigger and stronger. A meta-analysis of 28 clinical trials found that supplementing with 600 to 2000 mg of NAC per day significantly reduced biomarkers of oxidative stress and inflammation.[167]

Lastly, glutathione is essential for the proliferation of white blood cells and overall immune function.[168,169] One potential contributor to chronic fatigue is an overactive immune system resulting from chronic inflammation "stealing" NAC from muscle tissue and thereby limiting energy production in these tissues.[170]

Recommended Dose: 600 to 2000 mg per day, divided across 2 to 3 doses

Common Benefits: Supports antioxidant status and immune function, reduces oxidative stress, and improves mitochondrial function

Niacin Derivatives

In mitochondrial respiration, a molecule called *NAD+* is essential for energy generation. You can't turn carbohydrates or fats into cellular energy without it. People with chronic fatigue have lower levels of this molecule compared to healthy non-fatigued adults.[171] Accordingly, increasing NAD+ could be an effective way to restore mitochondrial function and bolster energy levels.

Since NAD+ is made from the essential vitamin niacin, there has been a growing interest in supplementing with niacin and its derivative, *nicotinamide riboside*, to increase NAD+ levels and improve mitochondrial function.

But while there has been a lot of hype surrounding these molecules, *the research in humans has not shown benefits.* Studies using 500 to 2000 mg per day of nicotinamide riboside in healthy adults,[172] elderly adults,[173,174] and obese adults[175,176,177,178] showed no appreciable effect on NAD+ concentrations in muscle tissue or several parameters of mitochondrial function, including energy production. A variety of health parameters were also unaffected, including energy expenditure, body composition, glycemic control, insulin sensitivity, exercise performance, and blood lipids.

Given the current state of the literature and the high price of these compounds, we do not feel a recommendation is warranted.

Panax Ginseng

Panax ginseng has been used medicinally for thousands of years in China, Korea, and Japan to alleviate physical and mental fatigue. While there are several types of ginseng on the market, *Panax ginseng* is considered the "true" ginseng.

At a fundamental level, *Panax ginseng* works to protect mitochondria from oxidative damage and improve energy production under conditions of oxidative stress.[179,180] Accordingly, a systematic review and meta-analysis of five studies in chronic fatigue patients found significant benefits of ginseng supplementation for reducing fatigue severity with 200 to 2000 mg per day.[181]

One study reported that supplementing with *Panax ginseng* for just one month led to a 20 percent reduction in fatigue severity compared to a placebo,[182] while another study reported a similar 20 percent fatigue reduction compared to a placebo over a month of supplementing with *Panax ginseng*, along with increased levels of internal antioxidants like glutathione and reduced biomarkers of oxidative stress.[183]

Recommended Dose: 200 to 2000 milligrams per day, divided across 2 to 3 doses

Common Benefits: Protects against oxidative stress and reduces fatigue severity

PQQ

Pyrroloquinoline quinone (PQQ) is a potent stimulator of pathways involved in mitochondrial biogenesis and antioxidant defenses.[184,185] In particular, it stimulates pathways shared by exercise training and is believed to potentiate and enhance activity-induced benefits on mitochondria.[186]

Supplementing with 20 mg of PQQ daily was shown to reduce fatigue and increase vigor by 20 percent in adults complaining of poor sleep and energy levels.[187] This study also reported improved mood, sleep quality, and overall quality of life. In another study of healthy adults, just three days of supplementing with 20 to 30 mg of PQQ reduced inflammation and improved markers of mitochondrial respiration.[188]

Recommended Dose: 10 to 30 mg per day

Common Benefits: Facilitates mitochondrial biogenesis and energy production, reduces fatigue, increases vigor, and improves sleep quality

Quercetin

Quercetin is a well-known bioflavonoid found in many fruits and vegetables, particularly onions and apples. It is a potent antioxidant and anti-inflammatory molecule that affects an array of mitochondrial processes, including mitochondrial biogenesis, mitochondrial energy production, and the protection of mitochondria from oxidative stress.[189,190]

Several meta-analyses of clinical trials have reported that 500 to 1000 mg of quercetin taken daily can improve endurance exercise performance and maximal oxygen consumption,[191,192] and, in those with metabolic dysfunction, reduce markers of inflammation,[193,194] improve blood lipids,[195,196,197] and lower blood pressure.[198,199]

Importantly, most studies use regular unenhanced quercetin. Yet a quercetin phytosome complex has vastly superior bioavailability, leading to quercetin levels 20-fold greater in the blood following supplementation.[200] In other words, 50 mg of the phytosome is equivalent to 1000 mg of regular quercetin.

Recommended Dose: 500 to 1000 mg per day, ideally in the phytosome form, which has greatly improved bioavailability compared to the unenhanced version

Common Benefits: Improves mitochondrial function and metabolic health

SLEEP SUPPORT AND RELAXATION

The following supplements can help you fall asleep more quickly, stay asleep, and wake up feeling refreshed and rejuvenated. Most supplements increase GABA signaling and have a sedative effect, thereby helping calm anxiety, promote relaxation, and smooth the transition from wake to sleep.

The benefits of these compounds will be greatest in those who are struggling with circadian dysregulation, insomnia, chronic fatigue, chronic stress, or an anxiety disorder. All supplements should be taken 30 to 60 minutes before bed.

Ashwagandha

Ashwagandha (*Withania somnifera*) is a nightshade revered in Ayurvedic medicine for its physical- and mental-enhancing effects.[201] Today, it's considered an adaptogen for similar reasons, able to increase a person's resilience to stress and help reduce anxiety.[202,203]

These effects are largely due to its constituent withanolide structures, which have several important neuroprotective effects within the brain, such as scavenging free radicals, reducing neuroinflammation, and promoting neurotransmitter signaling.[204] They also bind to and activate GABA receptors.[205]

Several studies have reported reductions in stress and anxiety following supplementation with 600 to 1000 mg per day of an Ashwagandha extract called KSM-66. The reductions ranged from 15 to 20 percent in otherwise healthy adults dealing with mild stress[206,207] to 40 to 70 percent in adults battling chronic mental stress,[208] to 50 percent in adults with an anxiety disorder.[209] These stress- and anxiety-reducing benefits also translate to improved sleep.[210,211,212]

Although the KSM-66 extract is the best researched, it is not the most potent. The concentration of withanolides in regular dried Ashwagandha root is less than 1 percent, at least 5 percent in the KSM-66 extract, but a whopping 35 percent in the Shoden extract (which is why we chose it for our mitochondrial formula, Energenesis).

To illustrate this difference, just 240 mg of the Shoden extract reduces anxiety by 60 percent in mildly stressed healthy adults, compared to a 15 to 20 percent reduction in anxiety with 600 mg of the KSM-66 extract.[213]

Recommended Dose: 600 mg per day of a KSM-66 extract or 150 to 240 mg per day of a Shoden extract, 30 to 60 minutes before bed

Common Benefits: Improves stress tolerance, enhances sleep quality, and lessens anxiety

CBD Oil

Cannabidiol (CBD) oil is considered to be the non-psychoactive component of cannabis plants (marijuana and hemp). It's currently being heavily researched as a therapeutic for anxiety, depression, addiction, epilepsy, neurodegeneration, chronic pain, and inflammatory diseases.[214,215] While research on CBD and sleep is still in its infancy, the results seem promising.[216]

The cannabinoid system is intimately tied to the sleep-wake cycle by inhibiting the arousal system in the brain and promoting a hypnotic-like state.[217,218] The sleep benefits of CBD have been shown in adults with sleep disorders at doses of 75 mg per night[219] and at 25 mg in children.[220] Another study involving 72 adults complaining of anxiety and poor sleep found that 25 to 175 mg of CBD nightly reduced anxiety by 31 to 38 percent and improved sleep quality by 15 to 28 percent after three months.[221]

Anecdotally, in *The Energy Blueprint* program, we've observed that individuals who seem to be resistant to other sleep aids, like melatonin and the variety of herbs already discussed, often have excellent results using CBD oil before bed. The only issue with CBD is that CBD research for sleep enhancement used high doses, which can be quite expensive and often unaffordable for many people. If you don't have the funds, then don't despair. Instead, try other supplements. Still, if you're interested in trying CBD and it's within reach financially, then we recommend experimenting with doses of 25 to 100 mg taken 30 to 60 minutes before bed.

Recommended Dose: 25 to 100 mg per day, 30 to 60 minutes before bed

Common Benefits: Improves sleep quality and lessens anxiety

Chamomile

Chamomile is a daisy-like flower traditionally brewed into tea and used to treat a variety of ailments, particularly those characterized by inflammation and oxidative stress.[222] It's also been used as a mild sedative to calm nerves and reduce anxiety.

You've likely seen it in teas and supplements that are advertised to help with sleep, and with good reason. A meta-analysis of six studies administering 400 to 2000 mg of chamomile before bed found it to significantly improve sleep quality.[223]

For those who are battling anxiety, there may be additional benefits. Several studies have reported that supplementing with 1100 to 1500 mg of chamomile can reduce feelings of anxiety and improve several other aspects of mental well-being.[224,225,226]

Recommended Dose: 1100 to 1500 mg per day, 30 to 60 minutes before bed

Common Benefits: Improves sleep quality and lessens anxiety

Lemon Balm

Lemon balm (*Melissa officinalis*) is a plant native to the Mediterranean basin and central Asia, where it was traditionally used for the treatment of mental disorders and central nervous system complaints.[227] Today it is commonly used to promote sedation and relaxation.

Several studies have found that taking 300 to 1600 mg of lemon balm promotes calmness in the hours following supplementation,[228,229] particularly when dealing with stressful situations.[230,231] These benefits extend to individuals battling anxiety as well, where supplementing with 600 mg per day has been shown to reduce a variety of anxiety manifestations and symptoms.[232]

Notably, insomnia was one of the most debilitating symptoms for anxious adults, and lemon balm supplementation reduced it by an average of 42 percent, with 85 percent of people dealing with insomnia experiencing a benefit. Other studies have found similar benefits for sleep when lemon balm is combined with valerian root.[233,234]

Recommended Dose: 300 to 1600 mg per day, 30 to 60 minutes before bed

Common Benefits: Improves sleep quality and lessens anxiety

Melatonin

When it comes to getting a good night's rest, no supplement beats melatonin. As we talked about in Chapter 2, melatonin is naturally secreted by our brain at night to help transition us from wakefulness to sleep.

Numerous meta-analyses have reported that supplementing with 1 to 12 mg of melatonin improves sleep quality in adults and children with a variety of health conditions, including:

- Primary sleep disorders like insomnia[235,236]
- Secondary sleep disorders resulting from other medical conditions[237]

- Neurodegenerative disorders like Alzheimer's disease[238,239]

- Neurodevelopmental conditions like autism and attention-deficit hyperactivity disorder[240,241]

Moreover, these doses of melatonin have also been shown to lower fasting glucose,[242] blood pressure,[243] systemic inflammation,[244] and oxidative stress,[245,246] suggesting that there are multiple health benefits above and beyond improved sleep quality with supplementation, including boosting energy and reducing the effects of chronic fatigue syndrome.[247]

All that said, there are anecdotal reports of melatonin interfering with sleep when taken in too high a dose. In *The Energy Blueprint* program, we've found that a subset of individuals (possibly as high as 20 percent of people) is *extremely* sensitive to even small doses of melatonin, where any more than 1 mg disturbs sleep.

While it is not yet well researched clinically, it's possible that individual differences in melatonin receptor distribution and density play a role.[248,249]

Thankfully, the solution is rather simple: start with a very low dose of melatonin and slowly work your way up to higher doses until you find your personal limit. You'll know when you hit your threshold if you wake up feeling groggy or experience any sleep difficulties for two to three nights (not just a one-off occurrence). Just 300 mcg of melatonin mimics what we could obtain with good sleep hygiene,[250] so this is a good dose to start with.

As a final point, supplementing with melatonin does not interfere with your own natural production at doses of 500 mcg,[251] 2 mg,[252] 5 mg,[253] or 50 mg.[254] However, keep in mind that if you regularly use melatonin to improve your sleep and then stop using it, many people report reduced sleep quality for several nights before things normalize.

Recommended Dose: 300 micrograms to 10 mg per day, 30 to 60 minutes before bed

Common Benefits: Improves sleep quality, quickens the time it takes to fall asleep, increases the ability to stay asleep through the night, and improves cardiometabolic health

Passionflower

For thousands of years, Native Americans have used passionflower (*Passiflora incarnata Linneaus*) as a sedative and treatment for anxiety.[255] It works primarily through activating GABA receptors in the brain that are responsible for relaxation.[256]

Whether taken as a pill, a tincture, or a tea, passionflower has been shown to improve sleep quality,[257,258] particularly the amount of time that is spent in deep, rejuvenating, slow-wave sleep,[259] and without any side effects common to sleep and anti-anxiety medications.[260]

These sleep benefits may be secondary to reductions in anxiety. Several studies have shown that supplementing with 360 to 700 mg of passionflower reduces anxiety in the 30 to 90 minutes after taking it.[261,262,263] At least one study has shown that passionflower's anti-anxiety effects are as potent as a benzodiazepine, with both reducing feelings of anxiety by half after just two weeks and by nearly 75 percent after four weeks.[264]

Recommended Dose: 360 to 700 mg per day, 30 to 60 minutes before bed

Common Benefits: Improves sleep quality and lessens anxiety

Theanine

Theanine is a naturally occurring amino acid found in tea that alters neurotransmitter signaling within the brain. After consumption, it crosses the blood-brain barrier, interferes with excitatory glutamate signaling, stimulates dopamine release, and promotes inhibitory neurotransmission, thereby helping to create a state of relaxation.[265,266]

In fact, electroencephalography (EEG) studies have shown that theanine shifts brain waves toward alpha oscillatory patterns indicative of a relaxed state, particularly in those with high levels of baseline anxiety.[267,268,269,270,271] Accordingly, several studies have found that theanine supplementation improves feelings of relaxation, tension, calmness, and anxiety in the hours following doses of 200 to 600 mg.[272,273] There is also evidence that theanine improves sleep quality, likely through its anti-anxiety and calming effects,[274,275] and can help offset the stimulatory effects of caffeine.[276,277]

Recommended Dose: 200 to 600 mg per day, 30 to 60 minutes before bed

Common Benefits: Enhances feelings of relaxation and calmness, lessens anxiety, and improves sleep quality

Valerian Root

Valerian root (*Valeriana officinalis*) is one of the best-researched and most common sleep aid supplements on the market, second only to melatonin. Valerian root's use as a sedative dates back to the first century C.E., and it was used to treat nervous disorders and insomnia in the Middle Ages.

More recently, a systematic review of 60 studies and a meta-analysis of 18 studies reported that supplementing with 450 to 1400 mg of valerian root was effective for both improving sleep quality and reducing anxiety, provided that the whole valerian root was used.[278] These benefits were observed in healthy adults, those suffering from insomnia, and those with conditions in which sleep is often impaired.

Recommended Dose: 450 to 1400 mg per day, 30 to 60 minutes before bed

Common Benefits: Improves sleep quality and lessens anxiety

GUT REPAIR

While nothing can replace the dietary strategies discussed in Chapter 4, when it comes to repairing our gut and improving its health, there are a handful of supplements that can provide additional support to the gut barrier and thereby help strengthen the gut's integrity.

Colostrum

Colostrum is the first form of milk made by moms following birth. It's enriched with many immunoglobulins (antibodies), growth factors, prebiotics, and specific proteins that are thought to promote babies' rapid growth and development while improving their immunity.[279]

These characteristics have garnered an interest in using colostrum to bolster gut health under a variety of conditions. Its prebiotics help facilitate the development of a healthy microbiome while its bioactive molecules work to support intestinal integrity.[280] For example, a meta-analysis of five randomized, controlled trials demonstrated that colostrum supplementation reduced the occurrence of infectious diarrhea by 70 percent.[281]

In healthy athletes supplementation with 10 to 20 grams of colostrum daily over two weeks reduced exercise-induced increases in intestinal permeability (due to the heat stress) by 70 to 80 percent compared to a placebo[282,283] and reduced markers of intestinal damage by 33 percent.[284] Even just 500 mg of colostrum has been shown to normalize intestinal permeability among athletes with elevated levels.[285]

Recommended Dose: 10 to 20 grams per day

Common Benefits: Enhances gut barrier integrity and improves leaky gut

Glutamine

Glutamine is the most abundant amino acid in the body and a favored source of energy for many cells that need to rapidly divide and proliferate, such as those of the immune system and intestinal tract. In particular, glutamine is believed to enhance gut barrier integrity through reducing inflammation and oxidative stress, increasing protein synthesis, and enhancing mitochondrial function.[286,287]

One of the established side effects of glutamine deprivation is an increase in intestinal permeability,[288] and glutamine supplementation in conditions of deficiency restores intestinal barrier function.[289] Given that these intestinal benefits are not seen with glutamine infusions, it's likely that your intestinal cells absorb and utilize most of the glutamine you get in your diet.[290]

To illustrate these points in a more real-world context, several studies have shown glutamine supplementation to be of benefit in athletes who commonly have to deal with leaky gut due to exercise-induced heat stress. In one such study, taking 45 grams of glutamine two hours before exercise halved the normal increase in intestinal permeability and lowered blood endotoxin levels by 18 percent.[291]

Now, 45 grams is a huge dose, equating to roughly 3 tablespoons of pure glutamine. Thankfully, a follow-up study testing lower doses found that using just one-third this dose, about 1 tablespoon of glutamine, was able to confer similar benefits.[292] And for clarity, these benefits don't seem to occur with other amino acids like the branched-chain amino acids.[293]

Recommended Dose: At least 15 grams (1 tablespoon) per day

Common Benefits: Improves gut barrier integrity and reduces intestinal permeability

Partially Hydrolyzed Guar Gum

Partially hydrolyzed guar gum (PHGG) is a water-soluble prebiotic fiber used in the treatment of gastrointestinal disorders such as

IBS, small-intestinal bacterial overgrowth, diarrhea, and constipation, including in medical settings.[294,295,296] It's a phenomenal supplemental prebiotic fiber that you can use to help create a healthy microbiome and foster gut health.

For example, in adults with chronic constipation, supplementing with 5 grams (1 teaspoon) of PHGG improved colon transit time by 20 percent after just one month, with the effects being greatest in those who were the most constipated.[297] The number of weekly bowel movements increased, less straining occurred, and abdominal pain decreased.

In adults with IBS, supplementing with both 5 and 10 grams of PHGG for three months reduced gastrointestinal symptoms by 37 percent and improved various parameters of quality of life, including a 17 percent increase in vitality.[298] In another, larger study of IBS patients, taking 6 grams of PHGG for three months reduced bloating and flatulence by 12 percent.[299]

These benefits come from its prebiotic effects. Studies have shown that PHGG preferentially increases the abundance of beneficial butyrate-producing bacteria like *Bifidobacterium* and *Ruminococcus*, along with overall microbial diversity and SCFA concentrations.[300,301]

Recommended Dose: 5 to 10 grams (1 to 2 teaspoons) per day

Common Benefits: Improves microbiome diversity, reduces constipation, and lowers sensitivity to bloating

Zinc Carnosine

Zinc is an essential mineral needed for cell turnover and repair, as well as the maintenance of the intestinal barrier. In particular, zinc is essential for maintaining the integrity of tight junctions between intestinal cells, the breakdown of which is fundamental to "leaky" gut.[302]

In adults with inflammatory bowel disease, low zinc status correlates with greater disease severity,[303] and normalization of zinc status through supplementation reduces intestinal symptoms through strengthening tight junctions.[304,305]

Although any type of zinc is going to provide benefits for gut health, zinc carnosine is unique. Early research found that zinc carnosine was able to promote intestinal repair processes and prevent a threefold increase in intestinal permeability in response to drug-induced injury.[306] Furthermore, in a study of healthy athletes, supplementing with 37.5 mg of zinc carnosine (providing just 9 mg of elemental zinc) twice per day for two weeks reduced exercise-induced increase in intestinal permeability by 70 percent.[307]

Recommended Dose: 37.5 mg of zinc carnosine (providing 9 mg of elemental zinc) twice per day

Common Benefits: Improves intestinal barrier function

BRAIN HEALTH AND COGNITIVE SUPPORT

What would you think if someone told you that taking a pill could help make you feel smarter, sharper, and more creative? What if they told you a pill could maintain those feelings throughout your life? Would you call BS?

Those pills exist!

They're called nootropics and include an array of compounds that either improve cognitive function—particularly executive function, memory, focus, and the ability to work under stressful conditions—or prevent cognitive decline.

While the best-known examples include synthetic drugs like Adderall, modafinil, and piracetam, there are numerous herbs and naturally occurring molecules that possess similar properties while being far safer, especially for long-term use.

These brain-boosting supplements work through a variety of mechanisms to improve brain health and functionality,[308,309,310] including:

- Increasing blood flow and nutrient delivery to brain cells

- Reducing neuroinflammation and oxidative stress

- Bolstering mitochondrial function and energy production

- Facilitating the removal of neurotoxins

- Promoting the growth of neurons

- Improving neuronal communication and synaptic plasticity

- Optimizing neurotransmitter levels

The following supplements are some of the most powerful brain-boosting compounds in existence. They can help you fight brain fog, become more vigilant, maintain cognitive performance, and ensure your mind is fully functional—which will contribute to improved energy levels too.

Bacopa Monnieri

Bacopa monnieri is an Ayurvedic swamp plant (Brahmi) traditionally used for enhancing memory and cognition, as well as a general brain tonic. Its bioactive constituents, the bacosides, generate numerous biological effects within the brain that facilitate this use.[311,312,313,314,315] These constituents:

- Reduce oxidative stress and increase antioxidant enzyme activity

- Reduce inflammation

- Protect nerves

- Reduce β-amyloid deposition

- Increase the growth of nerve endings to enhance neuronal communication

- Increase blood flow and the delivery of oxygen and nutrients

A variety of studies have shown that supplementing with 300 mg per day of bacopa (50 percent bacosides) improves working memory, information processing, learning rate, and other aspects of cognitive function in medical students,[316] healthy younger adults,[317,318] and healthy older adults.[319,320,321]

Recommended Dose: 300 to 600 mg per day

Common Benefits: Improves brain health, protects against neuro-degeneration, and enhances memory

Ginkgo Biloba

Ginkgo biloba possesses an array of qualities relevant to brain health and neurological function, with numerous studies showing that it is neuroprotective and an antioxidant, preserves brain receptors susceptible to age-related loss, counteracts cognitive impairment, enhances neuronal plasticity, and improves memory.[322]

Numerous interventions have been conducted with ginkgo biloba supplementation, usually in the form of a 50:1 concentrated extract called EGb-761, and systematic reviews of this evidence have found that it improves cognitive performance and quality of life in older adults experiencing cognitive decline but doesn't have much of a benefit in young and cognitively healthy adults.[323,324]

Recommended Dose: 240 mg per day, ideally EGb-761 extract

Common Benefits: Helps prevent cognitive decline and neurodegeneration

Lion's Mane Mushroom

Lion's mane mushroom (also called *yamabushitake* or *Hericium erinaceus*) is a medicinal mushroom that has been extensively studied for its neurohealth properties.[325,326] Research has shown that lion's mane:

- Stimulates the production of nerve growth factor (NGF),[327,328,329] which promotes neuronal growth, development, and regeneration[330]

- Restores levels of key neurotransmitters serotonin, noradrenaline, and dopamine in the brain (that are often suppressed due to chronic stress)[331]

- Reduces neuroinflammation[332,333]

- Stimulates the expression of brain-derived neurotrophic factor (BDNF),[334] which has neuroprotective effects, plays a role in neuronal development, and helps in the formation of neuronal connections that are important for memory and cognition[335]

Studies in mice have demonstrated that these effects ultimately lend lion's mane cognitive-enhancing,[336] neuroprotective,[337] and mood-stabilizing properties.[338]

In men with mild cognitive impairment, 3000 mg per day was found to improve cognitive function by 12 percent over 16 weeks compared to a placebo.[339] In overweight and obese adults, 1500 mg per day for 8 weeks was found to reduce feelings of anxiety by 27 percent and feelings of depression by 39 percent.[340]

Recommended Dose: 1500 to 3000 mg per day of plain powder (or lower dose of a more potent extract)

Common Benefits: Reduces neuroinflammation, improves cognitive function, improves mood

Magnesium Taurate (or Threonate)

Magnesium is an essential mineral required for over 300 enzymes to function properly,[341] including those necessary for mitochondrial function and energy production.[342,343] Within the brain, magnesium is required for optimal nerve transmission and protection against neurotoxicity.[344,345]

Individuals with neurodegenerative disorders such as Parkinson's disease[346,347] and Alzheimer's disease[348,349,350] have lower brain concentrations of magnesium than healthy adults, and studies in mice suggest that elevating brain magnesium concentrations can provide neuroprotective effects and enhance cognitive function.[351,352]

But not all forms of magnesium have the same ability to enter the brain. Studies have shown that magnesium taurate increases brain magnesium concentrations 10 to 20 percent more than a variety of other forms.[353,354]

Recommended Dose: 200 mg (minimum) to 400 mg per day, ideally of magnesium taurate

Common Benefits: Improves cognitive function and lowers risk of neurodegeneration

Rhodiola Rosea

Rhodiola rosea is a medicinal herb traditionally used for enhancing mental performance and resilience to stress,[355] resulting from its interactions with genes, signaling pathways, and molecular networks within the brain to alter emotional behavior.[356]

It's an incredibly powerful adaptogen, with effects noticed soon after supplementation. In one study of over 100 adults dealing with chronic stress, supplementing with 400 mg per day of *Rhodiola* reduced feelings of physical exhaustion, difficulty concentrating, and anxiety after as few as three days, nearly *cutting them in half* after just one week.[357]

Similarly, in adults with chronic fatigue, 400 mg of *Rhodiola* per day improved every aspect of fatigue after just one week, with further improvements seen after eight weeks.[358] Ultimately, 83 percent of the participants reported "very much" or "much" improved conditions, with fatigue, stress, anxiety, and brain fog being *cut in half.*

Several other studies have also shown that supplementing with 100 to 400 mg of *Rhodiola* improves physical and mental energy, reduces stress, and ultimately improves quality of life in adults struggling with job burnout,[359] first-year medical students,[360] military cadets,[361] and adults with stress-related fatigue.[362] (This is why we made it one of the core ingredients in our brain formula, UltraBrain.)

Recommended Dose: 100 to 400 mg per day (ideally with 3 percent salidrosides and 1 percent rosavins)

Common Benefits: Improves stress resilience, reduces mental and physical fatigue, and enhances quality of life

Vitamin E Tocotrienols

Vitamin E tocotrienols are potent antioxidant molecules that incorporate into cell membranes and neutralize free radicals that would otherwise oxidize phospholipids.[363,364,365]

It's an incredibly important job, one that works synergistically with other antioxidants like vitamin C and glutathione to ensure the integrity of our cell membranes.[366]

Supplementation with tocotrienols significantly increases their concentration in critically important organs such as the brain, heart, and liver.[367] Moreover, the concentrations achieved within the brain are precisely around the concentrations needed to prevent brain damage and neurotoxicity from excessive glutamate and other toxicants.[368]

Because of their neuroprotective and antioxidant effects, an ever-growing body of research is looking into tocotrienol use for the prevention and treatment of Alzheimer's disease.[369] For example, a randomized, controlled trial of individuals with active white matter lesions of their brains, a sign of neurodegeneration, found that 400 mg per day of mixed tocotrienols completely halted the loss of white matter and further brain deterioration after two years.[370] Comparatively, the white matter loss of the placebo group had increased by 23 percent.

Recommended Dose: 100 to 400 mg per day

Common Benefits: Improves antioxidant defenses, protects mito-chondria, and prevents neurodegeneration

DOPAMINE BOOSTERS

Dopamine is involved in motivation and reward. Whenever we do something pleasurable, like eat cake, orgasm, or accomplish a goal, dopamine is released to help reinforce that behavior, motivating us to continue engaging in those behaviors.

Mucuna Pruriens

Arguably the best supplement to increase dopamine signaling within the brain is *Mucuna pruriens*, more commonly known as velvet bean. Mature seeds are about 4 percent L-DOPA, meaning that every gram of velvet beans provide about 40 mg of L-DOPA.[371]

L-DOPA is the only reliable way to increase dopamine synthesis, for two reasons:

1. Dopamine itself can't cross the blood-brain barrier, so supplementing with it would be futile.[372] L-DOPA can cross the blood-brain barrier with ease.

2. The rate-limiting step in dopamine synthesis is the conversion of tyrosine to L-DOPA because high levels of dopamine inhibit the enzyme responsible for this conversion.[373] Taking L-DOPA directly bypasses this negative feedback loop.

L-DOPA is the go-to molecule to increase dopamine synthesis in conditions that need it, including Parkinson's disease. And velvet beans might be the ideal way to get L-DOPA because they are not only more potent than isolated L-DOPA but also safer,[374] with a lower risk for adverse effects like dyskinesias than the standard drug treatment with L-DOPA.[375,376,377]

Recommended Dose: The dose of velvet bean will be variable depending on one's needs. Start with a low dose of 1 to 2 grams and work your way up until your symptoms of dopamine insufficiency are minimized (e.g., improved mood, motivation, energy levels, and mental clarity).

Common Benefits: Enhances motivation, improves mental clarity, and stabilizes moods

Tyrosine

If you are under a lot of stress, taking tyrosine may also be helpful because dopamine is the precursor to the stress hormones adrenaline and noradrenaline. If you are chronically stressed, then you can expect your dopamine to dwindle as it is further metabolized into these molecules.[378,379]

As dopamine levels fall, the conversion of tyrosine to L-DOPA picks up, but you need to ensure that you have sufficient tyrosine available to let that happen. Accordingly, supplementing with extra tyrosine can help offset this reduction in dopamine by allowing for its continued synthesis.[380]

Several clinical trials have shown that supplementing with 2 to 12 grams per day of tyrosine improves cognition, alertness, memory, and energy levels in stressful and demanding situations that would otherwise drain dopamine and impair the ability to think.[381,382]

Recommended Dose: 2 to 12 grams per day

Common Benefits: Enhances the ability to think and focus under stress

ACETYLCHOLINE BOOSTERS

Acetylcholine is involved in regulating muscle contractions of the heart, blood vessels, and skeletal muscle, as well as the ability to learn and remember. Disturbances in acetylcholine signaling have widespread consequences for cognitive function and physical function.

Alpha-GPC

Alpha-glycerophosphocholine (Alpha-GPC) is a highly bioavailable source of choline for the brain.[383] A systematic review of 14 clinical trials involving individuals with neurodegenerative disorders and dementia found that supplementation had consistently positive results on brain function,[384] being more effective than standard drug therapies.[385] The enhanced brain activity has been shown to translate into improvements in exercise performance, with 250 to 600 mg taken before exercise shown to improve strength and power output.[386,387,388,389] At least one comparative study has found that 400 mg of Alpha-GPC may be more effective than caffeine.[390]

Recommended Dose: 600 to 1200 mg per day

Common Benefits: Reduces risk of neurodegeneration, improves cognitive function, and enhances physical performance (due to better brain signaling)

CDP-Choline

Supplementing with CDP-choline has been shown to improve cognitive function in both healthy adults and those suffering from cognitive decline.

A Cochrane Systematic Review of 14 double-blind, placebo-controlled trials of older adults with cognitive deficits like dementia reported that 600 to 1000 mg per day of CDP-choline improved memory, corrected abnormal behaviors, and increased physicians' overall impression that participants had improved cognitive functioning.[391]

Several other studies have also shown benefits in older adults with dementia or Alzheimer's disease,[392,393] older adults with mild vascular dementia,[394] adolescents,[395] and healthy women.[396]

Recommended Dose: 500 to 1000 mg per day

Common Benefits: Enhances cognitive function

Huperzine A

Huperzine A is an alkaloid derived from the moss *Huperzia serrata,* which itself has been used in Traditional Chinese Medicine for centuries to treat neuronal- and cognitive-based illnesses.[397] It's a naturally occurring acetylcholinesterase inhibitor, meaning it prevents the breakdown of acetylcholine just as many Alzheimer's drugs do.[398]

At least 20 randomized controlled trials have evaluated the efficacy of Huperzine A in patients with Alzheimer's disease, with a meta-analysis showing improvements in cognitive function, daily living activity, and clinicians' overall impression that patients showed signs of cognitive improvement with doses of 200 to 800 mcg (average: 370 mcg) over 8 to 36 weeks.[399]

Other meta-analyses have reported that Huperzine A improves cognition in those with vascular dementia,[400] as well as in those with major depression.[401]

Recommended Dose: 200 to 800 micrograms per day

Common Benefits: Improves cognitive function

GABA BOOSTERS

GABA is the most potent inhibitory neurotransmitter in the brain and regulates many of the sedative actions required for relaxation. It is also critical for the regulation of neuronal communication, cognition, emotion, and memory.

Nearly all the GABA-boosting supplements were already discussed in the sleep supplements section. Passionflower, chamomile, lemon balm, and theanine all induce a state of relaxation that helps us calm down and get to bed, in part by increasing GABA signaling.

It's actually a rarity that we can supplement a neurotransmitter and have it not only survive digestion and absorption but also cross the blood-brain barrier and be integrated into our GABA system.

But that's the case with dietary GABA.

A systematic review of 14 studies concluded that 20 to 100 mg of GABA could reduce stress and increase feelings of calmness, while 100 to 300 mg could improve sleep quality.[402] However, it's important to note that some people can't tolerate GABA supplements and don't feel well when using them. Don't stress if GABA isn't working for you personally; instead try some of the other options found in the section on sleep supplements (page 193).

Recommended Dose: 100 to 500 mg per day

Common Benefits: Improves relaxation and sleep quality

SEROTONIN BOOSTERS

Serotonin heavily impacts how we feel, think, and behave, as well as numerous physiological processes involved in digestion and bowel motility, breathing, cardiovascular function, and sexual function. In particular, serotonin modulates mood, perception, reward, anger, aggression, appetite, memory, and attention.

5-HTP

One of the best supplements you can take to bolster serotonin production is 5-HTP, the intermediate molecule between tryptophan and serotonin. The conversion of tryptophan to 5-HTP is the bottleneck step for serotonin production, so supplementing with 5-HTP directly helps bypass this step and reliably increases serotonin levels in the brain.[403]

While research looking into how 5-HTP supplementation affects mood is limited, the data that is available shows it does effectively alleviate depression in those with clinical depression.[404,405] In particular, studies reveal that supplementing with a slow-release 5-HTP can help treat depression that has historically been resistant to standard drug therapies.[406]

Recommended Dose: 250 to 500 mg per day

Common Benefits: Improves mood; especially reduces depression

Saffron

Saffron is a medicinal and culinary spice that has been traded and used throughout Eurasia for thousands of years. Ancient Persians used saffron to treat a variety of ailments, including depression, and modern research has since supported this use. Studies indicate that saffron can:[407,408]

- Increase serotonin signaling
- Increase antioxidants
- Reduce neuroinflammation
- Protect neurons

Numerous meta-analyses of clinical trials have reported that 30 mg per day of saffron has a potency comparable to routinely prescribed antidepressant drugs but with fewer side effects in individuals with mild to moderate depression.[409,410,411,412] The largest of these meta-analyses found that saffron reduced levels of depression by an average of 52 percent, which was comparable to standard drug therapies.[413]

Recommended Dose: 30 mg per day

Common Benefits: Protects the brain against oxidative stress and reduces symptoms of depression (enhances mood)

CONCLUSION

All-Day Energy Starts . . . Now

Congratulations! You've made it to the end. You have in your hands some of the most powerful, evidence-based nutritional strategies you can use to beat fatigue, boost your mitochondria, and experience all-day energy.

Eat for Energy Nutritional Strategy Recap

We covered a lot of material in this book, so here's a handy summary of the nutritional strategies you can add to your daily life, starting today.

Circadian Alignment and Quality Sleep	• Eat within a 6- to 12-hour window. • Stack most of your calories in the morning and afternoon. • Avoid eating late at night, ideally having your last meal no later than 7 to 8 P.M. • Do not consume rapidly digestible carbs at dinner. • Be consistent with your mealtimes. • Limit your alcohol to no more than one drink per day. • Keep caffeine consumption to the morning or early afternoon at the latest.
Fat Loss and Muscle Gain	• Eat sufficient protein throughout the day, which is about 1.1 to 1.6 g/kg (0.5 to 0.7 g/lb) of protein if overweight or obese and 1.6 to 2.2 g/kg (0.7 to 1.0 g/lb) if normal weight (BMI > 25 for overweight and <25 for normal weight). • Eat sufficient protein at every meal, which is at least 30 grams of protein from high-quality sources like meat, soy, or protein powders. • Base each meal around an abundance of fibrous vegetables. • Eat as much wholesome, minimally processed food as possible. • Do not graze on food throughout the day, but instead eat 2 to 4 defined meals every 3 to 5 hours.
Intestinal Integrity and Microbiome Diversity	• Consume at least 30 grams of fiber per day, ideally from prebiotic-rich sources. • Consume a form of fermented food at least once per day. • Add resistant starches to your diet. • Incorporate more prebiotic vegetables into your meals.

Glycemic Control	• Eat within a 6- to 12-hour window. • Consume fibrous vegetables and sources of protein first in your meal, saving your starches for last. • Consume 1 to 2 tablespoons (15 to 30 mL) of vinegar before eating meals containing starch. • Consume at least 5 g of cinnamon per day. • If you have diabetes and are concomitantly working to lose fat mass, eat a low-carbohydrate diet. • Reduce your intake of digestible carbohydrates.
Brain Function	• Eat as much wholesome, minimally processed food as possible. • Incorporate more fish or seafood into your diet. • Up your berry intake, regularly incorporating it into your diet throughout the week. • Base each meal around fibrous vegetables. • Regularly consume nuts, beans, legumes, and whole grains. • Make leafy green vegetables a staple of your meals. • Consume adequate EPA and DHA (500 to 1000 mg per day). • Consume adequate lutein (10-plus mg per day). • Consume adequate choline, B_6, folate, and iron. • Ensure your diet provides you with adequate daily protein. • Drink enough water.

At its heart, this book is truly about transformation—about transforming what's happening to your body on a cellular level. Self-improvement, regaining your health, and restoring your energy aren't a race. I know that you want to feel more energized right now and to put your symptoms and all the stressors that have ravaged your body behind you at this very moment.

But the truth is, rebuilding your mitochondria will take time. Honor that. Honor your body's wisdom and the pace that it needs to go at to heal.

While many of my clients do report improvements within four weeks, this isn't a miraculous recovery. We're building a foundation they use to continue the steady progress to repair and return their mitochondria to the optimal energy producers they were designed to be. Some days you may feel like you've fallen back. And there may be weeks when the nutritional strategies you've adopted fall to the wayside.

It's okay. Just start fresh the next day. This is about embracing new ways of eating for energy that will remain with you throughout your life.

I understand that setting energy recovery goals like "I want to regain my energy in three months," is important and helpful for many people. I would never tell you "No setting goals," but please make them realistic and achievable. Choose time frames that you can achieve, and at the same time, recognize that regaining your energy and healing your mitochondria are fluid and dynamic processes.

As humans, we have a tendency to weigh the negatives more heavily than the positives. And when it comes to judging, we often give more weight to our perceived failures than our successes.

This isn't some psychological "woo-woo"—we have neuroscientific evidence for a *negativity bias*. Amazingly, our brain can respond more rapidly to negative rather than positive stimuli.[1,2]

Thus we can identify negativity faster than any positive transformation. Meaning that if you aren't achieving your goals "fast" enough or in exactly the way you imagined, then you're likely to get down on yourself, possibly feeling frustrated, defeated, depressed, anxious, or afraid that your energy will never return.

Fighting negativity bias is a losing battle. So instead of waging war against it, or allowing those intense emotions to drag you down, recognize the emotion. Recognize that the negativity bias ingrained in all humans has appeared, and then use your prefrontal cortex of rational thought to remind yourself that your thoughts are normal, that it's human nature to perceive the negative . . . and that these thoughts are *changeable*.

If it helps, keep a journal. Write down three to five positives or daily wins that you might have overlooked, like that you're eating more protein with every meal, or you've closed your window of eating, or you've added more servings of leafy green or fibrous vegetables to your daily diet, or you're consuming more probiotics, or you've stopped eating four hours before sleep.

As an ancient Chinese proverb states, this energy journey of a thousand miles begins with a single step. Small daily victories add up, and it's those little wins that lead to radical transformation.

Find a pace that works for you, that's comfortable, and that you can sustain. Maybe you add a new strategy every two weeks, or maybe it's one every month, or maybe it's one every six to eight weeks. There is no "right" pace, only what's right for you. I want you to pick changes that you can stick with, that aren't too difficult, time consuming, or overwhelming.

Slow and steady improvements are better than none.

I know it's easier said than done, but try to relax, and dare I say, have fun. You are on the road to recovering your energy, and that's a powerful place to be. Focus on eating healthy, whole foods, mostly plants, get enough protein at every meal, and go easy on yourself. Be kind and cheer yourself on for just taking these steps in the right direction.

Your energy will return.

No matter where you are in life, how old you are, or how long you've lived with fatigue, I know that by rebuilding and restoring your mitochondria, by reducing cell danger stressors, and by utilizing the nutritional strategies in this book, you can regain your energy and your life.

APPENDIX

Best Protein Sources

Meats, Poultry, and Seafood—4 ounces raw (about 3 ounces cooked)

Poultry, light meat (chicken or turkey breast)	27 g
Poultry, dark meat (drumstick, thigh, wing, or back)	23 g
Lean beef (top/bottom round, eye of round, sirloin tip, top sirloin, 95/5 ground beef)	25 g
Pork (chop, loin)	24 g
Fatty fish (salmon, sardines, mackerel)	23 g
White fish (cod, halibut, pollack, tuna)	20 g
Shellfish (crab, shrimp, lobster)	20 g
Game meat (bison, kangaroo, elk, venison, lamb, boar)	24 g

Dairy

Milk, 8 fluid ounces or 1 cup (skim, 1%, 2%, whole)	8 g
Greek yogurt, 1 cup	23 g
Cottage cheese, 1 cup	25 g
Hard cheeses, 1 ounce or 1/4 cup (cheddar, Gouda, parmesan)	7 g
Soft cheeses, 1 ounce or 1/4 cup (brie, Havarti, cream cheese)	6 g

Eggs

Whole chicken egg, 1 large	6 g
Whole duck egg, 1 large	9 g
Egg whites, 1 cup	26 g
Whole quail egg, 1 large	1 g
Roe, fish eggs, 1 tbsp	4 g

Soy Products—1 cup cooked

Edamame (in pod)	11 g
Edamame (shelled)	18 g
Soybeans	30 g
Soy milk	6 g
Soy nuts	37 g
Tofu (soft)	18 g
Tofu (firm)	23 g
Miso	35 g
Natto	34 g
Tempeh	33 g

Legumes—1 cup cooked

Kidney beans	15 g
Aduki beans	17 g
Lentils	18 g
Split peas	16 g
Lima beans	15 g
Black beans	15 g
Chickpeas	14 g
Black-eyed peas	13 g
Pinto beans	12 g

Nuts and Seeds

Peanuts, 1/4 cup	9 g
Almonds, 1/4 cup	6 g
Pistachios, 1/4 cup	6 g
Cashews, 1/4 cup	5 g
Walnuts, 1/4 cup	5 g
Hazelnuts, 1/4 cup	4 g
Hemp seeds, 3 tbsp	10 g
Pumpkin seeds, 1/4 cup	9 g
Sunflower seeds, 1/4 cup	9 g
Chia seeds, 1/4 cup	4 g
Peanut butter, 2 tbsp	8 g
Other nut butters, 2 tbsp	5 g

Grains and Starches—1 cup cooked

Amaranth	9 g
Quinoa	8 g
Oat bran	7 g
Wild rice	7 g
Oatmeal	6 g
Buckwheat	6 g
Brown rice	5 g
White rice	4 g
Barley	4 g
Potatoes	4 g
Sweet potatoes	4 g

Recommended Protein Intake by Weight

Protein Intake			
Weight (lbs)	Weight (kg)	1.1 g/kg	1.6 g/kg
100	45	50	73
110	50	55	80
120	55	60	87
130	59	65	95
140	64	70	102
150	68	75	109
160	73	80	116
170	77	85	124
180	82	90	131
190	86	95	138
200	91	100	145
210	95	105	153
220	100	110	160
230	105	115	167
240	109	120	175
250	114	125	182
260	118	130	189
270	123	135	196
280	127	140	204
290	132	145	211
300	136	150	218

ENDNOTES

Introduction

1. Lim E-J, Ahn Y-C, Jang E-S, Lee S-W, Lee S-H, Son C-G. Systematic review and meta-analysis of the prevalence of chronic fatigue syndrome/myalgic encephalomyelitis (CFS/ME). J Transl Med. 2020;18:100. https://pubmed .ncbi.nlm.nih.gov/32093722/

2. NSC Fatigue Reports, National Safety Council, https://www.nsc.org/ workplace/safety-topics/fatigue/fatigue-reports

3. Kroenke K, Wood DR, Mangelsdorff AD, Meier NJ, Powell JB. Chronic fatigue in primary care. Prevalence, patient characteristics, and outcome. JAMA. 1988;260:929–34. https://pubmed.ncbi.nlm.nih.gov/3398197/

4. Hammond EC. Some preliminary findings on physical complaints from a prospective study of 1,064,004 men and women. Am J Public Health Nations Health. 1964;54:11–23. https://pubmed.ncbi.nlm.nih.gov/14117648/

5. Katz DL, Frates EP, Bonnet JP, Gupta SK, Vartiainen E, Carmona RH. Lifestyle as medicine: the case for a true health initiative. Am J Health Promot. 2018;32:1452–58. https://journals.sagepub.com/doi/ abs/10.1177/0890117117705949

PART I

Chapter 1

1. Filler K, Lyon D, Bennett J, McCain N, Elswick R, Lukkahatai N, et al. Association of mitochondrial dysfunction and fatigue: a review of the literature. BBA Clin. 2014;1:12–23. https://pubmed.ncbi.nlm.nih.gov/ 25147756/

2. Naviaux RK, Naviaux JC, Li K, Bright AT, Alaynick WA, Wang L, et al. Metabolic features of chronic fatigue syndrome. Proc Natl Acad Sci U S A. 2016;113:E5472–80. https://www.pnas.org/content/113/37/E5472

3. Naviaux RK. Metabolic features of the cell danger response. Mitochondrion. 2014;16:7–17. https://pubmed.ncbi.nlm.nih.gov/23981537/

4. Naviaux. Metabolic features of the cell danger response.

5. Open Medicine Foundation. "Dr. Naviaux has published a ground-breaking study 'Metabolic Features of Chronic Fatigue Syndrome.' Below are answers regarding his results." September 9, 2016. https://www.omf.ngo/

updated-metabolic-features-of-chronic-fatigue-syndrome-q-a-with-robert
-naviaux-md/

6. Naviaux, R (n.d.). Mitochondrial disease research. Naviaux Lab. Retrieved from
    https://naviauxlab.ucsd.edu/science-item/mitochondrial-disease-research/

Chapter 2

1. Consensus Conference Panel, Watson NF, Badr MS, Belenky G, Bliwise DL,
    Buxton OM, et al. Joint consensus statement of the American Academy of
    Sleep Medicine and Sleep Research Society on the recommended amount
    of sleep for a healthy adult: methodology and discussion. J Clin Sleep Med.
    2015;11:931–52. https://pubmed.ncbi.nlm.nih.gov/26235159/

2. Ford ES, Cunningham TJ, Croft JB. Trends in self-reported sleep duration
    among US adults from1985 to 2012. Sleep. 2015;38:829–32. https://pubmed
    .ncbi.nlm.nih.gov/25669182/

3. Ohayon MM. Epidemiology of insomnia: what we know and what we still
    need to learn. Sleep Med Rev. 2002;6:97–111. https://pubmed.ncbi.nlm.nih
    .gov/12531146/

4. Bertisch SM, Herzig SJ, Winkelman JW, Buettner C. National use of prescrip-
    tion medications for insomnia: NHANES 1999–2010. Sleep. 2014;37:343–49.
    https://pubmed.ncbi.nlm.nih.gov/24497662/

5. Zimmet P, Alberti KGMM, Stern N, Bilu C, El-Osta A, Einat H, et al. The Cir-
    cadian Syndrome: is the Metabolic Syndrome and much more! J Intern Med.
    2019;286:181–91. https://pubmed.ncbi.nlm.nih.gov/31081577/

6. Engin A. Circadian rhythms in diet-induced obesity. Adv Exp Med Biol.
    2017;960:19–52. https://pubmed.ncbi.nlm.nih.gov/28585194/

7. Perelis M, Ramsey KM, Marcheva B, Bass J. Circadian transcription from beta
    cell function to diabetes pathophysiology. J Biol Rhythms. 2016;31:323–36.
    https://pubmed.ncbi.nlm.nih.gov/27440914/

8. Thosar SS, Butler MP, Shea SA. Role of the circadian system in cardiovascular
    disease. J Clin Invest. 2018;128:2157–67. https://pubmed.ncbi.nlm.nih.gov/
    29856365/

9. Khaper N, Bailey CDC, Ghugre NR, Reitz C, Awosanmi Z, Waines R, et al.
    Implications of disturbances in circadian rhythms for cardiovascular health:
    a new frontier in free radical biology. Free Radic Biol Med. 2018;119:85–92.
    https://pubmed.ncbi.nlm.nih.gov/29146117/

10. Musiek ES. Circadian clock disruption in neurodegenerative diseases: cause
    and effect? Front Pharmacol. 2015;6:29. https://www.frontiersin.org/
    articles/10.3389/fphar.2015.00029/full

11. Hood S, Amir S. Neurodegeneration and the circadian clock. Front Aging
    Neurosci. 2017;9:170. https://pubmed.ncbi.nlm.nih.gov/28611660/

12. Asarnow LD, Soehner AM, Harvey AG. Circadian rhythms and psychiatric
    illness. Curr Opin Psychiatry. 2013;26:566–71. https://pubmed.ncbi.nlm.nih
    .gov/24060916/

13. Karatsoreos IN. Links between circadian rhythms and psychiatric disease. Front Behav Neurosci. 2014;8:162. https://pubmed.ncbi.nlm.nih.gov/24834040/

14. McAlpine CS, Swirski FK. Circadian influence on metabolism and inflammation in atherosclerosis. Circ Res. 2016;119:131–41. https://pubmed.ncbi.nlm.nih.gov/27340272/

15. Wilking M, Ndiaye M, Mukhtar H, Ahmad N. Circadian rhythm connections to oxidative stress: implications for human health. Antioxid Redox Signal. 2013;19:192–208. https://www.ncbi.nlm.nih.gov/pmc/articles/PMC3689169/

16. Sardon Puig L, Valera-Alberni M, Cantó C, Pillon NJ. Circadian rhythms and mitochondria: connecting the dots. Front Genet. 2018;9:452. https://pubmed.ncbi.nlm.nih.gov/30349557/

17. Savvidis C, Koutsilieris M. Circadian rhythm disruption in cancer biology. Mol Med. 2012;18:1249–60. https://pubmed.ncbi.nlm.nih.gov/22811066/

18. Poggiogalle E, Jamshed H, Peterson CM. Circadian regulation of glucose, lipid, and energy metabolism in humans. Metabolism. 2018;84:11–27. https://pubmed.ncbi.nlm.nih.gov/29195759/

19. Tanioka M, Yamada H, Doi M, Bando H, Yamaguchi Y, Nishigori C, et al. Molecular clocks in mouse skin. J Invest Dermatol. 2009;129:1225–31. https://pubmed.ncbi.nlm.nih.gov/19037239/

20. Mendoza J. Circadian clocks: setting time by food. J Neuroendocrinol. 2007;19:127–37. https://pubmed.ncbi.nlm.nih.gov/17214875/

21. Goel N, Basner M, Rao H, Dinges DF. Circadian rhythms, sleep deprivation, and human performance. Prog Mol Biol Transl Sci. 2013;119:155–90. https://pubmed.ncbi.nlm.nih.gov/23899598/

22. Sardon Puig L. Circadian rhythms and mitochondria.

23. Wrede JE, Mengel-From J, Buchwald D, Vitiello MV, Bamshad M, Noonan C, et al. Mitochondrial DNA copy number in sleep duration discordant monozygotic twins. Sleep. 2015;38:1655–58. https://www.ncbi.nlm.nih.gov/pmc/articles/PMC4576340/

24. Peek CB, Affinati AH, Ramsey KM, Kuo H-Y, Yu W, Sena LA, et al. Circadian clock NAD+ cycle drives mitochondrial oxidative metabolism in mice. Science. 2013;342:1243417. https://pubmed.ncbi.nlm.nih.gov/24051248/

25. Jacobi D, Liu S, Burkewitz K, Kory N, Knudsen NH, Alexander RK, et al. Hepatic Bmal1 regulates rhythmic mitochondrial dynamics and promotes metabolic fitness. Cell Metab. 2015;22:709–20. https://pubmed.ncbi.nlm.nih.gov/26365180/

26. Neufeld-Cohen A, Robles MS, Aviram R, Manella G, Adamovich Y, Ladeuix B, et al. Circadian control of oscillations in mitochondrial rate-limiting enzymes and nutrient utilization by PERIOD proteins. Proc Natl Acad Sci U S A. 2016;113:E1673–82. https://pubmed.ncbi.nlm.nih.gov/26862173/

27. Kohsaka A, Das P, Hashimoto I, Nakao T, Deguchi Y, Gouraud SS, et al. The circadian clock maintains cardiac function by regulating mitochondrial metabolism in mice. PLoS One. 2014;9:e112811. https://pubmed.ncbi.nlm.nih.gov/25389966/

28. Schmitt K, Grimm A, Dallmann R, Oettinghaus B, Restelli LM, Witzig M, et al. Circadian control of DRP1 activity regulates mitochondrial dynamics and bioenergetics. Cell Metab. 2018;27:657–66.e5. https://pubmed.ncbi.nlm.nih.gov/29478834/

29. Peek. Circadian clock NAD.

30. Jacobi. Hepatic Bmal1 regulates.

31. Kohsaka. The circadian clock maintains cardiac function.

32. Andrews JL, Zhang X, McCarthy JJ, McDearmon EL, Hornberger TA, Russell B, et al. CLOCK and BMAL1 regulate MyoD and are necessary for maintenance of skeletal muscle phenotype and function. Proc Natl Acad Sci U S A. 2010;107:19090–5. https://pubmed.ncbi.nlm.nih.gov/20956306/

33. Rey G, Reddy AB. Protein acetylation links the circadian clock to mitochondrial function. Proc. Natl. Acad. Sci. U. S. A. 2013. p. 3210–1. https://www.ncbi.nlm.nih.gov/pmc/articles/PMC3587251/

34. Jacobi. Hepatic Bmal1 regulates.

35. Magnone MC, Langmesser S, Bezdek AC, Tallone T, Rusconi S, Albrecht U. The Mammalian circadian clock gene per2 modulates cell death in response to oxidative stress. Front Neurol. 2014;5:289. https://pubmed.ncbi.nlm.nih.gov/25628599/

36. de Goede P, Wefers J, Brombacher EC, Schrauwen P, Kalsbeek A. Circadian rhythms in mitochondrial respiration. J Mol Endocrinol. 2018;60:R115–30. https://www.ncbi.nlm.nih.gov/pmc/articles/PMC5854864/

37. Gomes LC, Scorrano L. Mitochondrial morphology in mitophagy and macroautophagy. Biochim Biophys Acta. 2013;1833:205–12. https://pubmed.ncbi.nlm.nih.gov/22406072/

38. Srinivasan V, Spence DW, Pandi-Perumal SR, Brown GM, Cardinali DP. Melatonin in mitochondrial dysfunction and related disorders. Int J Alzheimers Dis. 2011;2011:326320. https://pubmed.ncbi.nlm.nih.gov/21629741/

39. Zhang H-M, Zhang Y. Melatonin: a well-documented antioxidant with conditional pro-oxidant actions. J Pineal Res. 2014;57:131–46. https://pubmed.ncbi.nlm.nih.gov/25060102/

40. Tan D-X, Hardeland R, Manchester LC, Poeggeler B, Lopez-Burillo S, Mayo JC, et al. Mechanistic and comparative studies of melatonin and classic antioxidants in terms of their interactions with the ABTS cation radical. J Pineal Res. 2003;34:249–59. https://onlinelibrary.wiley.com/doi/pdf/10.1034/j.1600-079X.2003.00037.x

41. Tan D-X, Manchester LC, Terron MP, Flores LJ, Reiter RJ. One molecule, many derivatives: a never-ending interaction of melatonin with reactive oxygen and nitrogen species? J Pineal Res. 2007;42:28–42. https://pubmed.ncbi.nlm.nih.gov/17198536/

42. Rodriguez C, Mayo JC, Sainz RM, Antolín I, Herrera F, Martín V, et al. Regulation of antioxidant enzymes: a significant role for melatonin. J Pineal Res. 2004;36:1–9. https://pubmed.ncbi.nlm.nih.gov/14675124/

43. Sofic E, Rimpapa Z, Kundurovic Z, Sapcanin A, Tahirovic I, Rustembegovic A, et al. Antioxidant capacity of the neurohormone melatonin. J Neural Transm. 2005;112:349–58. https://pubmed.ncbi.nlm.nih.gov/15666035/

44. Reiter RJ, Rosales-Corral S, Tan DX, Jou MJ, Galano A, Xu B. Melatonin as a mitochondria-targeted antioxidant: one of evolution's best ideas. Cell Mol Life Sci. 2017;74:3863–81. https://pubmed.ncbi.nlm.nih.gov/28864909/

45. Lowes DA, Webster NR, Murphy MP, Galley HF. Antioxidants that protect mitochondria reduce interleukin-6 and oxidative stress, improve mitochondrial function, and reduce biochemical markers of organ dysfunction in a rat model of acute sepsis. Br J Anaesth. 2013;110:472–80. https://pubmed.ncbi.nlm.nih.gov/23381720/

46. Coto-Montes A, Boga JA, Rosales-Corral S, Fuentes-Broto L, Tan D-X, Reiter RJ. Role of melatonin in the regulation of autophagy and mitophagy: a review. Mol Cell Endocrinol. 2012;361:12–23. https://pubmed.ncbi.nlm.nih.gov/22575351/

47. Reiter. Melatonin as a mitochondria-targeted antioxidant.

48. Tan. Mitochondria and chloroplasts as the original sites of melatonin synthesis.

49. Reiter RJ, Tan DX, Galano A. Melatonin: exceeding expectations. Physiology. 2014;29:325–33. https://pubmed.ncbi.nlm.nih.gov/25180262/

50. Xie L, Kang H, Xu Q, Chen MJ, Liao Y, Thiyagarajan M, et al. Sleep drives metabolite clearance from the adult brain. Science. 2013;342:373–77. https://pubmed.ncbi.nlm.nih.gov/24136970/

51. Jessen NA, Munk ASF, Lundgaard I, Nedergaard M. The glymphatic system: a beginner's guide. Neurochem Res. 2015;40:2583–99. https://pubmed.ncbi.nlm.nih.gov/25947369/

52. Glassford JAG. The neuroinflammatory etiopathology of myalgic encephalomyelitis/chronic fatigue syndrome (ME/CFS). Front Physiol. 2017;8:88. https://pubmed.ncbi.nlm.nih.gov/28261110/

53. Weeke J, Gundersen HJ. Circadian and 30 minutes variations in serum TSH and thyroid hormones in normal subjects. Acta Endocrinol . 1978;89:659–72. https://pubmed.ncbi.nlm.nih.gov/716774/

54. Ikegami K, Refetoff S, Van Cauter E, Yoshimura T. Interconnection between circadian clocks and thyroid function. Nat Rev Endocrinol. 2019;15:590–600. https://pubmed.ncbi.nlm.nih.gov/31406343/

55. Spiegel K, Leproult R, Van Cauter E. Impact of sleep debt on metabolic and endocrine function. Lancet. 1999;354:1435–39. https://pubmed.ncbi.nlm.nih.gov/10543671/

56. Holl RW, Hartman ML, Veldhuis JD, Taylor WM, Thorner MO. Thirty-second sampling of plasma growth hormone in man: correlation with sleep stages. J Clin Endocrinol Metab. 1991;72:854–61. https://pubmed.ncbi.nlm.nih.gov/2005213/

57. Berwaerts J, Moorkens G, Abs R. Secretion of growth hormone in patients with chronic fatigue syndrome. Growth Horm IGF Res. 1998;8 Suppl B:127–29. https://pubmed.ncbi.nlm.nih.gov/10990147/

58. Cadegiani FA, Kater CE. Adrenal fatigue does not exist: a systematic review. BMC Endocr Disord. 2016;16:48. https://pubmed.ncbi.nlm.nih .gov/27557747/

59. Kumari M, Badrick E, Chandola T, Adam EK, Stafford M, Marmot MG, et al. Cortisol secretion and fatigue: associations in a community based cohort. Psychoneuroendocrinology. 2009;34:1476–85. https://pubmed.ncbi.nlm.nih .gov/19497676/

60. Abbruzzese EA, Klingmann A, Ehlert U. The influence of the chronotype on the awakening response of cortisol in the morning. Adv Soc Sci Res J. 2014;1:115–21. https://journals.scholarpublishing.org/index.php/ASSRJ/ article/view/519

61. Edwards S, Evans P, Hucklebridge F, Clow A. Association between time of awakening and diurnal cortisol secretory activity. Psychoneuroendocrinology. 2001;26:613–22. https://pubmed.ncbi.nlm.nih.gov/11403981/

62. Kudielka BM, Federenko IS, Hellhammer DH, Wüst S. Morningness and eveningness: the free cortisol rise after awakening in "early birds" and "night owls." Biol Psychol. 2006;72:141–6. https://pubmed.ncbi.nlm.nih .gov/16236420/

63. Oginska H, Fafrowicz M, Golonka K, Marek T, Mojsa-Kaja J, Tucholska K. Chronotype, sleep loss, and diurnal pattern of salivary cortisol in a simulated daylong driving. Chronobiol Int. 2010;27:959–74. https://pubmed.ncbi.nlm .nih.gov/20636209/

64. Bozic J, Galic T, Supe-Domic D, Ivkovic N, Ticinovic Kurir T, Valic Z, et al. Morning cortisol levels and glucose metabolism parameters in moderate and severe obstructive sleep apnea patients. Endocrine. 2016;53:730–39. https:// pubmed.ncbi.nlm.nih.gov/27000083/

65. Späth-Schwalbe E, Schöller T, Kern W, Fehm HL, Born J. Nocturnal adrenocorticotropin and cortisol secretion depends on sleep duration and decreases in association with spontaneous awakening in the morning. J Clin Endocrinol Metab. 1992;75:1431–35. https://pubmed.ncbi.nlm.nih. gov/1334495/

66. Leese G, Chattington P, Fraser W, Vora J, Edwards R, Williams G. Short-term night-shift working mimics the pituitary-adrenocortical dysfunction in chronic fatigue syndrome. J Clin Endocrinol Metab. 1996;81:1867–70. https://scholar.google.com/scholar?q=J+Clin+Endocrinol+Metab.+1996%3B8 1:1867%E2%80%9370.&hl=en&as_sdt=0&as_vis=1&oi=scholart

67. Mirick DK, Bhatti P, Chen C, Nordt F, Stanczyk FZ, Davis S. Night shift work and levels of 6-sulfatoxymelatonin and cortisol in men. Cancer Epidemiol Biomarkers Prev. 2013;22:1079–87. https://pubmed.ncbi.nlm.nih .gov/23563887/

68. Almoosawi S, Vingeliene S, Gachon F, Voortman T, Palla L, Johnston JD, et al. Chronotype: implications for epidemiologic studies on chrono-nutrition and cardiometabolic health. Adv Nutr. 2019;10:30–42. https://pubmed.ncbi .nlm.nih.gov/30500869/

69. Kant AK, Graubard BI. 40-year trends in meal and snack eating behaviors of American adults. J Acad Nutr Diet. 2015;115:50–63. https://pubmed.ncbi .nlm.nih.gov/25088521/

70. Gill S, Panda S. A smartphone app reveals erratic diurnal eating patterns in humans that can be modulated for health benefits. Cell Metab. 2015;22:789–98. https://pubmed.ncbi.nlm.nih.gov/26411343/

71. Queiroz J do N, Macedo RCO, Tinsley GM, Reischak-Oliveira A. Time-restricted eating and circadian rhythms: the biological clock is ticking. Crit Rev Food Sci Nutr. 2020;1–13. https://pubmed.ncbi.nlm.nih.gov/32662279/

72. Melkani GC, Panda S. Time-restricted feeding for prevention and treatment of cardiometabolic disorders. J Physiol. 2017;595:3691–700. https://pubmed .ncbi.nlm.nih.gov/28295377/

73. St-Onge M-P, Ard J, Baskin ML, Chiuve SE, Johnson HM, Kris-Etherton P, et al. Meal timing and frequency: implications for cardiovascular disease prevention: a scientific statement from the American Heart Association. Circulation. 2017;135:e96–121. https://pubmed.ncbi.nlm.nih.gov/28137935/

74. Chaix A, Manoogian ENC, Melkani GC, Panda S. Time-restricted eating to prevent and manage chronic metabolic diseases. Annu Rev Nutr. 2019;39:291–315. https://pubmed.ncbi.nlm.nih.gov/31180809/

75. Adafer R, Messaadi W, Meddahi M, Patey A, Haderbache A, Bayen S, et al. Food timing, circadian rhythm and chrononutrition: a systematic review of time-restricted eating's effects on human health. Nutrients. 2020;12. http:// dx.doi.org/10.3390/nu12123770

76. Lettieri-Barbato D, Cannata SM, Casagrande V, Ciriolo MR, Aquilano K. Time-controlled fasting prevents aging-like mitochondrial changes induced by persistent dietary fat overload in skeletal muscle. PLoS One. 2018;13:e0195912. https://pubmed.ncbi.nlm.nih.gov/29742122/

77. Sutton EF, Beyl R, Early KS, Cefalu WT, Ravussin E, Peterson CM. Early time-restricted feeding improves insulin sensitivity, blood pressure, and oxidative stress even without weight loss in men with prediabetes. Cell Metab. 2018;27:1212–21.e3. https://pubmed.ncbi.nlm.nih.gov/29754952/

78. Kahleova H, Belinova L, Malinska H, Oliyarnyk O, Trnovska J, Skop V, et al. Eating two larger meals a day (breakfast and lunch) is more effective than six smaller meals in a reduced-energy regimen for patients with type 2 diabetes: a randomised crossover study. Diabetologia. 2014;57:1552–60. https:// pubmed.ncbi.nlm.nih.gov/24838678/

79. Moro T, Tinsley G, Bianco A, Marcolin G, Pacelli QF, Battaglia G, et al. Effects of eight weeks of time-restricted feeding (16/8) on basal metabolism, maximal strength, body composition, inflammation, and cardiovascular risk factors in resistance-trained males. J Transl Med. 2016;14:290. https://pubmed .ncbi.nlm.nih.gov/27737674/

80. Tinsley GM, Moore ML, Graybeal AJ, Paoli A, Kim Y, Gonzales JU, et al. Time-restricted feeding plus resistance training in active females: a randomized trial. Am J Clin Nutr. 2019;110:628–40. https://pubmed.ncbi.nlm.nih .gov/31268131/

81. Gill S. A smartphone app reveals erratic diurnal eating patterns in humans that can be modulated for health benefits. Cel Metab. 2015;22:789–98. https://www.ncbi.nlm.nih.gov/pmc/articles/PMC4635036/

82. Bass J, Takahashi JS. Circadian integration of metabolism and energetics. Science. 2010;330:1349–54. https://pubmed.ncbi.nlm.nih.gov/21127246/

83. Damiola F, Le Minh N, Preitner N, Kornmann B, Fleury-Olela F, Schibler U. Restricted feeding uncouples circadian oscillators in peripheral tissues from the central pacemaker in the suprachiasmatic nucleus. Genes Dev. 2000;14:2950–61. https://pubmed.ncbi.nlm.nih.gov/11114885/

84. Stokkan KA, Yamazaki S, Tei H, Sakaki Y, Menaker M. Entrainment of the circadian clock in the liver by feeding. Science. 2001;291:490–93. https://pubmed.ncbi.nlm.nih.gov/11161204/

85. Bonham MP, Bonnell EK, Huggins CE. Energy intake of shift workers compared to fixed day workers: A systematic review and meta-analysis. Chronobiol Int. 2016;33:1086–1100. https://pubmed.ncbi.nlm.nih.gov/27303804/

86. Cayanan EA, Eyre NAB, Lao V, Comas M, Hoyos CM, Marshall NS, et al. Is 24-hour energy intake greater during night shift compared to non-night shift patterns? A systematic review. Chronobiol Int. 2019;36:1599–1612. https://pubmed.ncbi.nlm.nih.gov/31571507/

87. Zhang Y, Papantoniou K. Night shift work and its carcinogenicity. Lancet Oncol. 2019. e550. https://pubmed.ncbi.nlm.nih.gov/31578992/

88. Hatori M, Vollmers C, Zarrinpar A, DiTacchio L, Bushong EA, Gill S, et al. Time-restricted feeding without reducing caloric intake prevents metabolic diseases in mice fed a high-fat diet. Cell Metab. 2012;15:848–60. https://pubmed.ncbi.nlm.nih.gov/22608008/

89. Sherman H, Genzer Y, Cohen R, Chapnik N, Madar Z, Froy O. Timed high-fat diet resets circadian metabolism and prevents obesity. FASEB J. 2012;26:3493–502. https://pubmed.ncbi.nlm.nih.gov/22593546/

90. Ye Y, Xu H, Xie Z, Wang L, Sun Y, Yang H, et al. Time-restricted feeding reduces the detrimental effects of a high-fat diet, possibly by modulating the circadian rhythm of hepatic lipid metabolism and gut microbiota. Front Nutr. 2020;7:596285. https://pubmed.ncbi.nlm.nih.gov/33425971/

91. Moran-Ramos S, Baez-Ruiz A, Buijs RM, Escobar C. When to eat? The influence of circadian rhythms on metabolic health: are animal studies providing the evidence? Nutr Res Rev. 2016;29:180–93. https://pubmed.ncbi.nlm.nih.gov/27364352/

92. Ravussin E, Beyl RA, Poggiogalle E, Hsia DS, Peterson CM. Early time-restricted feeding reduces appetite and increases fat oxidation but does not affect energy expenditure in humans. Obesity. 2019;27:1244–54. https://pubmed.ncbi.nlm.nih.gov/31339000/

93. Jamshed H, Beyl RA, Della Manna DL, Yang ES, Ravussin E, Peterson CM. Early time-restricted feeding improves 24-hour glucose levels and affects markers of the circadian clock, aging, and autophagy in humans. Nutrients. 2019;11. http://dx.doi.org/10.3390/nu11061234.

94. Adib-Hajbaghery M, Mousavi SN. The effects of chamomile extract on sleep quality among elderly people: A clinical trial. Complement Ther Med. 2017;35:109–14. https://pubmed.ncbi.nlm.nih.gov/29154054/

95. Thomas EA, Higgins J, Bessesen DH, McNair B, Cornier M-A. Usual breakfast eating habits affect response to breakfast skipping in overweight women. Obesity. 2015;23:750–59. https://pubmed.ncbi.nlm.nih.gov/25755093/

96. St-Onge M-P, Mikic A, Pietrolungo CE. Effects of diet on sleep quality. Adv Nutr. 2016;7:938–49. https://pubmed.ncbi.nlm.nih.gov/27633109/

97. Ekman AC, Leppäluoto J, Huttunen P, Aranko K, Vakkuri O. Ethanol inhibits melatonin secretion in healthy volunteers in a dose-dependent randomized double blind cross-over study. J Clin Endocrinol Metab. 1993;77:780–83. https://pubmed.ncbi.nlm.nih.gov/8370699/

98. Röjdmark S, Wikner J, Adner N, Andersson DE, Wetterberg L. Inhibition of melatonin secretion by ethanol in man. Metabolism. 1993;42:1047–51. https://pubmed.ncbi.nlm.nih.gov/8345809/

99. Rupp TL, Acebo C, Carskadon MA. Evening alcohol suppresses salivary melatonin in young adults. Chronobiol Int. 2007;24:463–70. https://pubmed.ncbi.nlm.nih.gov/17612945/

100. Ebrahim IO, Shapiro CM, Williams AJ, Fenwick PB. Alcohol and sleep I: effects on normal sleep. Alcohol Clin Exp Res. 2013;37:539–49. https://pubmed.ncbi.nlm.nih.gov/23347102/

101. Ribeiro JA, Sebastião AM. Caffeine and adenosine. J Alzheimers Dis. 2010;20 Suppl 1:S3–15. https://pubmed.ncbi.nlm.nih.gov/20164566/

102. Childs E, de Wit H. Subjective, behavioral, and physiological effects of acute caffeine in light, nondependent caffeine users. Psychopharmacology. 2006;185:514–23. https://pubmed.ncbi.nlm.nih.gov/16541243/

103. Tarnopolsky M, Cupido C. Caffeine potentiates low frequency skeletal muscle force in habitual and nonhabitual caffeine consumers. J Appl Physiol. 2000;89:1719–24. https://pubmed.ncbi.nlm.nih.gov/11053318/

104. Astorino TA, Rohmann RL, Firth K. Effect of caffeine ingestion on one-repetition maximum muscular strength. Eur J Appl Physiol. 2008;102:127–32. https://pubmed.ncbi.nlm.nih.gov/17851681/

105. Bell DG, McLellan TM. Exercise endurance 1, 3, and 6 h after caffeine ingestion in caffeine users and nonusers. J Appl Physiol. 2002;93:1227–34. https://pubmed.ncbi.nlm.nih.gov/12235019/

106. Bell DG, McLellan TM. Effect of repeated caffeine ingestion on repeated exhaustive exercise endurance. Med Sci Sports Exerc. 2003;35:1348–54. https://pubmed.ncbi.nlm.nih.gov/12900689/

107. O'Callaghan F, Muurlink O, Reid N. Effects of caffeine on sleep quality and daytime functioning. Risk Manag Healthc Policy. 2018;11:263–71. https://pubmed.ncbi.nlm.nih.gov/30573997/

108. Bchir F, Dogui M, Ben Fradj R, Arnaud MJ, Saguem S. Differences in pharmacokinetic and electroencephalographic responses to caffeine in sleep-sensitive and non-sensitive subjects. C R Biol. 2006;329:512–19. https://pubmed.ncbi.nlm.nih.gov/16797457/

109. Robertson D, Wade D, Workman R, Woosley RL, Oates JA. Tolerance to the humoral and hemodynamic effects of caffeine in man. J Clin Invest. 1981;67:1111–17. https://www.ncbi.nlm.nih.gov/pmc/articles/PMC370671/

110. Marangos PJ, Boulenger JP, Patel J. Effects of chronic caffeine on brain adenosine receptors: regional and ontogenetic studies. Life Sci. 1984;34:899–907. https://pubmed.ncbi.nlm.nih.gov/6321875/

Chapter 3

1. Hales CM, Fryar CD, Carroll MD, Freedman DS, Ogden CL. Trends in obesity and severe obesity prevalence in US youth and adults by sex and age. 2007–2008 to 2015–2016. JAMA. 2018;319:1723–25. https://pubmed.ncbi.nlm.nih.gov/29570750/

2. The prevalence of overfat adults and children in the US. Front Public Health. 2017;5:290. https://pubmed.ncbi.nlm.nih.gov/29164096/

3. Hart BL. Biological basis of the behavior of sick animals. Neurosci Biobehav Rev. 1988;12:123–37. https://pubmed.ncbi.nlm.nih.gov/3050629/

4. GBD 2015 Obesity Collaborators, Afshin A, Forouzanfar MH, Reitsma MB, Sur P, Estep K, et al. Health effects of overweight and obesity in 195 countries over 25 years. N Engl J Med. 2017;377:13–27. https://pubmed.ncbi.nlm.nih.gov/28604169/

5. Dobbs R, Sawers C, Thompson F, Manyika J, Woetzel J, Child P, et al. Overcoming obesity: an initial economic analysis. McKinsey Global Institute; 2014 Nov. https://www.mckinsey.com/~/media/McKinsey/Business%20Functions/Economic%20Studies%20TEMP/Our%20Insights/How%20the%20world%20could%20better%20fight%20obesity/MGI_Overcoming_obesity_Full_report.ashx.

6. Biener A, Cawley J, Meyerhoefer C. The high and rising costs of obesity to the US health care system. J Gen Intern Med. 2017;32:6–8. https://pubmed.ncbi.nlm.nih.gov/28271429/

7. Finkelstein EA, Trogdon JG, Cohen JW, Dietz W. Annual medical spending attributable to obesity: payer-and service-specific estimates. Health Aff. 2009;28:w822–31. https://pubmed.ncbi.nlm.nih.gov/19635784/

8. Ul-Haq Z, Mackay DF, Fenwick E, Pell JP. Meta-analysis of the association between body mass index and health-related quality of life among adults, assessed by the SF-36. Obesity. 2013;21:E322–27. https://pubmed.ncbi.nlm.nih.gov/23592685/

9. Galland-Decker C, Marques-Vidal P, Vollenweider P. Prevalence and factors associated with fatigue in the Lausanne middle-aged population: a population-based, cross-sectional survey. BMJ Open. 2019;9:e027070. https://bmjopen.bmj.com/content/bmjopen/9/8/e027070.full.pdf

10. Katz DA, McHorney CA, Atkinson RL. Impact of obesity on health-related quality of life in patients with chronic illness. J Gen Intern Med. 2000;15:789–96. https://pubmed.ncbi.nlm.nih.gov/11119171/

11. Lacourt TE, Vichaya EG, Chiu GS, Dantzer R, Heijnen CJ. The high costs of low-grade inflammation: persistent fatigue as a consequence of reduced

cellular-energy availability and non-adaptive energy expenditure. Front Behav Neurosci. 2018;12:78. https://pubmed.ncbi.nlm.nih.gov/29755330/

12. Miller AH, Haroon E, Raison CL, Felger JC. Cytokine targets in the brain: impact on neurotransmitters and neurocircuits. Depress Anxiety. 2013;30:297–306. https://pubmed.ncbi.nlm.nih.gov/23468190/

13. Capuron L, Miller AH. Immune system to brain signaling: neuropsycho-pharmacological implications. Pharmacol Ther. 2011;130:226–38. https://pubmed.ncbi.nlm.nih.gov/21334376/

14. Karshikoff B, Sundelin T, Lasselin J. Role of inflammation in human fatigue: relevance of multidimensional assessments and potential neuronal mechanisms. Front Immunol. 2017;8:21. https://pubmed.ncbi.nlm.nih.gov/28163706/

15. Pollmächer T, Haack M, Schuld A, Reichenberg A, Yirmiya R. Low levels of circulating inflammatory cytokines—do they affect human brain functions? Brain Behav Immun. 2002;16:525–32. https://pubmed.ncbi.nlm.nih.gov/12401466/

16. Lasselin J, Capuron L. Chronic low-grade inflammation in metabolic disorders: relevance for behavioral symptoms. Neuroimmunomodulation. 2014;21:95–101. https://pubmed.ncbi.nlm.nih.gov/24557041/

17. Hart. Biological basis of the behavior of sick animals.

18. van Horssen J, van Schaik P, Witte M. Inflammation and mitochondrial dysfunction: a vicious circle in neurodegenerative disorders? Neurosci Lett. 2019;710:132931. https://pubmed.ncbi.nlm.nih.gov/28668382/

19. Dela Cruz CS, Kang M-J. Mitochondrial dysfunction and damage associated molecular patterns (DAMPs) in chronic inflammatory diseases. Mitochondrion. 2018;41:37–44. https://www.ncbi.nlm.nih.gov/pmc/articles/PMC5988941/

20. Morris G, Maes M. Mitochondrial dysfunctions in myalgic encephalomyelitis/chronic fatigue syndrome explained by activated immuno-inflammatory, oxidative and nitrosative stress pathways. Metab Brain Dis. 2014;29:19–36. https://pubmed.ncbi.nlm.nih.gov/24557875/

21. Kominsky DJ, Campbell EL, Colgan SP. Metabolic shifts in immunity and inflammation. J Immunol. 2010;184:4062–68. https://pubmed.ncbi.nlm.nih.gov/20368286/

22. Wang H, Ye J. Regulation of energy balance by inflammation: common theme in physiology and pathology. Rev Endocr Metab Disord. 2015;16:47–54. https://pubmed.ncbi.nlm.nih.gov/25526866/

23. Lacourt. The high costs of low-grade inflammation.

24. Vgontzas AN, Bixler EO, Chrousos GP, Pejovic S. Obesity and sleep disturbances: meaningful sub-typing of obesity. Arch Physiol Biochem. 2008;114:224–36. https://www.researchgate.net/publication/23407878_Obesity_and_sleep_disturbances_Meaningful_sub-typing_of_obesity

25. Mullington JM, Simpson NS, Meier-Ewert HK, Haack M. Sleep loss and inflammation. Best Pract Res Clin Endocrinol Metab. 2010;24:775–84. https://pubmed.ncbi.nlm.nih.gov/21112025/

26. Kizaki T, Sato S, Shirato K, Sakurai T, Ogasawara J, Izawa T, et al. Effect of circadian rhythm on clinical and pathophysiological conditions and inflammation. Crit Rev Immunol. 2015;35:261–75. https://pubmed.ncbi.nlm.nih.gov/26757391/

27. Global BMI Mortality Collaboration, Di Angelantonio E, Bhupathiraju S, Wormser D, Gao P, Kaptoge S, et al. Body-mass index and all-cause mortality: individual-participant-data meta-analysis of 239 prospective studies in four continents. Lancet. 2016;388:776–86. https://pubmed.ncbi.nlm.nih.gov/27423262/

28. Flegal KM, Shepherd JA, Looker AC, Graubard BI, Borrud LG, Ogden CL, et al. Comparisons of percentage body fat, body mass index, waist circumference, and waist-stature ratio in adults. Am J Clin Nutr. 2009;89:500–508. https://pubmed.ncbi.nlm.nih.gov/19116329/

29. Argilés JM, Campos N, Lopez-Pedrosa JM, Rueda R, Rodriguez-Mañas L. Skeletal muscle regulates m\Metabolism via interorgan crosstalk: roles in health and disease. J Am Med Dir Assoc. 2016;17:789–96. https://pubmed.ncbi.nlm.nih.gov/27324808/

30. Wolfe RR. The underappreciated role of muscle in health and disease. Am J Clin Nutr. 2006;84:475–82. https://pubmed.ncbi.nlm.nih.gov/16960159/

31. Cao L, Morley JE. Sarcopenia is recognized as an independent condition by an international classification of disease, tenth revision, clinical modification (ICD-10-CM) code. J Am Med Dir Assoc. 2016;17:675–77. https://pubmed.ncbi.nlm.nih.gov/27470918/

32. Janssen I, Heymsfield SB, Ross R. Low relative skeletal muscle mass (sarcopenia) in older persons is associated with functional impairment and physical disability. J Am Geriatr Soc. 2002;50:889–96. https://pubmed.ncbi.nlm.nih.gov/12028177/

33. Patino-Hernandez D, David-Pardo DG, Borda MG, Pérez-Zepeda MU, Cano-Gutiérrez C. Association of fatigue with sarcopenia and its elements: a secondary analysis of SABE-Bogotá. Gerontol Geriatr Med. 2017;3:2333721417703734. https://pubmed.ncbi.nlm.nih.gov/28474000/

34. Neefjes ECW, van den Hurk RM, Blauwhoff-Buskermolen S, van der Vorst MJDL, Becker-Commissaris A, de van der Schueren MAE, et al. Muscle mass as a target to reduce fatigue in patients with advanced cancer. J Cachexia Sarcopenia Muscle. 2017;8:623–29. https://www.ncbi.nlm.nih.gov/pmc/articles/PMC5566642/

35. Blissmer B, Riebe D, Dye G, Ruggiero L, Greene G, Caldwell M. Health-related quality of life following a clinical weight loss intervention among overweight and obese adults: intervention and 24 month follow-up effects. Health Qual Life Outcomes. 2006;4:43. https://pubmed.ncbi.nlm.nih.gov/16846509/

36. Williamson DA, Rejeski J, Lang W, Van Dorsten B, Fabricatore AN, Toledo K, et al. Impact of a weight management program on health-related quality of life in overweight adults with type 2 diabetes. Arch Intern Med. 2009;169:163–71. https://pubmed.ncbi.nlm.nih.gov/19171813/

37. Sarwer DB, Moore RH, Diewald LK, Chittams J, Berkowitz RI, Vetter M, et al. The impact of a primary care-based weight loss intervention on the quality of life. Int J Obes. 2013;37 Suppl 1:S25–30. https://pubmed.ncbi.nlm.nih .gov/23921778/

38. Pearl RL, Wadden TA, Tronieri JS, Berkowitz RI, Chao AM, Alamuddin N, et al. Short- and long-term changes in health-related quality of life with weight loss: results from a randomized controlled trial. Obesity. 2018;26:985–91. https://pubmed.ncbi.nlm.nih.gov/29676530/

39. 37. Kolotkin RL, Norquist JM, Crosby RD, Suryawanshi S, Teixeira PJ, Heyms-field SB, et al. One-year health-related quality of life outcomes in weight loss trial participants: comparison of three measures. Health Qual Life Outcomes. 2009;7:53. https://pubmed.ncbi.nlm.nih.gov/19505338/

40. Kaukua J, Pekkarinen T, Sane T, Mustajoki P. Health-related quality of life in WHO class II-III obese men losing weight with very-low-energy diet and behaviour modification: a randomised clinical trial. Int J Obes Relat Metab Disord. 2002;26:487–95. https://pubmed.ncbi.nlm.nih.gov/12075575/

41. Franz MJ, VanWormer JJ, Crain AL, Boucher JL, Histon T, Caplan W, et al. Weight-loss outcomes: a systematic review and meta-analysis of weight-loss clinical trials with a minimum 1-year follow-up. J Am Diet Assoc. 2007;107:1755–67. https://pubmed.ncbi.nlm.nih.gov/17904936/

42. Journel M, Chaumontet C, Darcel N, Fromentin G, Tomé D. Brain responses to high-protein diets. Adv Nutr. 2012;3:322–29. https://academic.oup.com/advances/article/3/3/322/4591532

43. Tappy L. Thermic effect of food and sympathetic nervous system activity in humans. Reprod Nutr Dev. 1996;36:391–97. https://pubmed.ncbi.nlm.nih .gov/8878356/

44. Wycherley TP, Moran LJ, Clifton PM, Noakes M, Brinkworth GD. Effects of energy-restricted high-protein, low-fat compared with standard-protein, low-fat diets: a meta-analysis of randomized controlled trials. Am J Clin Nutr. 2012;96:1281–98. https://pubmed.ncbi.nlm.nih.gov/23097268/

45. Kim JE, O'Connor LE, Sands LP, Slebodnik MB, Campbell WW. Effects of dietary protein intake on body composition changes after weight loss in older adults: a systematic review and meta-analysis. Nutr Rev. 2016;74:210–24. https://pubmed.ncbi.nlm.nih.gov/26883880/

46. Santesso N, Akl EA, Bianchi M, Mente A, Mustafa R, Heels-Ansdell D, et al. Effects of higher- versus lower-protein diets on health outcomes: a systematic review and meta-analysis. Eur J Clin Nutr. 2012;66:780–88. https://pubmed .ncbi.nlm.nih.gov/22510792/

47. Jäger R, Kerksick CM, Campbell BI, Cribb PJ, Wells SD, Skwiat TM, et al. International Society of Sports Nutrition position stand: protein and exercise. J Int Soc Sports Nutr. 2017;14:20. https://pubmed.ncbi.nlm.nih .gov/28642676/

48. Thomas DT, Erdman KA, Burke LM. American College of Sports Medicine joint position statement. Nutrition and athletic performance. Med Sci Sports Exerc. 2016;48:543–68. https://pubmed.ncbi.nlm.nih.gov/26891166/

49. Morton RW, Murphy KT, McKellar SR, Schoenfeld BJ, Henselmans M, Helms E, et al. A systematic review, meta-analysis and meta-regression of the effect of protein supplementation on resistance training-induced gains in muscle mass and strength in healthy adults. Br J Sports Med. 2018;52:376–84. https://pubmed.ncbi.nlm.nih.gov/28698222/

50. Moore DR, Churchward-Venne TA, Witard O, Breen L, Burd NA, Tipton KD, et al. Protein ingestion to stimulate myofibrillar protein synthesis requires greater relative protein intakes in healthy older versus younger men. J Gerontol A Biol Sci Med Sci. 2015;70:57–62. https://pubmed.ncbi.nlm.nih.gov/25056502/

51. Burd NA, Gorissen SH, van Loon LJC. Anabolic resistance of muscle protein synthesis with aging. Exerc Sport Sci Rev. 2013;41:169–73. https://pubmed.ncbi.nlm.nih.gov/23558692/

52. Rogerson D. Vegan diets: practical advice for athletes and exercisers. J Int Soc Sports Nutr. 2017;14:36. https://pubmed.ncbi.nlm.nih.gov/28924423/

53. Moughan PJ, Gilani S, Rutherfurd SM, Tome D. True ileal amino acid digestibility coefficients for application in the calculation of Digestible Indispensable Amino Acid Score (DIAAS) in human nutrition. FAO; 2012 Feb. http://www.fao.org/ag/humannutrition/36216 -04a2f02ec02eafd4f457dd2c9851b4c45.pdf

54. Sarwar Gilani G, Wu Xiao C, Cockell KA. Impact of antinutritional factors in food proteins on the digestibility of protein and the bioavailability of amino acids and on protein quality. Br J Nutr. 2012;108 Suppl 2:S315–32. https://pubmed.ncbi.nlm.nih.gov/23107545/

55. van Vliet S, Burd NA, van Loon LJC. The skeletal muscle anabolic response to plant- versus animal-based protein consumption. J Nutr. 2015;145:1981–91. https://pubmed.ncbi.nlm.nih.gov/26224750/

56. Rolls BJ. The relationship between dietary energy density and energy intake. Physiol Behav. 2009;97:609–15. https://pubmed.ncbi.nlm.nih.gov/19303887/

57. Rolls BJ. Dietary energy density: Applying behavioural science to weight management. Nutr Bull. 2017;42:246–53. https://pubmed.ncbi.nlm.nih.gov/29151813/

58. Roe LS, Meengs JS, Rolls BJ. Salad and satiety. The effect of timing of salad consumption on meal energy intake. Appetite. 2012;58:242–48. https://pubmed.ncbi.nlm.nih.gov/22008705/

59. Ello-Martin JA, Roe LS, Ledikwe JH, Beach AM, Rolls BJ. Dietary energy density in the treatment of obesity: a year-long trial comparing 2 weight-loss diets. Am J Clin Nutr. 2007;85:1465–77. https://www.ncbi.nlm.nih.gov/pmc/articles/PMC2018610/

60. Sampey BP, Vanhoose AM, Winfield HM, Freemerman AJ, Muehlbauer MJ, Fueger PT, et al. Cafeteria diet is a robust model of human metabolic syndrome with liver and adipose inflammation: comparison to high-fat diet. Obesity. 2011;19:1109–17. https://pubmed.ncbi.nlm.nih.gov/21331068/

61. Martire SI, Maniam J, South T, Holmes N, Westbrook RF, Morris MJ. Extended exposure to a palatable cafeteria diet alters gene expression in brain regions

implicated in reward, and withdrawal from this diet alters gene expression in brain regions associated with stress. Behav Brain Res. 2014;265:132–41. https://pubmed.ncbi.nlm.nih.gov/24583192/

62. Hashim SA, Van Itallie TB. Studies in normal and obese subjects with a monitored food dispensing device. Ann N Y Acad Sci. 1965;131:654–61. https://pubmed.ncbi.nlm.nih.gov/5216999/

63. Hall KD, Ayuketah A, Brychta R, Cai H, Cassimatis T, Chen KY, et al. Ultra-processed diets cause excess calorie intake and weight gain: an inpatient randomized controlled trial of ad libitum food intake. Cell Metab. 2019;30:67–77.e3. https://pubmed.ncbi.nlm.nih.gov/31105044/

64. Areta JL, Burke LM, Ross ML, Camera DM, West DWD, Broad EM, et al. Timing and distribution of protein ingestion during prolonged recovery from resistance exercise alters myofibrillar protein synthesis. J Physiol. 2013;591:2319–31. https://pubmed.ncbi.nlm.nih.gov/23459753/

65. Ostendorf DM, Caldwell AE, Creasy SA, Pan Z, Lyden K, Bergouignan A, et al. Physical activity energy expenditure and total daily energy expenditure in successful weight loss maintainers. Obesity. 2019;27:496–504. https://pubmed.ncbi.nlm.nih.gov/30801984/

66. Poehlman ET, Melby CL, Badylak SF. Resting metabolic rate and postprandial thermogenesis in highly trained and untrained males. Am J Clin Nutr. 1988;47:793–98. https://pubmed.ncbi.nlm.nih.gov/3284328/

67. Burke CM, Bullough RC, Melby CL. Resting metabolic rate and postprandial thermogenesis by level of aerobic fitness in young women. Eur J Clin Nutr. 1993;47:575–85. https://pubmed.ncbi.nlm.nih.gov/8404794/

68. Bell C, Day DS, Jones PP, Christou DD, Petitt DS, Osterberg K, et al. High energy flux mediates the tonically augmented beta-adrenergic support of resting metabolic rate in habitually exercising older adults. J Clin Endocrinol Metab. 2004;89:3573–78. https://pubmed.ncbi.nlm.nih.gov/15240648/

69. Bullough RC, Gillette CA, Harris MA, Melby CL. Interaction of acute changes in exercise energy expenditure and energy intake on resting metabolic rate. Am J Clin Nutr. 1995;61:473–81. https://pubmed.ncbi.nlm.nih.gov/7872209/

70. Paris HL, Foright RM, Werth KA, Larson LC, Beals JW, Cox-York K, et al. Increasing energy flux to decrease the biological drive toward weight regain after weight loss—a proof-of-concept pilot study. Clin Nutr ESPEN. 2016;11:e12–20. https://pubmed.ncbi.nlm.nih.gov/28531421/

71. Santos HG, Chiavegato LD, Valentim DP, Padula RS. Effectiveness of a progressive resistance exercise program for industrial workers during breaks on perceived fatigue control: a cluster randomized controlled trial. BMC Public Health. 2020;20:849. https://bmcpublichealth.biomedcentral.com/articles/10.1186/s12889-020-08994-x

72. Sundstrup E, Jakobsen MD, Brandt M, Jay K, Aagaard P, Andersen LL. Strength training improves fatigue resistance and self-rated health in workers with chronic pain: a randomized controlled trial. Biomed Res Int. 2016;2016:4137918. https://pubmed.ncbi.nlm.nih.gov/27830144/

73. Katz DL, Meller S. Can we say what diet is best for health? Annu Rev Public Health. 2014;35:83–103. https://pubmed.ncbi.nlm.nih.gov/24641555/

Chapter 4

1. Carabotti M, Scirocco A, Maselli MA, Severi C. The gut-brain axis: interactions between enteric microbiota, central and enteric nervous systems. Ann Gastroenterol Hepatol . 2015;28:203–9. https://www.ncbi.nlm.nih.gov/pmc/articles/PMC4367209/

2. Konturek PC, Harsch IA, Konturek K, Schink M, Konturek T, Neurath MF, et al. Gut-liver axis: how do gut bacteria influence the liver? Med Sci (Basel). 2018;6. http://dx.doi.org/10.3390/medsci6030079

3. Przewłócka K, Folwarski M, Kaźmierczak-Siedlecka K, Skonieczna-Żydecka K, Kaczor JJ. Gut-muscle axis exists and may affect skeletal muscle adaptation to training. Nutrients. 2020;12. http://dx.doi.org/10.3390/nu12051451

4. Konrad D, Wueest S. The gut-adipose-liver axis in the metabolic syndrome. Physiology. 2014;29:304–13. https://pubmed.ncbi.nlm.nih.gov/25180260/

5. Zaiss MM, Jones RM, Schett G, Pacifici R. The gut-bone axis: how bacterial metabolites bridge the distance. J Clin Invest. 2019;129:3018–28. https://pubmed.ncbi.nlm.nih.gov/31305265/

6. Gracey E, Vereecke L, McGovern D, Fröhling M, Schett G, Danese S, et al. Revisiting the gut-joint axis: links between gut inflammation and spondyloarthritis. Nat Rev Rheumatol. 2020;16:415–33. https://pubmed.ncbi.nlm.nih.gov/32661321/

7. Barcik W, Boutin RCT, Sokolowska M, Brett Finlay B. The role of lung and gut microbiota in the pathology of asthma. Immunity. 2020; 52: 241–55. https://www.ncbi.nlm.nih.gov/pmc/articles/PMC7128389/

8. Carding S, Verbeke K, Vipond DT, Corfe BM, Owen LJ. Dysbiosis of the gut microbiota in disease. Microb Ecol Health Dis. 2015;26:26191. https://pubmed.ncbi.nlm.nih.gov/25651997/

9. Mitev K, Taleski V. Association between the gut microbiota and obesity. Open Access Maced J Med Sci. 2019;7:2050–56. https://pubmed.ncbi.nlm.nih.gov/31406553/

10. Sharma S, Tripathi P. Gut microbiome and type 2 diabetes: where we are and where to go? J Nutr Biochem. 2019;63:101–8. https://pubmed.ncbi.nlm.nih.gov/30366260/

11. Fernandes R, Viana SD, Nunes S, Reis F. Diabetic gut microbiota dysbiosis as an inflammaging and immunosenescence condition that fosters progression of retinopathy and nephropathy. Biochim Biophys Acta Mol Basis Dis. 2019;1865:1876–97. https://pubmed.ncbi.nlm.nih.gov/30287404/

12. Lau K, Srivatsav V, Rizwan A, Nashed A, Liu R, Shen R, et al. Bridging the gap between gut microbial dysbiosis and cardiovascular diseases. Nutrients. 2017;9. http://dx.doi.org/10.3390/nu9080859

13. Spielman LJ, Gibson DL, Klegeris A. Unhealthy gut, unhealthy brain: the role of the intestinal microbiota in neurodegenerative diseases. Neurochem Int. 2018;120:149–63. https://pubmed.ncbi.nlm.nih.gov/30114473/

14. Haran JP, McCormick BA. Aging, frailty, and the microbiome: how dysbiosis influences human aging and disease. G Gastroenterology. 2021;160:507–23. https://pubmed.ncbi.nlm.nih.gov/33307030/

15. Sender R, Fuchs S, Milo R. Are we really vastly outnumbered? Revisiting the ratio of bacterial to host cells in humans. Cell. 2016;164:337–40. https://pubmed.ncbi.nlm.nih.gov/26824647/

16. Liang D, Leung RKK, Guan W, et al. Involvement of gut microbiome in human health and disease: brief overview, knowledge gaps and research opportunities. Gut Pathog. 2018;10:3. https://doi.org/10.1186/s13099-018-0230-4

17. Sender. Are we really vastly outnumbered?

18. Du Preez S, Corbitt M, Cabanas H, Eaton N, Staines D, Marshall-Gradisnik S. A systematic review of enteric dysbiosis in chronic fatigue syndrome/myalgic encephalomyelitis. Syst Rev. 2018;7:241. https://www.ncbi.nlm.nih.gov/pmc/articles/PMC6302292/

19. Lobionda S, Sittipo P, Kwon HY, Lee YK. The role of gut microbiota in intestinal inflammation with respect to diet and extrinsic stressors. Microorganisms. 2019;7. http://dx.doi.org/10.3390/microorganisms7080271

20. Zeng MY, Inohara N, Nuñez G. Mechanisms of inflammation-driven bacterial dysbiosis in the gut. Mucosal Immunol. 2017;10:18–26. https://pubmed.ncbi.nlm.nih.gov/27554295/

21. Fasano A. All disease begins in the (leaky) gut: role of zonulin-mediated gut permeability in the pathogenesis of some chronic inflammatory diseases. F1000Res [Internet]. 2020;9. http://dx.doi.org/10.12688/f1000research.20510.1

22. Sturgeon C, Fasano A. Zonulin, a regulator of epithelial and endothelial barrier functions, and its involvement in chronic inflammatory diseases. Tissue Barriers. 2016;4:e1251384. https://pubmed.ncbi.nlm.nih.gov/28123927/

23. Fasano A. Leaky gut and autoimmune diseases. Clin Rev Allergy Immunol. 2012;42:71–78. https://pubmed.ncbi.nlm.nih.gov/22109896/

24. Michielan A, D'Incà R. Intestinal permeability in inflammatory bowel disease: pathogenesis, clinical evaluation, and therapy of leaky gut. Mediators Inflamm. 2015;2015:628157. https://pubmed.ncbi.nlm.nih.gov/26582965/

25. Lerner A, Jeremias P, Matthias T. Gut-thyroid axis and celiac disease. Endocr Connect. 2017;6:R52–58. https://www.ncbi.nlm.nih.gov/pmc/articles/PMC5435852/

26. Turner JR. Intestinal mucosal barrier function in health and disease. Nat Rev Immunol. 2009;9:799–809. https://pubmed.ncbi.nlm.nih.gov/19855405/

27. Vancamelbeke M, Vermeire S. The intestinal barrier: a fundamental role in health and disease. Expert Rev Gastroenterol Hepatol. 2017;11:821–34. https://pubmed.ncbi.nlm.nih.gov/28650209/

28. Szentkuti L, Riedesel H, Enss ML, Gaertner K, Von Engelhardt W. Pre-epithelial mucus layer in the colon of conventional and germ-free rats. Histochem J. 1990;22:491–97. https://pubmed.ncbi.nlm.nih.gov/1702088/

29. Johansson MEV, Jakobsson HE, Holmén-Larsson J, Schütte A, Ermund A, Rodríguez-Piñeiro AM, et al. Normalization of host intestinal mucus layers requires long-term microbial colonization. Cell Host Microbe. 2015;18:582–92. https://pubmed.ncbi.nlm.nih.gov/26526499/

30. Ibid.

31. Marcobal A, Southwick AM, Earle KA, Sonnenburg JL. A refined palate: bacterial consumption of host glycans in the gut. Glycobiology. 2013;23:1038–46. https://pubmed.ncbi.nlm.nih.gov/23720460/

32. Desai MS, Seekatz AM, Koropatkin NM, Kamada N, Hickey CA, Wolter M, et al. A dietary fiber-deprived gut microbiota degrades the colonic mucus barrier and enhances pathogen susceptibility. Cell. 2016;167:1339–53.e21. https://pubmed.ncbi.nlm.nih.gov/27863247/

33. Martens EC, Neumann M, Desai MS. Interactions of commensal and pathogenic microorganisms with the intestinal mucosal barrier. Nat Rev Microbiol. 2018;16:457–70. https://pubmed.ncbi.nlm.nih.gov/29904082/

34. Engevik MA, Luk B, Chang-Graham AL, Hall A, Herrmann B, Ruan W, et al. *Bifidobacterium dentium* fortifies the intestinal mucus layer via autophagy and calcium signaling pathways. MBio. 2019;10. http://dx.doi.org/10.1128/mBio.01087-19

35. Morrison DJ, Preston T. Formation of short chain fatty acids by the gut microbiota and their impact on human metabolism. Gut Microbes. 2016;7:189–200. https://pubmed.ncbi.nlm.nih.gov/26963409/

36. Lewandowski ED, Kudej RK, White LT, O'Donnell JM, Vatner SF. Mitochondrial preference for short chain fatty acid oxidation during coronary artery constriction. Circulation. 2002;105:367–72. https://pubmed.ncbi.nlm.nih.gov/11804994/

37. Schönfeld P, Wojtczak L. Short- and medium-chain fatty acids in energy metabolism: the cellular perspective. J Lipid Res. 2016;57:943–54. https://pubmed.ncbi.nlm.nih.gov/27080715/

38. Mollica MP, Mattace Raso G, Cavaliere G, Trinchese G, De Filippo C, Aceto S, et al. Butyrate regulates liver mitochondrial function, efficiency, and dynamics in insulin-resistant obese mice. Diabetes. 2017;66:1405–18. https://pubmed.ncbi.nlm.nih.gov/28223285/

39. Gao Z, Yin J, Zhang J, Ward RE, Martin RJ, Lefevre M, et al. Butyrate improves insulin sensitivity and increases energy expenditure in mice. Diabetes. 2009;58:1509–17. https://pubmed.ncbi.nlm.nih.gov/19366864/

40. Henagan TM, Stefanska B, Fang Z, Navard AM, Ye J, Lenard NR, et al. Sodium butyrate epigenetically modulates high-fat diet-induced skeletal muscle mitochondrial adaptation, obesity and insulin resistance through nucleosome positioning. Br J Pharmacol. 2015;172:2782–98. https://pubmed.ncbi.nlm.nih.gov/25559882/

41. Donohoe DR, Garge N, Zhang X, Sun W, O'Connell TM, Bunger MK, et al. The microbiome and butyrate regulate energy metabolism and autophagy in the mammalian colon. Cell Metab. 2011;13:517–26. https://pubmed.ncbi .nlm.nih.gov/21531334/

42. Espín JC, Larrosa M, García-Conesa MT, Tomás-Barberán F. Biological significance of urolithins, the gut microbial ellagic Acid-derived metabolites: the evidence so far. Evid Based Complement Alternat Med. 2013;2013:270418. https://pubmed.ncbi.nlm.nih.gov/23781257/

43. Ferreira CM, Vieira AT, Vinolo MAR, Oliveira FA, Curi R, Martins F dos S. The central role of the gut microbiota in chronic inflammatory diseases. J Immunol Res. 2014;2014:689492. https://pubmed.ncbi.nlm.nih.gov/25309932/

44. Salguero MV, Al-Obaide MAI, Singh R, Siepmann T, Vasylyeva TL. Dysbiosis of Gram-negative gut microbiota and the associated serum lipopolysaccharide exacerbates inflammation in type 2 diabetic patients with chronic kidney disease. Exp Ther Med. 2019;18:3461–69. https://pubmed.ncbi.nlm.nih .gov/31602221/

45. Anderson G, Maes M. Gut dysbiosis dysregulates central and systemic homeostasis via suboptimal mitochondrial function: assessment, treatment and classification implications. Curr Top Med Chem. 2020;20:524–39. https://pubmed.ncbi.nlm.nih.gov/32003689/

46. McGivney A, Bradley SG. Action of bacterial endotoxin and lipid A on mitochondrial enzyme activities of cells in culture and subcellular fractions. Infect Immun. 1979;25:664–71. https://pubmed.ncbi.nlm.nih.gov/114491/

47. Mishra DP, Dhali A. Endotoxin induces luteal cell apoptosis through the mitochondrial pathway. Prostaglandins Other Lipid Mediat. 2007;83:75–88. https://pubmed.ncbi.nlm.nih.gov/17259074/

48. Frisard MI, Wu Y, McMillan RP, Voelker KA, Wahlberg KA, Anderson AS, et al. Low levels of lipopolysaccharide modulate mitochondrial oxygen consumption in skeletal muscle. Metabolism. 2015;64:416–27. https://www .ncbi.nlm.nih.gov/pmc/articles/PMC4501015/

49. Jeger V, Brandt S, Porta F, Jakob SM, Takala J, Djafarzadeh S. Dose response of endotoxin on hepatocyte and muscle mitochondrial respiration in vitro. Biomed Res Int. 2015;2015:353074. https://pubmed.ncbi.nlm.nih .gov/25649304/

50. Giloteaux L, Goodrich JK, Walters WA, Levine SM, Ley RE, Hanson MR. Reduced diversity and altered composition of the gut microbiome in individuals with myalgic encephalomyelitis/chronic fatigue syndrome. Microbiome. 2016;4:30. https://pubmed.ncbi.nlm.nih.gov/27338587/

51. Hwang C, Ross V, Mahadevan U. Micronutrient deficiencies in inflammatory bowel disease: from A to zinc. Inflamm Bowel Dis. 2012;18:1961–81. https:// pubmed.ncbi.nlm.nih.gov/22488830/

52. Joustra ML, Minovic I, Janssens KAM, Bakker SJL, Rosmalen JGM. Vitamin and mineral status in chronic fatigue syndrome and fibromyalgia syndrome: a systematic review and meta-analysis. PLoS One. 2017;12:e0176631. https:// pubmed.ncbi.nlm.nih.gov/28453534/

53. Maes M, Mihaylova I, Leunis J-C. Increased serum IgA and IgM against LPS of enterobacteria in chronic fatigue syndrome (CFS): indication for the involvement of gram-negative enterobacteria in the etiology of CFS and for the presence of an increased gut-intestinal permeability. J Affect Disord. 2007;99:237–40. https://pubmed.ncbi.nlm.nih.gov/17007934/

54. King DE, Mainous AG 3rd, Lambourne CA. Trends in dietary fiber intake in the United States, 1999–2008. J Acad Nutr Diet. 2012;112:642–48. https://pubmed.ncbi.nlm.nih.gov/22709768/

55. Eaton SB, Konner M. Paleolithic nutrition. A consideration of its nature and current implications. N Engl J Med. 1985;312:283–89. https://pubmed.ncbi.nlm.nih.gov/2981409/

56. Smits SA, Leach J, Sonnenburg ED, Gonzalez CG, Lichtman JS, Reid G, et al. Seasonal cycling in the gut microbiome of the Hadza hunter-gatherers of Tanzania. Science. 2017;357:802–6. https://pubmed.ncbi.nlm.nih.gov/28839072/

57. Hiel S, Bindels LB, Pachikian BD, Kalala G, Broers V, Zamariola G, et al. Effects of a diet based on inulin-rich vegetables on gut health and nutritional behavior in healthy humans. Am J Clin Nutr. 2019;109:1683–95. https://pubmed.ncbi.nlm.nih.gov/31108510/

58. Davani-Davari D, Negahdaripour M, Karimzadeh I, Seifan M, Mohkam M, Masoumi SJ, et al. Prebiotics: definition, types, sources, mechanisms, and clinical applications. Foods. 2019;8. http://dx.doi.org/10.3390/foods8030092.

59. Gibson GR, Hutkins R, Sanders ME, Prescott SL, Reimer RA, Salminen SJ, et al. Expert consensus document: The International Scientific Association for Probiotics and Prebiotics (ISAPP) consensus statement on the definition and scope of prebiotics. Nat Rev Gastroenterol Hepatol. 2017;14:491–502. https://pubmed.ncbi.nlm.nih.gov/28611480/

60. Birt DF, Boylston T, Hendrich S, Jane J-L, Hollis J, Li L, et al. Resistant starch: promise for improving human health. Adv Nutr. 2013;4:587–601. https://pubmed.ncbi.nlm.nih.gov/24228189/

61. Kalala G, Kambashi B, Everaert N, Beckers Y, Richel A, Pachikian B, et al. Characterization of fructans and dietary fibre profiles in raw and steamed vegetables. Int J Food Sci Nutr. 2018;69:682–89. https://pubmed.ncbi.nlm.nih.gov/29252035/

62. Kalala. Characterization of fructans and dietary fibre profiles.

63. Shen D, Bai H, Li Z, Yu Y, Zhang H, Chen L. Positive effects of resistant starch supplementation on bowel function in healthy adults: a systematic review and meta-analysis of randomized controlled trials. Int J Food Sci Nutr. 2017;68:149–57. https://pubmed.ncbi.nlm.nih.gov/27593182/

64. Fuentes-Zaragoza E, Sánchez-Zapata E, Sendra E, Sayas E, Navarro C, Fernández-López J, et al. Resistant starch as prebiotic: a review. Starke. Wiley; 2011;63:406–15. https://onlinelibrary.wiley.com/doi/full/10.1002/star.201000099

65. Montroy J, Berjawi R, Lalu MM, Podolsky E, Peixoto C, Sahin L, et al. The effects of resistant starches on inflammatory bowel disease in preclinical and

clinical settings: a systematic review and meta-analysis. BMC Gastroenterol. 2020;20:372. https://bmcgastroenterol.biomedcentral.com/articles/10.1186/s12876-020-01516-4

66. Patterson MA, Maiya M, Stewart ML. Resistant starch content in foods commonly consumed in the United States: a narrative review. J Acad Nutr Diet. 2020;120:230–44. https://pubmed.ncbi.nlm.nih.gov/32040399/

67. Falcomer AL, Riquette RFR, de Lima BR, Ginani VC, Zandonadi RP. Health benefits of green banana consumption: a systematic review. Nutrients. 2019;11. http://dx.doi.org/10.3390/nu11061222

68. Hald S, Schioldan AG, Moore ME, Dige A, Lærke HN, Agnholt J, et al. Effects of arabinoxylan and resistant starch on intestinal microbiota and short-chain fatty acids in subjects with metabolic syndrome: a randomised crossover study. PLoS One. 2016;11:e0159223. https://pubmed.ncbi.nlm.nih.gov/27434092/

69. Alfa MJ, Strang D, Tappia PS, Graham M, Van Domselaar G, Forbes JD, et al. A randomized trial to determine the impact of a digestion resistant starch composition on the gut microbiome in older and mid-age adults. Clin Nutr. 2018;37:797–807. https://pubmed.ncbi.nlm.nih.gov/28410921/

70. Zhang L, Ouyang Y, Li H, Shen L, Ni Y, Fang Q, et al. Metabolic phenotypes and the gut microbiota in response to dietary resistant starch type 2 in normal-weight subjects: a randomized crossover trial. Sci Rep. 2019;9:4736. https://www.nature.com/articles/s41598-018-38216-9

71. Raatz SK, Idso L, Johnson LK, Jackson MI, Combs GF Jr. Resistant starch analysis of commonly consumed potatoes: content varies by cooking method and service temperature but not by variety. Food Chem. 2016;208:297–300. https://pubmed.ncbi.nlm.nih.gov/27132853

72. Upadhyaya B, McCormack L, Fardin-Kia AR, Juenemann R, Nichenametla S, Clapper J, et al. Impact of dietary resistant starch type 4 on human gut microbiota and immunometabolic functions. Sci Rep. 2016;6:28797. https://www.nature.com/articles/srep28797

73. Hasjim J, Ai Y, Jane J-L. Novel applications of amylose-lipid complex as resistant starch type 5. In *Resistant Starch*. (Hoboken, NJ: Wiley, 2013) 79–94.

74. ACS. New low-calorie rice could help cut rising obesity rates. American Chemistry Society. 2015. https://www.acs.org/content/acs/en/pressroom/newsreleases/2015/march/new-low-calorie-rice-could-help-cut-rising-obesity-rates.html

75. Derrien M, van Hylckama Vlieg JET. Fate, activity, and impact of ingested bacteria within the human gut microbiota. Trends Microbiol. 2015;23:354–66. https://pubmed.ncbi.nlm.nih.gov/25840765/

76. Marco ML, Heeney D, Binda S, Cifelli CJ, Cotter PD, Foligné B, et al. Health benefits of fermented foods: microbiota and beyond. Curr Opin Biotechnol. 2017;44:94–102. https://pubmed.ncbi.nlm.nih.gov/27998788/

77. Mikelsaar M, Sepp E, Štšepetova J, Songisepp E, Mändar R. Biodiversity of intestinal lactic acid bacteria in the healthy population. Adv Exp Med Biol. 2016;932:1–64. https://pubmed.ncbi.nlm.nih.gov/27167411/

78. McFarland LV. Use of probiotics to correct dysbiosis of normal microbiota following disease or disruptive events: a systematic review. BMJ Open. 2014;4:e005047. https://pubmed.ncbi.nlm.nih.gov/25157183/

79. Magge S, Lembo A. Low-FODMAP diet for treatment of irritable bowel syndrome. Gastroenterol Hepatol. 2012;8:739–45. https://pubmed.ncbi.nlm.nih.gov/24672410/

80. Sonnenburg ED, Smits SA, Tikhonov M, Higginbottom SK, Wingreen NS, Sonnenburg JL. Diet-induced extinctions in the gut microbiota compound over generations. Nature. 2016;529:212–5

Chapter 5

1. Rowley WR, Bezold C, Arikan Y, Byrne E, Krohe S. Diabetes 2030: insights from yesterday, today, and future trends. Popul Health Manag. 2017;20:6–12. https://pubmed.ncbi.nlm.nih.gov/27124621/

2. Rao Kondapally Seshasai S, Kaptoge S, Thompson A, Di Angelantonio E, Gao P, Sarwar N, et al. Diabetes mellitus, fasting glucose, and risk of cause-specific death. N Engl J Med. 2011;364:829–41. https://www.nejm.org/doi/full/10.1056/nejmoa1008862

3. American Diabetes Association. Economic costs of diabetes in the U.S. in 2017. Diabetes Care. 2018;41:917–28. https://care.diabetesjournals.org/content/41/5/917

4. Ibid.

5. Einarson TR, Machado M, Henk Hemels ME. Blood glucose and subsequent cardiovascular disease: update of a meta-analysis. Curr Med Res Opin. 2011;27:2155–63. https://pubmed.ncbi.nlm.nih.gov/21973198/

6. Færch K, Alssema M, Mela DJ, Borg R, Vistisen D. Relative contributions of preprandial and postprandial glucose exposures, glycemic variability, and non-glycemic factors to HbA 1c in individuals with and without diabetes. Nutr Diabetes. 2018;8:38. https://www.nature.com/articles/s41387-018-0047-8

7. Suh S, Kim JH. Glycemic variability: how do we measure it and why is it important? Diabetes Metab J. 2015;39:273–82. https://pubmed.ncbi.nlm.nih.gov/26301188/

8. Zhou Z, Sun B, Huang S, Zhu C, Bian M. Glycemic variability: adverse clinical outcomes and how to improve it? Cardiovasc Diabetol. 2020;19:102. https://pubmed.ncbi.nlm.nih.gov/32622354/

9. Reno CM, Skinner A, Bayles J, Chen YS, Daphna-Iken D, Fisher SJ. Severe hypoglycemia-induced sudden death is mediated by both cardiac arrhythmias and seizures. Am J Physiol Endocrinol Metab. 2018;315:E240–49. https://www.ncbi.nlm.nih.gov/pmc/articles/PMC6139495/

10. Simpson EJ, Holdsworth M, Macdonald IA. Prevalence of self-reported symptoms attributed to hypoglycaemia within a general female population of the UK. J Psychosom Res. 2006;60:403–6. https://pubmed.ncbi.nlm.nih.gov/16581365/

11. Alwafi H, Alsharif AA, Wei L, Langan D, Naser AY, Mongkhon P, et al. Incidence and prevalence of hypoglycaemia in type 1 and type 2 diabetes individuals: A systematic review and meta-analysis. Diabetes Res Clin Pract. 2020;170:108522. https://pubmed.ncbi.nlm.nih.gov/33096187/

12. Edridge CL, Dunkley AJ, Bodicoat DH, Rose TC, Gray LJ, Davies MJ, et al. Prevalence and incidence of hypoglycaemia in 532,542 people with type 2 diabetes on oral therapies and insulin: a systematic review and meta-analysis of population based studies. PLoS One. 2015;10:e0126427. https://pubmed.ncbi.nlm.nih.gov/26061690/

13. Altuntaş Y. Postprandial reactive hypoglycemia. Sisli Etfal Hastan Tip Bul. 2019;53:215–20. https://pubmed.ncbi.nlm.nih.gov/32377086/

14. Longkumer C, Nath CK, Barman B, Ruram AA, Visi V, Yasir MD, et al. Idiopathic post prandial glucose lowering, a whistle blower for subclinical hypothyroidism and insulin resistance. A cross-sectional study in Tertiary Care Centre of northeast India. J Family Med Prim Care. 2020;9:4637–40. https://journals.lww.com/jfmpc/pages/default.aspx

15. Mergenthaler P, Lindauer U, Dienel GA, Meisel A. Sugar for the brain: the role of glucose in physiological and pathological brain function. Trends Neurosci. 2013;36:587–97. https://pubmed.ncbi.nlm.nih.gov/23968694/

16. Charles MA, Hofeldt F, Shackelford A, Waldeck N, Dodson LE Jr, Bunker D, et al. Comparison of oral glucose tolerance tests and mixed meals in patients with apparent idiopathic postabsorptive hypoglycemia: absence of hypoglycemia after meals. Diabetes. 1981;30:465–70. https://pubmed.ncbi.nlm.nih.gov/7227659/

17. Chalew SA, McLaughlin JV, Mersey JH, Adams AJ, Cornblath M, Kowarski AA. The use of the plasma epinephrine response in the diagnosis of idiopathic postprandial syndrome. JAMA. 1984;251:612–15. https://jamanetwork.com/journals/jama/article-abstract/391267

18. Cardoso S, Santos MS, Seiça R, Moreira PI. Cortical and hippocampal mitochondria bioenergetics and oxidative status during hyperglycemia and/or insulin-induced hypoglycemia. Biochim Biophys Acta. 2010;1802:942–51. https://hal.archives-ouvertes.fr/hal-00623292/document

19. Monnier L, Mas E, Ginet C, Michel F, Villon L, Cristol J-P, et al. Activation of oxidative stress by acute glucose fluctuations compared with sustained chronic hyperglycemia in patients with type 2 diabetes. JAMA. 2006;295:1681–87. https://pubmed.ncbi.nlm.nih.gov/16609090/

20. Saisho Y. Glycemic variability and oxidative stress: a link between diabetes and cardiovascular disease? Int J Mol Sci. 2014;15:18381–406. https://pubmed.ncbi.nlm.nih.gov/25314300/

21. Brownlee M. Biochemistry and molecular cell biology of diabetic complications. Nature. 2001;414:813–20. https://pubmed.ncbi.nlm.nih.gov/11742414/

22. Piconi L, Quagliaro L, Assaloni R, Da Ros R, Maier A, Zuodar G, et al. Constant and intermittent high glucose enhances endothelial cell apoptosis through mitochondrial superoxide overproduction. Diabetes Metab Res Rev. 2006;22:198–203. https://pubmed.ncbi.nlm.nih.gov/16453381/

23. Quagliaro L, Piconi L, Assaloni R, Da Ros R, Maier A, Zuodar G, et al. Intermittent high glucose enhances ICAM-1, VCAM-1 and E-selectin expression in human umbilical vein endothelial cells in culture: the distinct role of protein kinase C and mitochondrial superoxide production. Atherosclerosis. 2005;183:259–67. https://pubmed.ncbi.nlm.nih .gov/16285992/

24. Esposito K, Nappo F, Marfella R, Giugliano G, Giugliano F, Ciotola M, et al. Inflammatory cytokine concentrations are acutely increased by hyperglycemia in humans: role of oxidative stress. Circulation. 2002;106:2067–72. https://pubmed.ncbi.nlm.nih.gov/12379575/

25. Watt C, Sanchez-Rangel E, Hwang JJ. Glycemic variability and CNS inflammation: reviewing the connection. Nutrients. 2020;12. http://dx.doi .org/10.3390/nu12123906

26. Kosse C, Gonzalez A, Burdakov D. Predictive models of glucose control: roles for glucose-sensing neurones. Acta Physiol. 2015;213:7–18. https://pubmed .ncbi.nlm.nih.gov/25131833/

27. Drivsholm T, de Fine Olivarius N, Nielsen ABS, Siersma V. Symptoms, signs and complications in newly diagnosed type 2 diabetic patients, and their relationship to glycaemia, blood pressure and weight. Diabetologia. 2005;48:210–14. https://pubmed.ncbi.nlm.nih.gov/15650820/

28. Kaikini AA, Kanchan DM, Nerurkar UN, Sathaye S. Targeting mitochondrial dysfunction for the treatment of diabetic complications: pharmacological interventions through natural products. Pharmacogn Rev. 2017;11:128–35. https://www.ncbi.nlm.nih.gov/pmc/articles/PMC5628518/

29. Sivitz WI, Yorek MA. Mitochondrial dysfunction in diabetes: from molecular mechanisms to functional significance and therapeutic opportunities. Antioxid Redox Signal. 2010;12:537–77. https://pubmed.ncbi.nlm.nih .gov/19650713/

30. Fritschi C, Quinn L. Fatigue in patients with diabetes: a review. J Psychosom Res. 2010;69:33–41. https://www.ncbi.nlm.nih.gov/pmc/articles/ PMC2905388/

31. Kalra S, Sahay R. Diabetes fatigue syndrome. Diabetes Ther. 2018;9:1421–29. https://pubmed.ncbi.nlm.nih.gov/29869049/

32. Taylor R, Holman RR. Normal weight individuals who develop type 2 diabetes: the personal fat threshold. Clin Sci . 2015;128:405–10. https:// pubmed.ncbi.nlm.nih.gov/25515001/

33. Haczeyni F, Bell-Anderson KS, Farrell GC. Causes and mechanisms of adipocyte enlargement and adipose expansion. Obes Rev. 2018;19:406–20. https://pubmed.ncbi.nlm.nih.gov/29243339/

34. Lafontan M. Adipose tissue and adipocyte dysregulation. Diabetes Metab. 2014;40:16–28. https://pubmed.ncbi.nlm.nih.gov/24139247/

35. Haider N, Larose L. Harnessing adipogenesis to prevent obesity. Adipocyte. 2019;8:98–104. https://pubmed.ncbi.nlm.nih.gov/30848691/

36. Hafidi ME, Buelna-Chontal M, Sánchez-Muñoz F, Carbó R. Adipogenesis: a necessary but harmful strategy. Int J Mol Sci. 2019;20. http://dx.doi.org/10.3390/ijms20153657

37. Kim JI, Huh JY, Sohn JH, Choe SS, Lee YS, Lim CY, et al. Lipid-overloaded enlarged adipocytes provoke insulin resistance independent of inflammation. Mol Cell Biol. 2015;35:1686–99. https://pubmed.ncbi.nlm.nih.gov/25733684/

38. Burhans MS, Hagman DK, Kuzma JN, Schmidt KA, Kratz M. Contribution of adipose tissue inflammation to the development of type 2 diabetes mellitus. Compr Physiol. 2018;9:1–58. https://pubmed.ncbi.nlm.nih.gov/30549014/

39. Frayn KN. Adipose tissue as a buffer for daily lipid flux. Diabetologia. 2002;45:1201–10. https://pubmed.ncbi.nlm.nih.gov/12242452/

40. Taylor R. Calorie restriction for long-term remission of type 2 diabetes. Clin Med. 2019;19:37–42. https://www.ncbi.nlm.nih.gov/pmc/articles/PMC6399621/

41. Taylor R, Al-Mrabeh A, Sattar N. Understanding the mechanisms of reversal of type 2 diabetes. Lancet Diabetes Endocrinol. 2019;7:726–36. https://pubmed.ncbi.nlm.nih.gov/31097391/

42. Taylor R. Calorie restriction and reversal of type 2 diabetes. Expert Rev Endocrinol Metab. 2016;11:521–28. https://pubmed.ncbi.nlm.nih.gov/30058916/

43. Lim EL, Hollingsworth KG, Aribisala BS, Chen MJ, Mathers JC, Taylor R. Reversal of type 2 diabetes: normalisation of beta cell function in association with decreased pancreas and liver triacylglycerol. Diabetologia. 2011;54:2506–14. https://pubmed.ncbi.nlm.nih.gov/21656330/

44. Steven S, Hollingsworth KG, Al-Mrabeh A, Avery L, Aribisala B, Caslake M, et al. Very low-calorie diet and 6 months of weight stability in type 2 diabetes: pathophysiological changes in responders and nonresponders. Diabetes Care. 2016;39:808–15. https://pubmed.ncbi.nlm.nih.gov/27002059/

45. Lean ME, Leslie WS, Barnes AC, Brosnahan N, Thom G, McCombie L, et al. Primary care-led weight management for remission of type 2 diabetes (DiRECT): an open-label, cluster-randomised trial. Lancet. 2018;391:541–51. https://pubmed.ncbi.nlm.nih.gov/29221645/

46. Taylor R, Al-Mrabeh A, Zhyzhneuskaya S, Peters C, Barnes AC, Aribisala BS, et al. Remission of human type 2 diabetes requires decrease in liver and pancreas fat content but is dependent upon capacity for β cell recovery. Cell Metab. 2018;28:547–56.e3. https://pubmed.ncbi.nlm.nih.gov/30078554

47. DiNicolantonio JJ, McCarty M. Autophagy-induced degradation of Notch1, achieved through intermittent fasting, may promote beta cell neogenesis: implications for reversal of type 2 diabetes. Open Heart. 2019;6:e001028. https://pubmed.ncbi.nlm.nih.gov/31218007/

48. Cheng C-W, Villani V, Buono R, Wei M, Kumar S, Yilmaz OH, et al. Fasting-mimicking diet promotes ngn3-driven β-cell regeneration to reverse diabetes. Cell. 2017;168:775–88.e12. https://pubmed.ncbi.nlm.nih.gov/28235195/

49. Sainsbury E, Kizirian NV, Partridge SR, Gill T, Colagiuri S, Gibson AA. Effect of dietary carbohydrate restriction on glycemic control in adults with diabetes: A systematic review and meta-analysis. Diabetes Res Clin Pract. 2018;139:239–52. https://pubmed.ncbi.nlm.nih.gov/29522789/

50. Goldenberg JZ, Day A, Brinkworth GD, Sato J, Yamada S, Jönsson T, et al. Efficacy and safety of low and very low carbohydrate diets for type 2 diabetes remission: systematic review and meta-analysis of published and unpublished randomized trial data. BMJ. 2021;372:m4743. https://pubmed.ncbi.nlm.nih.gov/33441384/

51. Davies MJ, D'Alessio DA, Fradkin J, Kernan WN, Mathieu C, Mingrone G, et al. Management of hyperglycemia in type 2 diabetes, 2018. A consensus report by the American Diabetes Association (ADA) and the European Association for the Study of Diabetes (EASD). Diabetes Care. 2018;41:2669–701. https://pubmed.ncbi.nlm.nih.gov/30291106/

52. Evert AB, Dennison M, Gardner CD, Garvey WT, Lau KHK, MacLeod J, et al. Nutrition therapy for adults with diabetes or prediabetes: a consensus report. Diabetes Care. 2019;42:731–54. https://pubmed.ncbi.nlm.nih.gov/31000505/

53. Hutchison AT, Wittert GA, Heilbronn LK. Matching meals to body clocks—impact on weight and glucose metabolism. Nutrients. 2017;9. http://dx.doi.org/10.3390/nu9030222

54. Potter GDM, Skene DJ, Arendt J, Cade JE, Grant PJ, Hardie LJ. Circadian rhythm and sleep disruption: causes, metabolic consequences, and countermeasures. Endocr Rev. 2016;37:584–608. https://pubmed.ncbi.nlm.nih.gov/27763782/

55. Kurose T, Yabe D, Inagaki N. Circadian rhythms and diabetes. J Diabetes Investig. 2011;2:176–77. https://pubmed.ncbi.nlm.nih.gov/24843479/

56. Marcheva B, Ramsey KM, Buhr ED, Kobayashi Y, Su H, Ko CH, et al. Disruption of the clock components CLOCK and BMAL1 leads to hypoinsulinaemia and diabetes. Nature. 2010;466:627–31. https://pubmed.ncbi.nlm.nih.gov/20562852/

57. Leproult R, Holmbäck U, Van Cauter E. Circadian misalignment augments markers of insulin resistance and inflammation, independently of sleep loss. Diabetes. 2014;63:1860–69. https://pubmed.ncbi.nlm.nih.gov/24458353/

58. Koren D, O'Sullivan KL, Mokhlesi B. Metabolic and glycemic sequelae of sleep disturbances in children and adults. Curr Diab Rep. 2015;15:562. https://www.ncbi.nlm.nih.gov/pmc/articles/PMC4467532/

59. Anothaisintawee T, Reutrakul S, Van Cauter E, Thakkinstian A. Sleep disturbances compared to traditional risk factors for diabetes development: Systematic review and meta-analysis. Sleep Med Rev. 2016;30:11–24. https://pubmed.ncbi.nlm.nih.gov/26687279/

60. Poggiogalle E, Jamshed H, Peterson CM. Circadian regulation of glucose, lipid, and energy metabolism in humans. Metabolism. 2018;84:11–27. https://pubmed.ncbi.nlm.nih.gov/29195759/

61. Jarrett RJ, Baker IA, Keen H, Oakley NW. Diurnal variation in oral glucose tolerance: blood sugar and plasma insulin levels morning, afternoon, and evening. Br Med J. 1972;1:199–201. https://www.ncbi.nlm.nih.gov/pmc/articles/PMC1789199/

62. Grabner W, Matzkies F, Prestele H, Rose A, Daniel U, Phillip J, et al. [Diurnal variation of glucose tolerance and insulin secretion in man (author's transl)]. Klin Wochenschr. 1975;53:773–78. https://pubmed.ncbi.nlm.nih.gov/1165623/

63. Van Cauter E, Shapiro ET, Tillil H, Polonsky KS. Circadian modulation of glucose and insulin responses to meals: relationship to cortisol rhythm. Am J Physiol. 1992;262:E467–75. https://pubmed.ncbi.nlm.nih.gov/1566835/

64. Sutton EF, Beyl R, Early KS, Cefalu WT, Ravussin E, Peterson CM. Early time-restricted feeding improves insulin sensitivity, blood pressure, and oxidative stress even without weight loss in men with prediabetes. Cell Metab. 2018;27:1212–21.e3. https://pubmed.ncbi.nlm.nih.gov/29754952/

65. Kahleova H, Belinova L, Malinska H, Oliyarnyk O, Trnovska J, Skop V, et al. Eating two larger meals a day (breakfast and lunch) is more effective than six smaller meals in a reduced-energy regimen for patients with type 2 diabetes: a randomised crossover study. Diabetologia. 2014;57:1552–60. https://pubmed.ncbi.nlm.nih.gov/24838678/

66. Jakubowicz D, Wainstein J, Ahrén B, Bar-Dayan Y, Landau Z, Rabinovitz HR, et al. High-energy breakfast with low-energy dinner decreases overall daily hyperglycaemia in type 2 diabetic patients: a randomised clinical trial. Diabetologia. 2015;58:912–19. https://pubmed.ncbi.nlm.nih.gov/25724569/

67. Arnason TG, Bowen MW, Mansell KD. Effects of intermittent fasting on health markers in those with type 2 diabetes: A pilot study. World J Diabetes. 2017;8:154–64. https://pubmed.ncbi.nlm.nih.gov/28465792/

68. Thomas EA, Higgins J, Bessesen DH, McNair B, Cornier M-A. Usual breakfast eating habits affect response to breakfast skipping in overweight women. Obesity. 2015;23:750–59. https://pubmed.ncbi.nlm.nih.gov/25755093/

69. Farshchi HR, Taylor MA, Macdonald IA. Regular meal frequency creates more appropriate insulin sensitivity and lipid profiles compared with irregular meal frequency in healthy lean women. Eur J Clin Nutr. 2004;58:1071–77. https://pubmed.ncbi.nlm.nih.gov/15220950/

70. Farshchi HR, Taylor MA, Macdonald IA. Beneficial metabolic effects of regular meal frequency on dietary thermogenesis, insulin sensitivity, and fasting lipid profiles in healthy obese women. Am J Clin Nutr. 2005;81:16–24. https://pubmed.ncbi.nlm.nih.gov/15640455/

71. Shishehbor F, Mansoori A, Shirani F. Vinegar consumption can attenuate postprandial glucose and insulin responses; a systematic review and meta-analysis of clinical trials. Diabetes Res Clin Pract. 2017;127:1–9. https://pubmed.ncbi.nlm.nih.gov/28292654/

72. Lim J, Henry CJ, Haldar S. Vinegar as a functional ingredient to improve postprandial glycemic control-human intervention findings and molecular mechanisms. Mol Nutr Food Res. 2016;60:1837–49. https://pubmed.ncbi.nlm.nih.gov/27213723/

73. Liljeberg H, Björck I. Delayed gastric emptying rate may explain improved glycaemia in healthy subjects to a starchy meal with added vinegar. Eur J Clin Nutr. 1998;52:368–71. https://pubmed.ncbi.nlm.nih.gov/9630389/

74. Hlebowicz J, Darwiche G, Björgell O, Almér L-O. Effect of apple cider vinegar on delayed gastric emptying in patients with type 1 diabetes mellitus: a pilot study. BMC Gastroenterol. 2007;7:46. https://pubmed.ncbi.nlm.nih.gov/18093343/

75. Ogawa N, Satsu H, Watanabe H, Fukaya M, Tsukamoto Y, Miyamoto Y, et al. Acetic acid suppresses the increase in disaccharidase activity that occurs during culture of caco-2 cells. J Nutr. 2000;130:507–13. https://pubmed.ncbi.nlm.nih.gov/10702577/

76. Noh Y-H, Lee D-B, Lee Y-W, Pyo Y-H. In vitro inhibitory effects of organic acids identified in commercial vinegars on α-amylase and α-glucosidase. Prev Nutr Food Sci. 2020;25:319–24. https://www.ncbi.nlm.nih.gov/pmc/articles/PMC7541927/

77. Sakakibara S, Yamauchi T, Oshima Y, Tsukamoto Y, Kadowaki T. Acetic acid activates hepatic AMPK and reduces hyperglycemia in diabetic KK-A(y) mice. Biochem Biophys Res Commun. 2006;344:597–604. https://pubmed.ncbi.nlm.nih.gov/16630552/

78. Yamashita H, Maruta H, Jozuka M, Kimura R, Iwabuchi H, Yamato M, et al. Effects of acetate on lipid metabolism in muscles and adipose tissues of type 2 diabetic Otsuka Long-Evans Tokushima Fatty (OLETF) rats. Biosci Biotechnol Biochem. 2009;73:570–76. https://pubmed.ncbi.nlm.nih.gov/19270372/

79. Fushimi T, Sato Y. Effect of acetic acid feeding on the circadian changes in glycogen and metabolites of glucose and lipid in liver and skeletal muscle of rats. Br J Nutr. 2005;94:714–19. https://pubmed.ncbi.nlm.nih.gov/16277773/

80. Mitrou P, Petsiou E, Papakonstantinou E, Maratou E, Lambadiari V, Dimitriadis P, et al. Vinegar consumption increases insulin-stimulated glucose uptake by the forearm muscle in humans with type 2 diabetes. J Diabetes Res. 2015;2015:175204. https://pubmed.ncbi.nlm.nih.gov/26064976/

81. Sakakibara S, Murakami R, Takahashi M, Fushimi T, Murohara T, Kishi M, et al. Vinegar intake enhances flow-mediated vasodilatation via upregulation of endothelial nitric oxide synthase activity. Biosci Biotechnol Biochem. 2010;74:1055–61. https://pubmed.ncbi.nlm.nih.gov/20460711/

82. Mitrou P, Petsiou E, Papakonstantinou E, Maratou E, Lambadiari V, Dimitriadis P, et al. The role of acetic acid on glucose uptake and blood flow rates in the skeletal muscle in humans with impaired glucose tolerance. Eur J Clin Nutr. 2015;69:734–39. https://www.nature.com/articles/ejcn2014289

83. Lambadiari V, Mitrou P, Maratou E, Raptis A, Raptis SA, Dimitriadis G. Increases in muscle blood flow after a mixed meal are impaired at all stages of type 2 diabetes. Clin Endocrinol. 2012;76:825–30. https://pubmed.ncbi.nlm.nih.gov/21950653/

84. Aykın E, Budak NH, Güzel-Seydim ZB. Bioactive components of mother vinegar. J Am Coll Nutr. 2015;34:80–89. https://pubmed.ncbi.nlm.nih.gov/25648676/

85. Imai S, Kajiyama S. Eating order diet reduced the postprandial glucose and glycated hemoglobin levels in Japanese patients with type 2 diabetes. J Rehabil Health Sci. 2010;8:1–7. https://www.rehab.osakafu-u.ac.jp/osakafu-content/uploads/sites/103/2015/12/jrhs_008_2010_01.pdf

86. Shukla AP, Iliescu RG, Thomas CE, Aronne LJ. Food order has a significant impact on postprandial glucose and insulin levels. Diabetes Care. 2015;38:e98–99. https://care.diabetesjournals.org/content/38/7/e98

87. Shukla AP, Andono J, Touhamy SH, Casper A, Iliescu RG, Mauer E, et al. Carbohydrate-last meal pattern lowers postprandial glucose and insulin excursions in type 2 diabetes. BMJ Open Diabetes Res Care. 2017;5:e000440. https://pubmed.ncbi.nlm.nih.gov/28989726/

88. Shukla AP, Dickison M, Coughlin N, Karan A, Mauer E, Truong W, et al. The impact of food order on postprandial glycaemic excursions in prediabetes. Diabetes Obes Metab. 2019;21:377–81. https://pubmed.ncbi.nlm.nih.gov/30101510/

89. Imai S, Fukui M, Ozasa N, Ozeki T, Kurokawa M, Komatsu T, et al. Eating vegetables before carbohydrates improves postprandial glucose excursions. Diabet Med. 2013;30:370–72. https://pubmed.ncbi.nlm.nih.gov/23167256/

90. Kuwata H, Iwasaki M, Shimizu S, Minami K, Maeda H, Seino S, et al. Meal sequence and glucose excursion, gastric emptying and incretin secretion in type 2 diabetes: a randomised, controlled crossover, exploratory trial. Diabetologia. 2016;59:453–61. https://pubmed.ncbi.nlm.nih.gov/26704625/

91. Imai S, Matsuda M, Hasegawa G, Fukui M, Obayashi H, Ozasa N, et al. A simple meal plan of "eating vegetables before carbohydrate" was more effective for achieving glycemic control than an exchange-based meal plan in Japanese patients with type 2 diabetes. Asia Pac J Clin Nutr. 2011;20:161–68. https://pubmed.ncbi.nlm.nih.gov/21669583/

92. Tricò D, Filice E, Trifirò S, Natali A. Manipulating the sequence of food ingestion improves glycemic control in type 2 diabetic patients under free-living conditions. Nutr Diabetes. 2016;6:e226. https://www.ncbi.nlm.nih.gov/pmc/articles/PMC5022147/

93. Allen RW, Schwartzman E, Baker WL, Coleman CI, Phung OJ. Cinnamon use in type 2 diabetes: an updated systematic review and meta-analysis. Ann Fam Med. 2013;11:452–59. https://pubmed.ncbi.nlm.nih.gov/24019277/

94. Wang J, Wang S, Yang J, Henning SM, Ezzat-Zadeh Z, Woo S-L, et al. Acute effects of cinnamon spice on post-prandial glucose and insulin in normal weight and overweight/obese subjects: a pilot study. Front Nutr. 2020;7:619782. https://pubmed.ncbi.nlm.nih.gov/33553233/

95. Magistrelli A, Chezem JC. Effect of ground cinnamon on postprandial blood glucose concentration in normal-weight and obese adults. J Acad Nutr Diet. 2012;112:1806–9. https://pubmed.ncbi.nlm.nih.gov/23102179/

96. Kizilaslan N, Erdem NZ. The effect of different amounts of cinnamon consumption on blood glucose in healthy adult individuals. Int J Food Sci. 2019;2019:4138534. https://pubmed.ncbi.nlm.nih.gov/30949494/

97. Solomon TPJ, Blannin AK. Effects of short-term cinnamon ingestion on in vivo glucose tolerance. Diabetes Obes Metab. 2007;9:895–901. https://pubmed.ncbi.nlm.nih.gov/17924872

98. Kim W, Khil LY, Clark R, Bok SH, Kim EE, Lee S, et al. Naphthalenemethyl ester derivative of dihydroxyhydrocinnamic acid, a component of cinnamon, increases glucose disposal by enhancing translocation of glucose transporter 4. Diabetologia. 2006;49:2437–48. https://link.springer.com/article/10.1007/s00125-006-0373-6

Chapter 6

1. Maksoud R, du Preez S, Eaton-Fitch N, Thapaliya K, Barnden L, Cabanas H, et al. A systematic review of neurological impairments in myalgic encephalomyelitis/ chronic fatigue syndrome using neuroimaging techniques. PLoS One. 2020;15:e0232475. https://pubmed.ncbi.nlm.nih.gov/32353033/

2. Rangaraju V, Calloway N, Ryan TA. Activity-driven local ATP synthesis is required for synaptic function. Cell. 2014;156:825–35. https://pubmed.ncbi.nlm.nih.gov/24529383/

3. Attwell D, Laughlin SB. An energy budget for signaling in the grey matter of the brain. J Cereb Blood Flow Metab. 2001;21:1133–45. https://pubmed.ncbi.nlm.nih.gov/11598490/

4. Grimm A, Eckert A. Brain aging and neurodegeneration: from a mitochondrial point of view. J Neurochem. 2017;143:418–31. https://pubmed.ncbi.nlm.nih.gov/28397282/

5. Abbott NJ, Patabendige AAK, Dolman DEM, Yusof SR, Begley DJ. Structure and function of the blood-brain barrier. Neurobiol Dis. 2010;37:13–25. https://pubmed.ncbi.nlm.nih.gov/19664713/

6. Bested AC, Saunders PR, Logan AC. Chronic fatigue syndrome: neurological findings may be related to blood--brain barrier permeability. Med Hypotheses. 2001;57:231–37. https://pubmed.ncbi.nlm.nih.gov/11461179/

7. Wang Y. Leaky blood-brain barrier: a double whammy for the brain. Epilepsy Curr. 2020. p. 165–67. https://pubmed.ncbi.nlm.nih.gov/32550839/

8. Senatorov VV Jr, Friedman AR, Milikovsky DZ, Ofer J, Saar-Ashkenazy R, Charbash A, et al. Blood-brain barrier dysfunction in aging induces hyperactivation of TGFβ signaling and chronic yet reversible neural dysfunction. Sci Transl Med. 2019;11. http://dx.doi.org/10.1126/scitranslmed.aaw8283

9. Milikovsky DZ, Ofer J, Senatorov VV Jr, Friedman AR, Prager O, Sheintuch L, et al. Paroxysmal slow cortical activity in Alzheimer's disease and epilepsy is associated with blood-brain barrier dysfunction. Sci Transl Med. 2019;11. http://dx.doi.org/10.1126/scitranslmed.aaw8954

10. Davis JM, Bailey SP. Possible mechanisms of central nervous system fatigue during exercise. Med Sci Sports Exerc. 1997;29:45–57. https://pubmed.ncbi.nlm.nih.gov/9000155/

11. Roelands B, de Koning J, Foster C, Hettinga F, Meeusen R. Neurophysiological determinants of theoretical concepts and mechanisms involved in pacing. Sports Med. 2013;43:301–11. https://pubmed.ncbi.nlm.nih.gov/23456493/

12. Rattray B, Argus C, Martin K, Northey J, Driller M. Is it time to turn our attention toward central mechanisms for post-exertional recovery strategies and performance? Front Physiol. 2015;6:79. https://www.frontiersin.org/articles/10.3389/fphys.2015.00079/full

13. Cordeiro LMS, Rabelo PCR, Moraes MM, Teixeira-Coelho F, Coimbra CC, Wanner SP, et al. Physical exercise-induced fatigue: the role of serotonergic

and dopaminergic systems. Braz J Med Biol Res. 2017;50:e6432. https://pubmed.ncbi.nlm.nih.gov/29069229/

14. Noakes TD. Fatigue is a brain-derived emotion that regulates the exercise behavior to ensure the protection of whole body homeostasis. Front Physiol. 2012;3:82. https://pubmed.ncbi.nlm.nih.gov/22514538/

15. Taylor JL, Amann M, Duchateau J, Meeusen R, Rice CL. Neural contributions to muscle fatigue: from the brain to the muscle and back again. Med Sci Sports Exerc. 2016;48:2294–2306. https://pubmed.ncbi.nlm.nih.gov/27003703/

16. Kent-Braun JA, Sharma KR, Weiner MW, Massie B, Miller RG. Central basis of muscle fatigue in chronic fatigue syndrome. Neurology. 1993;43:125–31. https://pubmed.ncbi.nlm.nih.gov/8423875/

17. Schillings ML, Kalkman JS, van der Werf SP, van Engelen BGM, Bleijenberg G, Zwarts MJ. Diminished central activation during maximal voluntary contraction in chronic fatigue syndrome. Clin Neurophysiol. 2004;115:2518–24. https://pubmed.ncbi.nlm.nih.gov/15465441/

18. Robinson RL, Stephenson JJ, Dennehy EB, Grabner M, Faries D, Palli SR, et al. The importance of unresolved fatigue in depression: costs and comorbidities. Psychosomatics. 2015;56:274–85. https://pubmed.ncbi.nlm.nih.gov/25596022/

19. Barroso J, Bengtson AM, Gaynes BN, McGuinness T, Quinlivan EB, Ogle M, et al. Improvements in depression and changes in fatigue: results from the SLAM DUNC depression treatment trial. AIDS Behav. 2016;20:235–42. https://www.researchgate.net/publication/283493669_Improvements_in_Depression_and_Changes_in_Fatigue_Results_from_the_SLAM_DUNC_Depression_Treatment_Trial

20. Madill PV. Chronic fatigue syndrome and the cholinergic hypothesis (letter). JAMA. 2004;292:2723. https://jamanetwork.com/journals/jama/article-abstract/199941

21. Spence VA, Khan F, Kennedy G, Abbot NC, Belch JJF. Acetylcholine mediated vasodilatation in the microcirculation of patients with chronic fatigue syndrome. Prostaglandins Leukot Essent Fatty Acids. 2004;70:403–7. https://pubmed.ncbi.nlm.nih.gov/15041034/

22. Sam C, Bordoni B. *Physiology, Acetylcholine.* StatPearls. (Treasure Island, FL: StatPearls Publishing, 2020). https://www.ncbi.nlm.nih.gov/books/NBK557825/

23. Bartus RT, Dean RL 3rd, Beer B, Lippa AS. The cholinergic hypothesis of geriatric memory dysfunction. Science. 1982;217:408–14. https://pubmed.ncbi.nlm.nih.gov/7046051/

24. Craig LA, Hong NS, McDonald RJ. Revisiting the cholinergic hypothesis in the development of Alzheimer's disease. Neurosci Biobehav Rev. 2011;35:1397–409. https://pubmed.ncbi.nlm.nih.gov/21392524/

25. Wise RA, Robble MA. Dopamine and addiction. Annu Rev Psychol. 2020;71:79–106. https://www.annualreviews.org/doi/abs/10.1146/annurev-psych-010418-103337

26. Dobryakova E, Genova HM, DeLuca J, Wylie GR. The dopamine imbalance hypothesis of fatigue in multiple sclerosis and other neurological disorders. Front Neurol. 2015;6:52. https://www.frontiersin.org/articles/10.3389/fneur.2015.00052/full

27. Ledinek AH, Sajko MC, Rot U. Evaluating the effects of amantadin, modafinil and acetyl-L-carnitine on fatigue in multiple sclerosis--result of a pilot randomized, blind study. Clin Neurol Neurosurg. 2013;115 Suppl 1:S86–89. https://pubmed.ncbi.nlm.nih.gov/24321164/

28. Berger M, Gray JA, Roth BL. The expanded biology of serotonin. Annu Rev Med. 2009;60:355–66. https://pubmed.ncbi.nlm.nih.gov/19630576/

29. Ibid.

30. Aghajanian GK, Marek GJ. Serotonin and hallucinogens. Neuropsychopharmacology. 1999;21:16S–23S. https://pubmed.ncbi.nlm.nih .gov/10432484/

31. Lin S-H, Lee L-T, Yang YK. Serotonin and mental disorders: a concise review on molecular neuroimaging evidence. Clin Psychopharmacol Neurosci. 2014;12:196–202. https://pubmed.ncbi.nlm.nih.gov/25598822/

32. Yohn CN, Gergues MM, Samuels BA. The role of 5-HT receptors in depression. Mol Brain. 2017;10:28. https://pubmed.ncbi.nlm.nih.gov/28646910/

33. Cowen PJ, Browning M. What has serotonin to do with depression? World Psychiatry. 2015;14:158–60. https://www.ncbi.nlm.nih.gov/pmc/articles/PMC4471964/

34. Yamamoto S, Ouchi Y, Onoe H, Yoshikawa E, Tsukada H, Takahashi H, et al. Reduction of serotonin transporters of patients with chronic fatigue syndrome. Neuroreport. 2004;15:2571–74. https://pubmed.ncbi.nlm.nih .gov/15570154/

35. Hesse S, Moeller F, Petroff D, Lobsien D, Luthardt J, Regenthal R, et al. Altered serotonin transporter availability in patients with multiple sclerosis. Eur J Nucl Med Mol Imaging. 2014;41:827–35. https://link.springer.com/article/10.1007/s00259-013-2636-z

36. The GKH, Verkes RJ, Fekkes D, Bleijenberg G, van der Meer JWM, Buitelaar JK. Tryptophan depletion in chronic fatigue syndrome, a pilot cross-over study. BMC Res Notes. 2014;7:650. https://www.mendeley.com/catalogue/a6c5f395-3633-3eb4-b1a3-1007b7206cfa/

37. Prober DA. Discovery of hypocretin/orexin ushers in a new era of sleep research. Trends Neurosci. 2018;41:70–72. https://pubmed.ncbi.nlm.nih .gov/29405929/

38. Mahlios J, De la Herrán-Arita AK, Mignot E. The autoimmune basis of narcolepsy. Curr Opin Neurobiol. 2013;23:767–73. https://pubmed.ncbi.nlm .nih.gov/23725858/

39. Coleman PJ, Gotter AL, Herring WJ, Winrow CJ, Renger JJ. The discovery of suvorexant, the first orexin receptor drug for insomnia. Annu Rev Pharmacol Toxicol. 2017;57:509–33. https://pubmed.ncbi.nlm.nih.gov/27860547/

40. Chieffi S, Carotenuto M, Monda V, Valenzano A, Villano I, Precenzano F, et al. Orexin system: the key for a healthy life. Front Physiol. 2017;8:357. https://pubmed.ncbi.nlm.nih.gov/28620314/

41. Hao Y-Y, Yuan H-W, Fang P-H, Zhang Y, Liao Y-X, Shen C, et al. Plasma orexin-A level associated with physical activity in obese people. Eat Weight Disord. 2017;22:69–77. https://pubmed.ncbi.nlm.nih.gov/27038345/

42. Ibid.

43. Kotz CM, Teske JA, Levine JA, Wang C. Feeding and activity induced by orexin A in the lateral hypothalamus in rats. Regul Pept. 2002;104:27–32. https://pubmed.ncbi.nlm.nih.gov/11830273/

44. Gottesmann C. GABA mechanisms and sleep. Neuroscience. 2002;111:231–39. https://pubmed.ncbi.nlm.nih.gov/11983310/

45. Abdou AM, Higashiguchi S, Horie K, Kim M, Hatta H, Yokogoshi H. Relaxation and immunity enhancement effects of gamma-aminobutyric acid (GABA) administration in humans. Biofactors. 2006;26:201–8. https://pubmed.ncbi.nlm.nih.gov/16971751/

46. Möhler H. Role of GABAA receptors in cognition. Biochem Soc Trans. 2009;37:1328–33. https://pubmed.ncbi.nlm.nih.gov/19909270/

47. Losi G, Mariotti L, Carmignoto G. GABAergic interneuron to astrocyte signalling: a neglected form of cell communication in the brain. Philos Trans R Soc Lond B Biol Sci. 2014;369:20130609. https://www.ncbi.nlm.nih.gov/pmc/articles/PMC4173294/

48. Schmidt-Wilcke T, Fuchs E, Funke K, Vlachos A, Müller-Dahlhaus F, Puts NAJ, et al. GABA-from Inhibition to cognition: emerging concepts. Neuroscientist. 2018;24:501–15. https://pubmed.ncbi.nlm.nih.gov/29283020/

49. Sumner P, Edden RAE, Bompas A, Evans CJ, Singh KD. More GABA, less distraction: a neurochemical predictor of motor decision speed. Nat Neurosci. 2010;13:825–27. https://pubmed.ncbi.nlm.nih.gov/20512136/

50. Steenbergen L, Sellaro R, Stock A-K, Beste C, Colzato LS. γ-Aminobutyric acid (GABA) administration improves action selection processes: a randomised controlled trial. Sci Rep. 2015;5:12770. https://pubmed.ncbi.nlm.nih.gov/26227783/

51. Leonte A, Colzato LS, Steenbergen L, Hommel B, Akyürek EG. Supplementation of gamma-aminobutyric acid (GABA) affects temporal, but not spatial visual attention. Brain Cogn. 2018;120:8–16. https://pubmed.ncbi.nlm.nih.gov/29222993/

52. Cao G, Edden RAE, Gao F, Li H, Gong T, Chen W, et al. Reduced GABA levels correlate with cognitive impairment in patients with relapsing-remitting multiple sclerosis. Eur Radiol. 2018;28:1140–48. https://www.ncbi.nlm.nih.gov/pmc/articles/PMC5812783/

53. Sandberg K, Blicher JU, Dong MY, Rees G, Near J, Kanai R. Occipital GABA correlates with cognitive failures in daily life. Neuroimage. 2014;87:55–60. https://pubmed.ncbi.nlm.nih.gov/24188817/

54. Cook E, Hammett ST, Larsson J. GABA predicts visual intelligence. Neurosci Lett. 2016;632:50–54. https://pubmed.ncbi.nlm.nih.gov/27495012/

55. Wang Q, Zhang Z, Dong F, Chen L, Zheng L, Guo X, et al. Anterior insula GABA levels correlate with emotional aspects of empathy: a proton magnetic resonance spectroscopy study. PLoS One. 2014;9:e113845. https://pubmed.ncbi.nlm.nih.gov/25419976/

56. Luscher B, Shen Q, Sahir N. The GABAergic deficit hypothesis of major depressive disorder. Mol Psychiatry. 2011;16:383–406. https://pubmed.ncbi.nlm.nih.gov/21079608/

57. Filip M, Frankowska M. GABA(B) receptors in drug addiction. Pharmacol Rep. 2008;60:755–70. https://pubmed.ncbi.nlm.nih.gov/19211967/

58. Morris MC, Tangney CC, Wang Y, Sacks FM, Barnes LL, Bennett DA, et al. MIND diet slows cognitive decline with aging. Alzheimers Dement. 2015;11:1015–22. https://pubmed.ncbi.nlm.nih.gov/26086182/

59. Morris MC, Tangney CC, Wang Y, Sacks FM, Bennett DA, Aggarwal NT. MIND diet associated with reduced incidence of Alzheimer's disease. Alzheimers Dement. 2015;11:1007–14. https://pubmed.ncbi.nlm.nih.gov/25681666/

60. O'Brien JS. Stability of the myelin membrane. Science. 1965;147:1099–1107. https://pubmed.ncbi.nlm.nih.gov/14242030/

61. Svennerholm L. Distribution and fatty acid composition of phospho-glycerides in normal human brain. J Lipid Res. 1968;9:570–79. https://pubmed.ncbi.nlm.nih.gov/4302302/

62. Carver JD, Benford VJ, Han B, Cantor AB. The relationship between age and the fatty acid composition of cerebral cortex and erythrocytes in human subjects. Brain Res Bull. 2001;56:79–85. https://pubmed.ncbi.nlm.nih.gov/11704343/

63. Bradbury J. Docosahexaenoic acid (DHA): an ancient nutrient for the modern human brain. Nutrients. 2011;3:529–54. https://pubmed.ncbi.nlm.nih.gov/22254110/

64. Crawford MA, Bloom M, Broadhurst CL, Schmidt WF, Cunnane SC, Galli C, et al. Evidence for the unique function of docosahexaenoic acid during the evolution of the modern hominid brain. Lipids. 1999;34 Suppl:S39–S47. https://pubmed.ncbi.nlm.nih.gov/10419087/

65. Stark KD, Van Elswyk ME, Higgins MR, Weatherford CA, Salem N Jr. Global survey of the omega-3 fatty acids, docosahexaenoic acid and eicosapentaenoic acid in the blood stream of healthy adults. Prog Lipid Res. 2016;63:132–52. https://pubmed.ncbi.nlm.nih.gov/27216485/

66. Cole GM, Ma Q-L, Frautschy SA. Omega-3 fatty acids and dementia. Prostaglandins Leukot Essent Fatty Acids. 2009;81:213–21. https://pubmed.ncbi.nlm.nih.gov/19523795/

67. Sethom MM, Fares S, Bouaziz N, Melki W, Jemaa R, Feki M, et al. Polyunsaturated fatty acids deficits are associated with psychotic state and negative symptoms in patients with schizophrenia. Prostaglandins Leukot Essent Fatty Acids. 2010;83:131–36. https://pubmed.ncbi.nlm.nih.gov/20667702/

68. Su K-P, Matsuoka Y, Pae C-U. Omega-3 polyunsaturated fatty acids in prevention of mood and anxiety disorders. Clin Psychopharmacol Neurosci. 2015;13:129–37. https://pubmed.ncbi.nlm.nih.gov/26243838/

69. Astarita G, Jung K-M, Berchtold NC, Nguyen VQ, Gillen DL, Head E, et al. Deficient liver biosynthesis of docosahexaenoic acid correlates with cognitive impairment in Alzheimer's disease. PLoS One. 2010;5:e12538. https://pubmed.ncbi.nlm.nih.gov/20838618/

70. Yurko-Mauro K, Alexander DD, Van Elswyk ME. Docosahexaenoic acid and adult memory: a systematic review and meta-analysis. PLoS One. 2015;10:e0120391. https://pubmed.ncbi.nlm.nih.gov/25786262/

71. Sambra V, Echeverria F, Valenzuela A, Chouinard-Watkins R, Valenzuela R. Docosahexaenoic and arachidonic acids as neuroprotective nutrients throughout the life cycle. Nutrients. 2021;13. http://dx.doi.org/10.3390/nu13030986

72. Weiser MJ, Butt CM, Mohajeri MH. Docosahexaenoic acid and cognition throughout the lifespan. Nutrients. 2016;8:99. https://www.ncbi.nlm.nih.gov/pmc/articles/PMC4772061/

73. Li K, Huang T, Zheng J, Wu K, Li D. Effect of marine-derived n-3 polyunsaturated fatty acids on C-reactive protein, interleukin 6 and tumor necrosis factor α: a meta-analysis. PLoS One. 2014;9:e88103. https://pubmed.ncbi.nlm.nih.gov/24505395/

74. Joffre C, Rey C, Layé S. N-3 polyunsaturated fatty acids and the resolution of neuroinflammation. Front Pharmacol. 2019;10:1022. https://www.ncbi.nlm.nih.gov/pmc/articles/PMC6755339/

75. Castro-Marrero J, Zaragozá MC, Domingo JC, Martinez-Martinez A, Alegre J, von Schacky C. Low omega-3 index and polyunsaturated fatty acid status in patients with chronic fatigue syndrome/myalgic encephalomyelitis. Prostaglandins Leukot Essent Fatty Acids. 2018;139:20–24. https://pubmed.ncbi.nlm.nih.gov/30471769/

76. Maes M, Mihaylova I, Leunis J-C. In chronic fatigue syndrome, the decreased levels of omega-3 poly-unsaturated fatty acids are related to lowered serum zinc and defects in T cell activation. Neuro Endocrinol Lett. 2005;26:745–51. https://pubmed.ncbi.nlm.nih.gov/16380690/

77. Visioli F, Risé P, Barassi MC, Marangoni F, Galli C. Dietary intake of fish vs. formulations leads to higher plasma concentrations of n-3 fatty acids. Lipids. 2003;38:415–18. https://pubmed.ncbi.nlm.nih.gov/12848287/

78. Arterburn LM, Oken HA, Bailey Hall E, Hamersley J, Kuratko CN, Hoffman JP. Algal-oil capsules and cooked salmon: nutritionally equivalent sources of docosahexaenoic acid. J Am Diet Assoc. 2008;108:1204–9. https://pubmed.ncbi.nlm.nih.gov/18589030/

79. Yurko-Mauro K, Kralovec J, Bailey-Hall E, Smeberg V, Stark JG, Salem N Jr. Similar eicosapentaenoic acid and docosahexaenoic acid plasma levels achieved with fish oil or krill oil in a randomized double-blind four-week bioavailability study. Lipids Health Dis. 2015;14:99. https://pubmed.ncbi.nlm.nih.gov/26328782/

80. Su H, Liu R, Chang M, Huang J, Jin Q, Wang X. Effect of dietary alpha-linolenic acid on blood inflammatory markers: a systematic review and meta-analysis of randomized controlled trials. Eur J Nutr. 2018;57:877–91. https://pubmed.ncbi.nlm.nih.gov/28275869/

81. Plourde M, Cunnane SC. Extremely limited synthesis of long chain polyunsaturates in adults: implications for their dietary essentiality and use as supplements. Appl Physiol Nutr Metab. 2007;32:619–34. https://pubmed.ncbi.nlm.nih.gov/17622276/

82. Kris-Etherton PM, Taylor DS, Yu-Poth S, Huth P, Moriarty K, Fishell V, et al. Polyunsaturated fatty acids in the food chain in the United States. Am J Clin Nutr. 2000;71:179S–88S. https://pubmed.ncbi.nlm.nih.gov/10617969/

83. Umhau JC, Zhou W, Carson RE, Rapoport SI, Polozova A, Demar J, et al. Imaging incorporation of circulating docosahexaenoic acid into the human brain using positron emission tomography. J Lipid Res. 2009;50:1259–68. https://pubmed.ncbi.nlm.nih.gov/19112173/

84. Lukiw WJ, Bazan NG. Docosahexaenoic acid and the aging brain. J Nutr. 2008;138:2510–14. https://academic.oup.com/jn/article/138/12/2510/4670186

85. Craft NE, Haitema TB, Garnett KM, Fitch KA, Dorey CK. Carotenoid, tocopherol, and retinol concentrations in elderly human brain. J Nutr Health Aging. 2004;8:156–62. https://pubmed.ncbi.nlm.nih.gov/15129301/

86. Arnal E, Miranda M, Barcia J, Bosch-Morell F, Romero FJ. Lutein and docosahexaenoic acid prevent cortex lipid peroxidation in streptozotocin-induced diabetic rat cerebral cortex. Neuroscience. 2010;166:271–78. https://pubmed.ncbi.nlm.nih.gov/20036322/

87. Johnson EJ, Vishwanathan R, Johnson MA, Hausman DB, Davey A, Scott TM, et al. Relationship between serum and brain carotenoids, α-tocopherol, and retinol concentrations and cognitive performance in the oldest old from the Georgia centenarian study.J Aging Res. 2013;2013:951786. https://pubmed.ncbi.nlm.nih.gov/23840953/

88. Nouchi R, Suiko T, Kimura E, Takenaka H, Murakoshi M, Uchiyama A, et al. Effects of lutein and astaxanthin intake on the improvement of cognitive functions among healthy adults: a systematic review of randomized controlled trials. Nutrients. 2020;12. http://dx.doi.org/10.3390/nu12030617

89. Stringham NT, Holmes PV, Stringham JM. Effects of macular xanthophyll supplementation on brain-derived neurotrophic factor, pro-inflammatory cytokines, and cognitive performance. Physiol Behav. 2019;211:112650. https://pubmed.ncbi.nlm.nih.gov/31425700/

90. Chung H-Y, Rasmussen HM, Johnson EJ. Lutein bioavailability is higher from lutein-enriched eggs than from supplements and spinach in men. J Nutr. 2004;134:1887–93. https://pubmed.ncbi.nlm.nih.gov/15284371/

91. Burns-Whitmore BL, Haddad EH, Sabaté J, Jaceldo-Siegl K, Tanzman J, Rajaram S. Effect of n-3 fatty acid enriched eggs and organic eggs on serum lutein in free-living lacto-ovo vegetarians. Eur J Clin Nutr. 2010;64:1332–37. https://www.researchgate.net/publication/45389554_Effect_of_n-3_fatty_acid_enriched_eggs_and_organic_eggs_on_serum_lutein_in_free-living_lacto-ovo_vegetarians

92. Guilarte TR. Effect of vitamin B-6 nutrition on the levels of dopamine, dopamine metabolites, dopa decarboxylase activity, tyrosine, and GABA in the developing rat corpus striatum. Neurochem Res. 1989;14:571–78. https://pubmed.ncbi.nlm.nih.gov/2761676/

93. Nelson C, Erikson K, Piñero DJ, Beard JL. In vivo dopamine metabolism is altered in iron-deficient anemic rats. J Nutr. 1997;127:2282–88. https://pubmed.ncbi.nlm.nih.gov/9405575/

94. Kim J, Wessling-Resnick M. Iron and mechanisms of emotional behavior. J Nutr Biochem. 2014;25:1101–7. https://pubmed.ncbi.nlm.nih.gov/25154570/

95. Stahl SM. L-methylfolate: a vitamin for your monoamines. J Clin Psychiatry. 2008;69:1352–53. https://pubmed.ncbi.nlm.nih.gov/19193337/

96. Hurrell R, Egli I. Iron bioavailability and dietary reference values. Am J Clin Nutr. 2010;91:1461S–67S. https://pubmed.ncbi.nlm.nih.gov/20200263/

97. Reddy MB, Hurrell RF, Cook JD. Estimation of nonheme-iron bioavailability from meal composition. Am J Clin Nutr. 2000;71:937–43. https://pubmed.ncbi.nlm.nih.gov/10731500/

98. Stahl. L-methylfolate.

99. Gorelova V, Ambach L, Rébeillé F, Stove C, Van Der Straeten D. Folates in plants: research advances and progress in crop biofortification. Front Chem. 2017;5:21. https://pubmed.ncbi.nlm.nih.gov/28424769/

100. Wurtman RJ, Wurtman JJ. Carbohydrate craving, obesity and brain serotonin. Appetite. 1986;7 Suppl:99–103. https://pubmed.ncbi.nlm.nih.gov/3527063/

101. Chin EWM, Goh ELK. Modulating neuronal plasticity with choline. Neural Regeneration Res. 2019;14:1697–98. https://pubmed.ncbi.nlm.nih.gov/31169177/

PART II

Chapter 7

1. Heber D. Pomegranate Ellagitannins. In Benzie IFF, Wachtel-Galor S, editors. *Herbal Medicine: Biomolecular and Clinical Aspects* (Boca Raton, FL: CRC Press/Taylor & Francis, 2012).

2. Ismail T, Calcabrini C, Diaz AR, Fimognari C, Turrini E, Catanzaro E, et al. Ellagitannins in cancer chemoprevention and therapy. Toxins. 2016;8. http://dx.doi.org/10.3390/toxins8050151

3. Aviram M, Rosenblat M, Gaitini D, Nitecki S, Hoffman A, Dornfeld L, et al. Pomegranate juice consumption for 3 years by patients with carotid artery stenosis reduces common carotid intima-media thickness, blood pressure and LDL oxidation. Clin Nutr. 2004;23:423–33. https://pubmed.ncbi.nlm.nih.gov/15158307/

4. Davidson MH, Maki KC, Dicklin MR, Feinstein SB, Witchger M, Bell M, et al. Effects of consumption of pomegranate juice on carotid intima-media thickness in men and women at moderate risk for coronary heart disease. Am J Cardiol. 2009;104:936–42. https://pubmed.ncbi.nlm.nih .gov/19766760/

5. Basu A, Newman ED, Bryant AL, Lyons TJ, Betts NM. Pomegranate polyphenols lower lipid peroxidation in adults with type 2 diabetes but have no effects in healthy volunteers: a pilot study. J Nutr Metab. 2013;2013:708381. https://pubmed.ncbi.nlm.nih.gov/23936637/

6. Tan S, Yu CY, Sim ZW, Low ZS, Lee B, See F, et al. Pomegranate activates TFEB to promote autophagy-lysosomal fitness and mitophagy. Sci Rep. 2019;9:727. https://www.nature.com/articles/s41598-018-37400-1

7. Torregrosa-García A, Ávila-Gandía V, Luque-Rubia AJ, Abellán-Ruiz MS, Querol-Calderón M, López-Román FJ Pomegranate extract improves maximal performance of trained cyclists after an exhausting endurance trial: a randomised controlled trial. Nutrients. 2019;11. http://dx.doi.org/10.3390/ nu11040721

8. Krikorian R, Shidler MD, Nash TA, Kalt W, Vinqvist-Tymchuk MR, Shukitt-Hale B, et al. Blueberry supplementation improves memory in older adults. J Agric Food Chem. 2010;58:3996–4000. https://pubmed.ncbi.nlm.nih.gov/ 20047325/

9. Bowtell JL, Aboo-Bakkar Z, Conway ME, Adlam A-LR, Fulford J. Enhanced task-related brain activation and resting perfusion in healthy older adults after chronic blueberry supplementation. Appl Physiol Nutr Metab. 2017;42:773–79. https://pubmed.ncbi.nlm.nih.gov/28249119/

10. Whyte AR, Cheng N, Fromentin E, Williams CM. A randomized, double-blinded, placebo-controlled study to compare the safety and efficacy of low dose enhanced wild blueberry powder and wild blueberry extract (ThinkBlueTM) in maintenance of episodic and working memory in older adults. Nutrients. 2018;10. http://dx.doi.org/10.3390/nu10060660

11. Boespflug EL, Eliassen JC, Dudley JA, Shidler MD, Kalt W, Summer SS, et al. Enhanced neural activation with blueberry supplementation in mild cognitive impairment. Nutr Neurosci. 2018;21:297–305. https://pubmed .ncbi.nlm.nih.gov/28221821/

12. Bergland AK, Soennesyn H, Dalen I, Rodriguez-Mateos A, Berge RK, Giil LM, et al. Effects of anthocyanin supplementation on serum lipids, glucose, markers of inflammation and cognition in adults with increased risk of dementia—a pilot study. Front Genet. 2019;10:536. https://www.frontiersin .org/articles/10.3389/fgene.2019.00536/full

13. Whyte AR, Cheng N, Butler LT, Lamport DJ, Williams CM. Flavonoid-rich mixed berries maintain and improve cognitive function over a 6 h period in young healthy adults. Nutrients. 2019;11. http://dx.doi.org/10.3390/ nu11112685

14. Ma L, Sun Z, Zeng Y, Luo M, Yang J. Molecular mechanism and health role of functional ingredients in blueberry for chronic disease in human beings. Int J Mol Sci. 2018;19. http://dx.doi.org/10.3390/ijms19092785

15. Feio CA, Izar MC, Ihara SS, Kasmas SH, Martins CM, Feio MN, et al. *Euterpe oleracea* (açaí) modifies sterol metabolism and attenuates experimentally-induced atherosclerosis. J Atheroscler Thromb. 2012;19:237–45. https://www.jstage.jst.go.jp/article/jat/19/3/19_11205/_pdf

16. de Souza MO, Souza E Silva L, de Brito Magalhães CL, de Figueiredo BB, Costa DC, Silva ME, et al. The hypocholesterolemic activity of açaí (Euterpe oleracea Mart.) is mediated by the enhanced expression of the ATP-binding cassette, subfamily G transporters 5 and 8 and low-density lipoprotein receptor genes in the rat. Nutr Res. 2012;32:976–84. https://pubmed.ncbi.nlm.nih.gov/23244543/

17. de Souza MO, Silva M, Silva ME, Oliveira R de P, Pedrosa ML. Diet supplementation with acai (Euterpe oleracea Mart.) pulp improves biomarkers of oxidative stress and the serum lipid profile in rats. Nutrition. 2010;26:804–10. https://pubmed.ncbi.nlm.nih.gov/20022468/

18. Poulose SM, Fisher DR, Bielinski DF, Gomes SM, Rimando AM, Schauss AG, et al. Restoration of stressor-induced calcium dysregulation and autophagy inhibition by polyphenol-rich açaí (Euterpe spp.) fruit pulp extracts in rodent brain cells in vitro. Nutrition. 2014;30:853–62. https://pubmed.ncbi.nlm.nih.gov/24985004/

19. Poulose SM, Bielinski DF, Carey A, Schauss AG, Shukitt-Hale B. Modulation of oxidative stress, inflammation, autophagy and expression of Nrf2 in hippocampus and frontal cortex of rats fed with açaí-enriched diets. Nutr Neurosci. 2017;20:305–15. https://pubmed.ncbi.nlm.nih.gov/26750735/

20. Poulose SM, Fisher DR, Larson J, Bielinski DF, Rimando AM, Carey AN, et al. Anthocyanin-rich açaí (Euterpe oleracea Mart.) fruit pulp fractions attenuate inflammatory stress signaling in mouse brain BV-2 microglial cells. J Agric Food Chem. 2012;60:1084–93. https://pubmed.ncbi.nlm.nih.gov/22224493/

21. Carey AN, Miller MG, Fisher DR, Bielinski DF, Gilman CK, Poulose SM, et al. Dietary supplementation with the polyphenol-rich açaí pulps (Euterpe oleracea Mart. and Euterpe precatoria Mart.) improves cognition in aged rats and attenuates inflammatory signaling in BV-2 microglial cells. Nutr Neurosci. 2017;20:238–45. https://pubmed.ncbi.nlm.nih.gov/26618555/

22. Alessandra-Perini J, Rodrigues-Baptista KC, Machado DE, Nasciutti LE, Perini JA. Anticancer potential, molecular mechanisms and toxicity of Euterpe oleracea extract (açaí): a systematic review. PLoS One. 2018;13:e0200101. https://pubmed.ncbi.nlm.nih.gov/29966007/

23. de Freitas Carvalho MM, Lage NN, de Souza Paulino AH, Pereira RR, de Almeida LT, da Silva TF, et al. Effects of açai on oxidative stress, ER stress, and inflammation-related parameters in mice with high fat diet-fed induced NAFLD. Sci Rep. 2019;9:8107. https://www.nature.com/articles/s41598-019-44563-y?proof=tNature

24. Sadowska-Krępa E, Kłapcińska B, Podgórski T, Szade B, Tyl K, Hadzik A. Effects of supplementation with acai (Euterpe oleracea Mart.) berry-based juice blend on the blood antioxidant defence capacity and lipid profile in junior hurdlers. A pilot study. Biol Sport. 2015;32:161–68. https://pubmed.ncbi.nlm.nih.gov/26060341/

25. Carvalho-Peixoto J, Moura MRL, Cunha FA, Lollo PCB, Monteiro WD, Carvalho LMJ de, et al. Consumption of açai (Euterpe oleracea Mart.) functional beverage reduces muscle stress and improves effort tolerance in elite athletes: a randomized controlled intervention study. Appl Physiol Nutr Metab. 2015;40:725–33. https://cdnsciencepub.com/doi/abs/10.1139/ apnm-2014-0518?src=recsys&journalCode=apnm

26. Kim H, Simbo SY, Fang C, McAlister L, Roque A, Banerjee N, et al. Açaí (Euterpe oleracea Mart.) beverage consumption improves biomarkers for inflammation but not glucose- or lipid-metabolism in individuals with metabolic syndrome in a randomized, double-blinded, placebo-controlled clinical trial. Food Funct. 2018;9:3097–103. https://pubmed.ncbi.nlm.nih .gov/29850709/

27. Alqurashi RM, Galante LA, Rowland IR, Spencer JP, Commane DM. Consumption of a flavonoid-rich açai meal is associated with acute improvements in vascular function and a reduction in total oxidative status in healthy overweight men. Am J Clin Nutr. 2016;104:1227–35. https:// academic.oup.com/ajcn/article/104/5/1227/4564373

28. Burdulis D, Ivanauskas L, Dirse V, Kazlauskas S, Razukas A. Study of diversity of anthocyanin composition in bilberry (Vaccinium myrtillus L.) fruits. Medicina. 2007;43:971–77. https://pubmed.ncbi.nlm.nih.gov/18182842/

29. Lätti AK, Riihinen KR, Kainulainen PS. Analysis of anthocyanin variation in wild populations of bilberry (Vaccinium myrtillus L.) in Finland. J Agric Food Chem. 2008;56:190–96. https://pubmed.ncbi.nlm.nih.gov/18072741/

30. Colak N, Torun H, Gruz J, Strnad M, Hermosín-Gutiérrez I, Hayirlioglu-Ayaz S, et al. Bog bilberry phenolics, antioxidant capacity and nutrient profile. Food Chem. 2016;201:339–49. https://pubmed.ncbi.nlm.nih.gov/26868586/

31. Kolehmainen M, Mykkänen O, Kirjavainen PV, Leppänen T, Moilanen E, Adriaens M, et al. Bilberries reduce low-grade inflammation in individuals with features of metabolic syndrome. Mol Nutr Food Res. 2012;56:1501–10. https://pubmed.ncbi.nlm.nih.gov/22961907/

32. Karlsen A, Paur I, Bøhn SK, Sakhi AK, Borge GI, Serafini M, et al. Bilberry juice modulates plasma concentration of NF-kappaB related inflammatory markers in subjects at increased risk of CVD. Eur J Nutr. 2010;49:345–55. https://pubmed.ncbi.nlm.nih.gov/20119859/

33. Karlsen A, Retterstøl L, Laake P, Paur I, Bøhn SK, Sandvik L, et al. Anthocyanins inhibit nuclear factor-kappaB activation in monocytes and reduce plasma concentrations of pro-inflammatory mediators in healthy adults. J Nutr. 2007;137:1951–54. https://pubmed.ncbi.nlm.nih.gov/ 17634269/

34. Hoggard N, Cruickshank M, Moar K-M, Bestwick C, Holst JJ, Russell W, et al. A single supplement of a standardised bilberry (Vaccinium myrtillus L.) extract (36 % wet weight anthocyanins) modifies glycaemic response in individuals with type 2 diabetes controlled by diet and lifestyle. J Nutr Sci. 2013;2:e22. https://pubmed.ncbi.nlm.nih.gov/25191571/

35. Quispe-Fuentes I, Vega-Gálvez A, Aranda M. Evaluation of phenolic profiles and antioxidant capacity of maqui (Aristotelia chilensis) berries and their

relationships to drying methods. J Sci Food Agric. 2018;98:4168–76. https://pubmed.ncbi.nlm.nih.gov/29417999/

36. Davinelli S, Bertoglio JC, Zarrelli A, Pina R, Scapagnini G. A randomized clinical trial evaluating the efficacy of an anthocyanin-maqui berry extract (Delphinol®) on oxidative stress biomarkers. J Am Coll Nutr. 2015;34 Suppl 1:28–33. https://pubmed.ncbi.nlm.nih.gov/26400431/

37. Schreckinger ME, Lotton J, Lila MA, de Mejia EG. Berries from South America: a comprehensive review on chemistry, health potential, and commercialization. J Med Food. 2010;13:233–46. https://pubmed.ncbi.nlm.nih.gov/20170356/

38. Araya H, Clavijo C, Herrera C. [Antioxidant capacity of fruits and vegetables cultivated in Chile]. Arch Latinoam Nutr. 2006;56:361–65. https://www.researchgate.net/publication/51389391_Antioxidant_capacity_of_fruits_and_vegetables_cultivated_in_Chile

39. Cespedes CL, Pavon N, Dominguez M, Alarcon J, Balbontin C, Kubo I, et al. The chilean superfruit black-berry Aristotelia chilensis (Elaeocarpaceae), Maqui as mediator in inflammation-associated disorders. Food Chem Toxicol. 2017;108:438–50. https://pubmed.ncbi.nlm.nih.gov/28040469/

40. Watson RR, Schönlau F. Nutraceutical and antioxidant effects of a delphinidin-rich maqui berry extract Delphinol®: a review. Minerva Cardioangiol. 2015;63:1–12. https://pubmed.ncbi.nlm.nih.gov/25892567/

41. Vergara D, Ávila D, Escobar E, Carrasco-Pozo C, Sánchez A, Gotteland M. The intake of maqui (*Aristotelia chilensis*) berry extract normalizes H2O2 and IL-6 concentrations in exhaled breath condensate from healthy smokers—an explorative study. Nutr J. 2015;14:27. https://pubmed.ncbi.nlm.nih.gov/25889552/

42. Alvarado J, Schoenlau F, Leschot A, Salgad AM, Vigil Portales P. Delphinol® standardized maqui berry extract significantly lowers blood glucose and improves blood lipid profile in prediabetic individuals in three-month clinical trial. Panminerva Med. 2016;58:1–6. https://pubmed.ncbi.nlm.nih.gov/27820958/

43. Hitoe S, Tanaka J, Shimoda H. MaquiBrightTM standardized maqui berry extract significantly increases tear fluid production and ameliorates dry eye-related symptoms in a clinical pilot trial. Panminerva Med. 2014;56:1–6. https://pubmed.ncbi.nlm.nih.gov/25208615/

44. Yamashita S-I, Suzuki N, Yamamoto K, Iio S-I, Yamada T. Effects of MaquiBright® on improving eye dryness and fatigue in humans: A randomized, double-blind, placebo-controlled trial. Afr J Tradit Complement Altern Med. 2019;9:172–78. https://pubmed.ncbi.nlm.nih.gov/31193920/

45. Caldas APS, Coelho OGL, Bressan J. Cranberry antioxidant power on oxidative stress, inflammation and mitochondrial damage. Int J Food Prop. Taylor & Francis; 2018;21:582–92. https://www.tandfonline.com/doi/full/10.1080/10942912.2017.1409758

46. Blumberg JB, Basu A, Krueger CG, Lila MA, Neto CC, Novotny JA, et al. Impact of cranberries on gut microbiota and cardiometabolic health: proceedings of the cranberry health research conference 2015. Adv Nutr. 2016;7:759S–70S. https://www.ars.usda.gov/research/publications/publication/?seqNo115=325862

47. De Souza Schmidt Gonçalves AE, Lajolo FM, Genovese MI. Chemical composition and antioxidant/antidiabetic potential of Brazilian native fruits and commercial frozen pulps. J Agric Food Chem. 2010;58:4666–74. https://pubmed.ncbi.nlm.nih.gov/20337450/

48. Genovese MI, Da Silva Pinto M, De Souza Schmidt Gonçalves AE, Lajolo FM. Bioactive compounds and antioxidant capacity of exotic fruits and commercial frozen pulps from Brazil. Food Sci Technol Int. SAGE Publications Ltd STM; 2008;14:207–14. https://journals.sagepub.com/doi/10.1177/1082013208092151

49. Justi KC, Visentainer JV, Evelázio de Souza N, Matsushita M. Nutritional composition and vitamin C stability in stored camu-camu (Myrciaria dubia) pulp. Arch Latinoam Nutr. 2000;50:405–8. https://pubmed.ncbi.nlm.nih.gov/11464674/

50. Fracassetti D, Costa C, Moulay L, Tomás-Barberán FA. Ellagic acid derivatives, ellagitannins, proanthocyanidins and other phenolics, vitamin C and antioxidant capacity of two powder products from camu-camu fruit (Myrciaria dubia). Food Chem. 2013;139:578–88. https://pubmed.ncbi.nlm.nih.gov/23561148/

51. Langley PC, Pergolizzi JV Jr, Taylor R Jr, Ridgway C. Antioxidant and associated capacities of Camu camu (*Myrciaria dubia*): a systematic review. J Altern Complement Med. 2015;21:8–14. https://www.ncbi.nlm.nih.gov/pmc/articles/PMC4296744/

52. Fidelis M, do Carmo MAV, da Cruz TM, Azevedo L, Myoda T, Miranda Furtado M, et al. Camu-camu seed (Myrciaria dubia)—from side stream to anantioxidant, antihyperglycemic, antiproliferative, antimicrobial, antihemolytic, anti-inflammatory, and antihypertensive ingredient. Food Chem. 2020;310:125909. https://pubmed.ncbi.nlm.nih.gov/31816536/

53. Neri-Numa IA, Soriano Sancho RA, Pereira APA, Pastore GM. Small Brazilian wild fruits: nutrients, bioactive compounds, health-promotion properties and commercial interest. Food Res Int. 2018;103:345–60. https://pubmed.ncbi.nlm.nih.gov/29389624/

54. Nascimento OV, Boleti APA, Yuyama LKO, Lima ES. Effects of diet supplementation with Camu-camu (Myrciaria dubia HBK McVaugh) fruit in a rat model of diet-induced obesity. An Acad Bras Cienc. 2013;85:355–63. https://pubmed.ncbi.nlm.nih.gov/23460435/

55. Akachi T, Shiina Y, Kawaguchi T, Kawagishi H, Morita T, Sugiyama K. 1-methylmalate from camu-camu (*Myrciaria dubia*) suppressed D-galactosamine-induced liver injury in rats. Biosci Biotechnol Biochem. 2010;74:573–78. https://pubmed.ncbi.nlm.nih.gov/20208347/

56. Inoue T, Komoda H, Uchida T, Node K. Tropical fruit camu-camu (Myrciaria dubia) has anti-oxidative and anti-inflammatory properties. J Cardiol. 2008;52:127–32. https://pubmed.ncbi.nlm.nih.gov/18922386/

57. Balisteiro DM, Araujo RL de, Giacaglia LR, Genovese MI. Effect of clarified Brazilian native fruit juices on postprandial glycemia in healthy subjects. Food Res Int. 2017;100:196–203. https://pubmed.ncbi.nlm.nih.gov/28888441/

58. Miyashita T, Koizumi R, Myoda T, Sagane Y, Niwa K, Watanabe T, et al. Data on a single oral dose of camu camu (*Myrciaria dubia*) pericarp extract on flow-mediated vasodilation and blood pressure in young adult humans. Data Brief. 2018;16:993–99. https://europepmc.org/article/med/29322080

59. Yamamoto H, Morino K, Mengistu L, Ishibashi T, Kiriyama K, Ikami T, et al. Amla enhances mitochondrial spare respiratory capacity by increasing mitochondrial biogenesis and antioxidant systems in a murine skeletal muscle cell line. Oxid Med Cell Longev. 2016;2016:1735841. https://pubmed.ncbi.nlm.nih.gov/27340504/

60. Yokozawa T, Kim HY, Kim HJ, Tanaka T, Sugino H, Okubo T, et al. Amla (Emblica officinalis Gaertn.) attenuates age-related renal dysfunction by oxidative stress. J Agric Food Chem. 2007;55:7744–52. https://pubmed.ncbi.nlm.nih.gov/17715896/

61. Husain I, Zameer S, Madaan T, Minhaj A, Ahmad W, Iqubaal A, et al. Exploring the multifaceted neuroprotective actions of Emblica officinalis (Amla): a review. Metab Brain Dis. 2019;34:957–65. https://pubmed.ncbi.nlm.nih.gov/30848470/

62. Baliga MS, Dsouza JJ. Amla (Emblica officinalis Gaertn), a wonder berry in the treatment and prevention of cancer. Eur J Cancer Prev. 2011;20:225–39. https://pubmed.ncbi.nlm.nih.gov/21317655/

63. Krishnaveni M, Mirunalini S. Therapeutic potential of Phyllanthus emblica (amla): the ayurvedic wonder. J Basic Clin Physiol Pharmacol. 2010;21:93–105. https://pubmed.ncbi.nlm.nih.gov/20506691/

64. Akhtar MS, Ramzan A, Ali A, Ahmad M. Effect of Amla fruit (Emblica officinalis Gaertn.) on blood glucose and lipid profile of normal subjects and type 2 diabetic patients. Int J Food Sci Nutr. 2011;62:609–16. https://pubmed.ncbi.nlm.nih.gov/21495900/

65. Usharani P, Fatima N, Muralidhar N. Effects of Phyllanthus emblica extract on endothelial dysfunction and biomarkers of oxidative stress in patients with type 2 diabetes mellitus: a randomized, double-blind, controlled study. Diabetes Metab Syndr Obes. 2013;6:275–84. https://pubmed.ncbi.nlm.nih.gov/23935377/

66. Usharani P, Merugu PL, Nutalapati C. Evaluation of the effects of a standardized aqueous extract of Phyllanthus emblica fruits on endothelial dysfunction, oxidative stress, systemic inflammation and lipid profile in subjects with metabolic syndrome: a randomised, double blind, placebo controlled clinical study. BMC Complement Altern Med. 2019;19:97. https://pubmed.ncbi.nlm.nih.gov/31060549/

67. Kapoor MP, Suzuki K, Derek T, Ozeki M, Okubo T. Clinical evaluation of Emblica Officinalis Gatertn (Amla) in healthy human subjects: health benefits and safety results from a randomized, double-blind, crossover placebo-controlled study. Contemp Clin Trials Commun. 2020;17:100499. https://pubmed.ncbi.nlm.nih.gov/31890983/

68. Ciferri O. Spirulina, the edible microorganism. Microbiol Rev. 1983;47:551–78. https://www.ncbi.nlm.nih.gov/pmc/articles/PMC283708/

69. Nawrocka D, Kornicka K, Śmieszek A, Marycz K. Spirulina platensis improves mitochondrial function impaired by elevated oxidative stress in adipose-derived mesenchymal stromal cells (ASCs) and intestinal epithelial cells (IECs), and enhances insulin sensitivity in equine metabolic syndrome (EMS) horses. Mar Drugs. 2017;15. http://dx.doi.org/10.3390/md15080237

70. Oriquat GA, Ali MA, Mahmoud SA, Eid RMHM, Hassan R, Kamel MA. Improving hepatic mitochondrial biogenesis as a postulated mechanism for the antidiabetic effect of Spirulina platensis in comparison with metformin. Appl Physiol Nutr Metab. 2019;44:357–64. https://pubmed.ncbi.nlm.nih.gov/30208279/

71. Gao J, Zhao L, Wang J, Zhang L, Zhou D, Qu J, et al. C-phycocyanin ameliorates mitochondrial fission and fusion dynamics in ischemic cardiomyocyte damage. Front Pharmacol. 2019;10:733. https://pubmed.ncbi.nlm.nih.gov/31316386/

72. Liu Q, Huang Y, Zhang R, Cai T, Cai Y. Medical application of spirulina platensis derived C-phycocyanin. Evid Based Complement Alternat Med. 2016;2016:7803846. https://pubmed.ncbi.nlm.nih.gov/27293463/

73. McCarty MF. Clinical potential of Spirulina as a source of phycocyanobilin. J Med Food. 2007;10:566–70. https://pubmed.ncbi.nlm.nih.gov/18158824/

74. Huang H, Liao D, Pu R, Cui Y. Quantifying the effects of spirulina supplementation on plasma lipid and glucose concentrations, body weight, and blood pressure. Diabetes Metab Syndr Obes. 2018;11:729–42. https://www.ncbi.nlm.nih.gov/pmc/articles/PMC6241722/

75. Baigent C, Keech A, Kearney PM, Blackwell L, Buck G, Pollicino C, et al. Efficacy and safety of cholesterol-lowering treatment: prospective meta-analysis of data from 90,056 participants in 14 randomised trials of statins. Lancet. 2005;366:1267–78. https://pubmed.ncbi.nlm.nih.gov/16214597/

76. Jansen T, Daiber A. Direct antioxidant properties of bilirubin and biliverdin. Is there a role for biliverdin reductase? Front Pharmacol. 2012;3:30. https://pubmed.ncbi.nlm.nih.gov/22438843/

77. McDonagh AF. The biliverdin-bilirubin antioxidant cycle of cellular protection: missing a wheel? Free Radic Biol Med. 2010;49:814–20. https://pubmed.ncbi.nlm.nih.gov/20547221/

78. Inoguchi T, Sonoda N, Maeda Y. Bilirubin as an important physiological modulator of oxidative stress and chronic inflammation in metabolic syndrome and diabetes: a new aspect on old molecule. Diabetol Int. 2016;7:338–41. https://pubmed.ncbi.nlm.nih.gov/30603284/

79. Kundur AR, Singh I, Bulmer AC. Bilirubin, platelet activation and heart disease: a missing link to cardiovascular protection in Gilbert's syndrome? Atherosclerosis. 2015;239:73–84. https://pubmed.ncbi.nlm.nih.gov/25576848/

80. Kalafati M, Jamurtas AZ, Nikolaidis MG, Paschalis V, Theodorou AA, Sakellariou GK, et al. Ergogenic and antioxidant effects of spirulina supplementation in humans. Med Sci Sports Exerc. 2010;42:142–51. https://pubmed.ncbi.nlm.nih.gov/20010119/

81. Lu H-K, Hsieh C-C, Hsu J-J, Yang Y-K, Chou H-N. Preventive effects of Spirulina platensis on skeletal muscle damage under exercise-induced oxidative stress. Eur J Appl Physiol. 2006;98:220–26. https://pubmed.ncbi .nlm.nih.gov/16944194/

82. Johnson M, Hassinger L, Davis J, Devor ST, DiSilvestro RA. A randomized, double blind, placebo controlled study of spirulina supplementation on indices of mental and physical fatigue in men. Int J Food Sci Nutr. 2016;67:203–6. https://pubmed.ncbi.nlm.nih.gov/26888417/

83. Bito T, Okumura E, Fujishima M, Watanabe F. Potential of chlorella as a dietary supplement to promote human health. Nutrients. 2020;12. http:// dx.doi.org/10.3390/nu12092524

84. Panahi Y, Tavana S, Sahebkar A, Masoudi H, Madanchi N. Impact of adjunctive therapy with chlorella vulgaris extract on antioxidant status, pulmonary function, and clinical symptoms of patients with obstructive pulmonary diseases. Sci Pharm. 2012;80:719–30. https://pubmed.ncbi.nlm .nih.gov/23008817/

85. Panahi Y, Mostafazadeh B, Abrishami A, Saadat A, Beiraghdar F, Tavana S, et al. Investigation of the effects of Chlorella vulgaris supplementation on the modulation of oxidative stress in apparently healthy smokers. Clin Lab. 2013;59:579–87. https://pubmed.ncbi.nlm.nih.gov/23865357/

86. Fallah AA, Sarmast E, Habibian Dehkordi S, Engardeh J, Mahmoodnia L, Khaledifar A, et al. Effect of chlorella supplementation on cardiovascular risk factors: a meta-analysis of randomized controlled trials. Clin Nutr. 2018;37:1892–1901. https://pubmed.ncbi.nlm.nih.gov/29037431/

87. Merchant RE, Carmack CA, Wise CM. Nutritional supplementation with Chlorella pyrenoidosa for patients with fibromyalgia syndrome: a pilot study. Phytother Res. 2000;14:167–73. https://pubmed.ncbi.nlm.nih.gov/ 10815009/

88. Houghton CA, Fassett RG, Coombes JS. Sulforaphane and other nutrigenomic Nrf2 activators: can the clinician's expectation be matched by the reality? Oxid Med Cell Longev. 2016;2016:7857186. https://pubmed .ncbi.nlm.nih.gov/26881038/

89. Eagles SK, Gross AS, McLachlan AJ. The effects of cruciferous vegetable-enriched diets on drug metabolism: a systematic review and meta-analysis of dietary intervention trials in humans. Clin Pharmacol Ther. 2020;108:212–27. https://pubmed.ncbi.nlm.nih.gov/32086800/

90. Houghton. Sulforaphane and other nutrigenomic Nrf2 activators.

91. Conzatti A, Fróes FCT da S, Schweigert Perry ID, Souza CG de. Clinical and molecular evidence of the consumption of broccoli, glucoraphanin and sulforaphane in humans. Nutr Hosp. 2014;31:559–69. https://pubmed.ncbi .nlm.nih.gov/25617536/

92. López-Chillón MT, Carazo-Díaz C, Prieto-Merino D, Zafrilla P, Moreno DA, Villaño D. Effects of long-term consumption of broccoli sprouts on inflammatory markers in overweight subjects. Clin Nutr. 2019;38:745–52. https://pubmed.ncbi.nlm.nih.gov/29573889/

93. Amagase H, Petesch BL, Matsuura H, Kasuga S, Itakura Y. Intake of garlic and its bioactive components. J Nutr. 2001;131:955S–62S. https://pubmed.ncbi .nlm.nih.gov/11238796/

94. Moosavian SP, Arab A, Paknahad Z, Moradi S. The effects of garlic supplementation on oxidative stress markers: A systematic review and meta-analysis of randomized controlled trials. Complement Ther Med. 2020;50:102385. https://pubmed.ncbi.nlm.nih.gov/32444050/

95. Darooghegi Mofrad M, Milajerdi A, Koohdani F, Surkan PJ, Azadbakht L. Garlic supplementation reduces circulating C-reactive protein, tumor necrosis factor, and interleukin-6 in adults: a systematic review and meta-analysis of randomized controlled trials. J Nutr. 2019;149:605–18. https:// pubmed.ncbi.nlm.nih.gov/30949665/

96. Taghizadeh M, Hamedifard Z, Jafarnejad S. Effect of garlic supplementation on serum C-reactive protein level: A systematic review and meta-analysis of randomized controlled trials. Phytother Res. 2019;33:243–52. https:// pubmed.ncbi.nlm.nih.gov/30370629/

97. Shabani E, Sayemiri K, Mohammadpour M. The effect of garlic on lipid profile and glucose parameters in diabetic patients: a systematic review and meta-analysis. Prim Care Diabetes. 2019;13:28–42. https://pubmed.ncbi.nlm .nih.gov/30049636/

98. Sun Y-E, Wang W, Qin J. Anti-hyperlipidemia of garlic by reducing the level of total cholesterol and low-density lipoprotein: a meta-analysis. Medicine. 2018;97:e0255. https://www.ncbi.nlm.nih.gov/pmc/articles/PMC6392629/

99. Ried K. Garlic lowers blood pressure in hypertensive individuals, regulates serum cholesterol, and stimulates immunity: an updated meta-analysis and review. J Nutr. 2016;146:389S–96S. https://pubmed.ncbi.nlm.nih.gov/ 26764326/

100. Panjeshahin A, Mollahosseini M, Panbehkar-Jouybari M, Kaviani M, Mirzavandi F, Hosseinzadeh M. Effects of garlic supplementation on liver enzymes: a systematic review and meta-analysis of randomized controlled trials. Phytother Res. 2020;34:1947–55. https://pubmed.ncbi.nlm.nih.gov/ 32135032/

101. Khodaie L, Sadeghpoor O. Ginger from ancient times to the new outlook. Jundishapur J Nat Pharm Prod. 2015;10:e18402. https://www.ncbi.nlm.nih .gov/pmc/articles/PMC4377061/

102. Lete I, Allué J. The effectiveness of ginger in the prevention of nausea and vomiting during pregnancy and chemotherapy. Integr Med Insights. 2016;11:11–17. https://www.ncbi.nlm.nih.gov/pmc/articles/PMC4818021/

103. Ibid.

104. Chang WP, Peng YX. Does the oral administration of ginger reduce chemotherapy-induced nausea and vomiting?: a meta-analysis of 10 randomized controlled trials. Cancer Nurs. 2019;42:E14–23. https://pubmed .ncbi.nlm.nih.gov/30299420/

105. Xu Y, Yang Q, Wang X. Efficacy of herbal medicine (cinnamon/fennel/ ginger) for primary dysmenorrhea: a systematic review and meta-analysis of randomized controlled trials. J Int Med Res. 2020;48:300060520936179. https://pubmed.ncbi.nlm.nih.gov/32603204/

106. Jalali M, Mahmoodi M, Moosavian SP, Jalali R, Ferns G, Mosallanezhad A, et al. The effects of ginger supplementation on markers of inflammatory and oxidative stress: a systematic review and meta-analysis of clinical trials. Phytother Res. 2020;34:1723–33. https://clinicalnutritionespen.com/article/S2405-4577(21)00261-8/fulltext

107. Hasani H, Arab A, Hadi A, Pourmasoumi M, Ghavami A, Miraghajani M. Does ginger supplementation lower blood pressure? A systematic review and meta-analysis of clinical trials. Phytother Res. 2019;33:1639–47. https://pubmed.ncbi.nlm.nih.gov/30972845/

108. Pourmasoumi M, Hadi A, Rafie N, Najafgholizadeh A, Mohammadi H, Rouhani MH. The effect of ginger supplementation on lipid profile: a systematic review and meta-analysis of clinical trials. Phytomedicine. 2018;43:28–36. https://pubmed.ncbi.nlm.nih.gov/29747751/

109. Maharlouei N, Tabrizi R, Lankarani KB, Rezaianzadeh A, Akbari M, Kolahdooz F, et al. The effects of ginger intake on weight loss and metabolic profiles among overweight and obese subjects: a systematic review and meta-analysis of randomized controlled trials. Crit Rev Food Sci Nutr. 2019;59:1753–66. https://pubmed.ncbi.nlm.nih.gov/29393665/

110. Dillinger TL, Barriga P, Escárcega S, Jimenez M, Salazar Lowe D, Grivetti LE. Food of the gods: cure for humanity? A cultural history of the medicinal and ritual use of chocolate. J Nutr. 2000;130:2057S–72S. https://academic.oup.com/jn/article/130/8/2057S/4686320

111. Lippi D. Sin and pleasure: the history of chocolate in medicine. J Agric Food Chem. 2015;63:9936–41. https://pubs.acs.org/doi/10.1021/acs.jafc.5b00829

112. Lee KW, Kim YJ, Lee HJ, Lee CY. Cocoa has more phenolic phytochemicals and a higher antioxidant capacity than teas and red wine. J Agric Food Chem. 2003;51:7292–95. https://pubmed.ncbi.nlm.nih.gov/14640573/

113. Jafari Azad B, Daneshzad E, Meysamie AP, Koohdani F. Chronic and acute effects of cocoa products intake on arterial stiffness and platelet count and function: a systematic review and dose-response Meta-analysis of randomized clinical trials. Crit Rev Food Sci Nutr. 2021;61:357–79. https://pubmed.ncbi.nlm.nih.gov/32126803/

114. Sun Y, Zimmermann D, De Castro CA, Actis-Goretta L. Dose-response relationship between cocoa flavanols and human endothelial function: a systematic review and meta-analysis of randomized trials. Food Funct. 2019;10:6322–30. https://www.ncbi.nlm.nih.gov/pmc/articles/PMC7851825/

115. Mehrabani S, Arab A, Mohammadi H, Amani R. The effect of cocoa consumption on markers of oxidative stress: a systematic review and meta-analysis of interventional studies. Complement Ther Med. 2020;48:102240. https://pubmed.ncbi.nlm.nih.gov/31987247/

116. Ried K, Fakler P, Stocks NP. Effect of cocoa on blood pressure. Cochrane Database Syst Rev. 2017;4:CD008893. https://pubmed.ncbi.nlm.nih.gov/28439881/

117. Lin X, Zhang I, Li A, Manson JE, Sesso HD, Wang L, et al. Cocoa flavanol intake and biomarkers for cardiometabolic health: a systematic review and meta-analysis of randomized controlled trials. J Nutr. 2016;146:2325–33. https://pubmed.ncbi.nlm.nih.gov/27683874/

118. Barreca D, Nabavi SM, Sureda A, Rasekhian M, Raciti R, Silva AS, et al. Almonds (Prunus Dulcis Mill. D. A. Webb): a source of nutrients and health-promoting compounds. Nutrients. 2020;12. http://dx.doi.org/10.3390/nu12030672

119. Asbaghi O, Moodi V, Hadi A, Eslampour E, Shirinbakhshmasoleh M, Ghaedi E, et al. The effect of almond intake on lipid profile: a systematic review and meta-analysis of randomized controlled trials. Food Funct. 2021;12:1882–96. https://pubs.rsc.org/en/content/articlelanding/2021/fo/d0fo02878a

120. Eslampour E, Moodi V, Asbaghi O, Ghaedi E, Shirinbakhshmasoleh M, Hadi A, et al. The effect of almond intake on anthropometric indices: a systematic review and meta-analysis. Food Funct. 2020;11:7340–55. https://pubmed.ncbi.nlm.nih.gov/32857083/

121. Kamil A, Chen C-YO. Health benefits of almonds beyond cholesterol reduction. J Agric Food Chem. 2012;60:6694–702. https://pubmed.ncbi.nlm.nih.gov/22296169/

122. Ellis PR, Kendall CWC, Ren Y, Parker C, Pacy JF, Waldron KW, et al. Role of cell walls in the bioaccessibility of lipids in almond seeds. Am J Clin Nutr. 2004;80:604–13. https://pubmed.ncbi.nlm.nih.gov/15321799/

123. Cassady BA, Hollis JH, Fulford AD, Considine RV, Mattes RD. Mastication of almonds: effects of lipid bioaccessibility, appetite, and hormone response. Am J Clin Nutr. 2009;89:794–800. https://pubmed.ncbi.nlm.nih.gov/19144727/

124. Dhillon J, Li Z, Ortiz RM. Almond snacking for 8 wk increases alpha-diversity of the gastrointestinal microbiome and decreases *Bacteroides fragilis* abundance compared with an isocaloric snack in college freshmen. Curr Dev Nutr. 2019;3:nzz079. https://pubmed.ncbi.nlm.nih.gov/31528836/

125. Scott TM, Rasmussen HM, Chen O, Johnson EJ. Avocado consumption increases macular pigment density in older adults: a randomized, controlled trial. Nutrients. 2017;9. http://dx.doi.org/10.3390/nu9090919

126. Peou S, Milliard-Hasting B, Shah SA. Impact of avocado-enriched diets on plasma lipoproteins: a meta-analysis. J Clin Lipidol. 2016;10:161–71. https://pubmed.ncbi.nlm.nih.gov/26892133/

127. Schoeneck M, Iggman D. The effects of foods on LDL cholesterol levels: a systematic review of the accumulated evidence from systematic reviews and meta-analyses of randomized controlled trials. Nutr Metab Cardiovasc Dis. 2021;31:1325–38. https://pubmed.ncbi.nlm.nih.gov/33762150/

128. Sousa FH, Valenti VE, Pereira LC, Bueno RR, Prates S, Akimoto AN, et al. Avocado (Persea americana) pulp improves cardiovascular and autonomic recovery following submaximal running: a crossover, randomized, double-blind and placebo-controlled trial. Sci Rep. 2020;10:10703. https://pubmed.ncbi.nlm.nih.gov/32612186/

129. Wang L, Tao L, Hao L, Stanley TH, Huang K-H, Lambert JD, et al. A moderate-fat diet with one avocado per day increases plasma antioxidants and decreases the oxidation of small, dense LDL in adults with overweight and obesity: a randomized controlled trial. J Nutr. 2020;150:276–84. https://pubmed.ncbi.nlm.nih.gov/31616932/

130. Park E, Edirisinghe I, Burton-Freeman B. Avocado fruit on postprandial markers of cardio-metabolic risk: a randomized controlled dose response trial in overweight and obese men and women. Nutrients. 2018;10. http://dx.doi.org/10.3390/nu10091287

131. Di Mascio P, Kaiser S, Sies H. Lycopene as the most efficient biological carotenoid singlet oxygen quencher. Arch Biochem Biophys. 1989;274:532–38. https://pubmed.ncbi.nlm.nih.gov/2802626/

132. Terao J, Minami Y, Bando N. Singlet molecular oxygen-quenching activity of carotenoids: relevance to protection of the skin from photoaging. J Clin Biochem Nutr. 2011;48:57–62. https://www.jstage.jst.go.jp/article/jcbn/48/1/48_11-008FR/_article

133. Rizwan M, Rodriguez-Blanco I, Harbottle A, Birch-Machin MA, Watson REB, Rhodes LE. Tomato paste rich in lycopene protects against cutaneous photodamage in humans in vivo: a randomized controlled trial. Br J Dermatol. 2011;164:154–62. https://pubmed.ncbi.nlm.nih.gov/20854436/

134. Aust O, Stahl W, Sies H, Tronnier H, Heinrich U. Supplementation with tomato-based products increases lycopene, phytofluene, and phytoene levels in human serum and protects against UV-light-induced erythema. Int J Vitam Nutr Res. 2005;75:54–60. https://pubmed.ncbi.nlm.nih.gov/15830922/

135. Sokoloski L, Borges M, Bagatin E. Lycopene not in pill, nor in natura has photoprotective systemic effect. Arch Dermatol Res. 2015;307:545–49. https://pubmed.ncbi.nlm.nih.gov/26024575/

136. Aust. Supplementation with tomato-based products increases lycopene.

137. Engelmann NJ, Clinton SK, Erdman JW Jr. Nutritional aspects of phytoene and phytofluene, carotenoid precursors to lycopene. Adv Nutr. 2011;2:51–61. https://pubmed.ncbi.nlm.nih.gov/22211189/

138. Li N, Wu X, Zhuang W, Xia L, Chen Y, Wu C, et al. Tomato and lycopene and multiple health outcomes: umbrella review. Food Chem. 2021;343:128396. https://pubmed.ncbi.nlm.nih.gov/33131949/

139. Li H, Chen A, Zhao L, Bhagavathula AS, Amirthalingam P, Rahmani J, et al. Effect of tomato consumption on fasting blood glucose and lipid profiles: a systematic review and meta-analysis of randomized controlled trials. Phytother Res. 2020;34:1956–65. https://ur.booksc.eu/book/81562647/c24dd6

140. Rowles JL 3rd, Ranard KM, Applegate CC, Jeon S, An R, Erdman JW Jr. Processed and raw tomato consumption and risk of prostate cancer: a systematic review and dose-response meta-analysis. Prostate Cancer Prostatic Dis. 2018;21:319–36. https://pubmed.ncbi.nlm.nih.gov/29317772/

141. Rowles JL 3rd, Ranard KM, Smith JW, An R, Erdman JW Jr. Increased dietary and circulating lycopene are associated with reduced prostate cancer risk: a systematic review and meta-analysis. Prostate Cancer Prostatic Dis. 2017;20:361–77. https://pubmed.ncbi.nlm.nih.gov/28440323/

142. Lundberg JO, Weitzberg E, Gladwin MT. The nitrate-nitrite-nitric oxide pathway in physiology and therapeutics. Nat Rev Drug Discov. 2008;7:156–67. https://pubmed.ncbi.nlm.nih.gov/18167491/

143. Moncada S, Palmer RM, Higgs EA. Nitric oxide: physiology, pathophysiology, and pharmacology. Pharmacol Rev. 1991;43:109–42. https://pubmed.ncbi .nlm.nih.gov/1852778/

144. Bondonno CP, Croft KD, Hodgson JM. Dietary nitrate, nitric oxide, and cardiovascular health. Crit Rev Food Sci Nutr. 2016;56:2036–52. https:// pubmed.ncbi.nlm.nih.gov/25976309/

145. Hord NG, Tang Y, Bryan NS. Food sources of nitrates and nitrites: the physiologic context for potential health benefits. Am J Clin Nutr. 2009;90:1–10. https://pubmed.ncbi.nlm.nih.gov/19439460/

146. McMahon NF, Leveritt MD, Pavey TG. The effect of dietary·nitrate supplementation on endurance exercise performance in healthy adults: a systematic review and meta-analysis. Sports Med. 2017;47:735–56. https:// pubmed.ncbi.nlm.nih.gov/27600147/

147. Chang ST, Wasser SP. The role of culinary-medicinal mushrooms on human welfare with a pyramid model for human health. Int J Med Mushrooms. 2012;14:95–134. https://pubmed.ncbi.nlm.nih.gov/22506573/

148. Valverde ME, Hernández-Pérez T, Paredes-López O. Edible mushrooms: improving human health and promoting quality life. Int J Microbiol. 2015;2015:376387. https://pubmed.ncbi.nlm.nih.gov/25685150/

149. Jayachandran M, Xiao J, Xu B. A critical review on health promoting benefits of edible mushrooms through gut microbiota. Int J Mol Sci. 2017;18. http:// dx.doi.org/10.3390/ijms18091934

150. Volman JJ, Mensink RP, van Griensven LJLD, Plat J. Effects of alpha-glucans from Agaricus bisporus on ex vivo cytokine production by LPS and PHA-stimulated PBMCs; a placebo-controlled study in slightly hypercholesterolemic subjects. Eur J Clin Nutr. 2010;64:720–26. https:// pubmed.ncbi.nlm.nih.gov/20197785/

151. Jeong SC, Koyyalamudi SR, Pang G. Dietary intake of Agaricus bisporus white button mushroom accelerates salivary immunoglobulin A secretion in healthy volunteers. Nutrition. 2012;28:527–31. https://pubmed.ncbi.nlm .nih.gov/22113068/

152. Varshney J, Ooi JH, Jayarao BM, Albert I, Fisher J, Smith RL, et al. White button mushrooms increase microbial diversity and accelerate the resolution of Citrobacter rodentium infection in mice. J Nutr. 2013;143:526–32. https:// pubmed.ncbi.nlm.nih.gov/23343678/

153. Wu D, Pae M, Ren Z, Guo Z, Smith D, Meydani SN. Dietary supplementation with white button mushroom enhances natural killer cell activity in C57BL/6 mice. J Nutr. 2007;137:1472–77. https://pubmed.ncbi.nlm.nih.gov/ 17513409/

154. Jesenak M, Hrubisko M, Majtan J, Rennerova Z, Banovcin P. Anti-allergic effect of Pleuran (β-glucan from Pleurotus ostreatus) in children with recurrent respiratory tract infections. Phytother Res. 2014;28:471–74. https:// pubmed.ncbi.nlm.nih.gov/23744488/

155. Bergendiova K, Tibenska E, Majtan J. Pleuran (β-glucan from Pleurotus ostreatus) supplementation, cellular immune response and respiratory tract infections in athletes. Eur J Appl Physiol. 2011;111:2033–40. https:// pubmed.ncbi.nlm.nih.gov/21249381/

156. Bobovčák M, Kuniaková R, Gabriž J, Majtán J. Effect of Pleuran (β-glucan from Pleurotus ostreatus) supplementation on cellular immune response after intensive exercise in elite athletes. Appl Physiol Nutr Metab. 2010;35:755–62. https://pubmed.ncbi.nlm.nih.gov/21164546/

157. Ofek I, Pruzzo C, Spratt D. Functional foods: towards improving oral health. J Biomed Biotechnol. 2012;2012:618314. https://www.hindawi.com/journals/bmri/2012/618314/

158. Dai X, Stanilka JM, Rowe CA, Esteves EA, Nieves C Jr, Spaiser SJ, et al. Consuming lentinula edodes (shiitake) mushrooms daily improves human immunity: a randomized dietary intervention in healthy young adults. J Am Coll Nutr. 2015;34:478–87. https://pubmed.ncbi.nlm.nih.gov/25866155/

159. Mugnai C, Sossidou EN, Dal Bosco A, Ruggeri S, Mattioli S, Castellini C. The effects of husbandry system on the grass intake and egg nutritive characteristics of laying hens. J Sci Food Agric. 2014;94:459–67. https://pubmed.ncbi.nlm.nih.gov/23775487/

160. Ibid.

161. Lopez-Bote CJ, Sanz Arias R, Rey AI, Castaño A, Isabel B, Thos J. Effect of free-range feeding on n–3 fatty acid and α-tocopherol content and oxidative stability of eggs. Anim Feed Sci Technol. 1998;72:33–40. http://www.centerforfoodsafety.org/files/lopez-bote-1998_32145.pdf

162. Mugnai. The effects of husbandry system.

163. Lopez-Bote. Effect of free-range feeding on n–3 fatty acid.

164. Saito H, Cherasse Y, Suzuki R, Mitarai M, Ueda F, Urade Y. Zinc-rich oysters as well as zinc-yeast- and astaxanthin-enriched food improved sleep efficiency and sleep onset in a randomized controlled trial of healthy individuals. Mol Nutr Food Res. 2017;61. http://dx.doi.org/10.1002/mnfr.201600882

165. Ho HVT, Sievenpiper JL, Zurbau A, Blanco Mejia S, Jovanovski E, Au-Yeung F, et al. The effect of oat β-glucan on LDL-cholesterol, non-HDL-cholesterol and apoB for CVD risk reduction: a systematic review and meta-analysis of randomised-controlled trials. Br J Nutr. 2016;116:1369–82. https://pubmed.ncbi.nlm.nih.gov/27724985/

166. Bao L, Cai X, Xu M, Li Y. Effect of oat intake on glycaemic control and insulin sensitivity: a meta-analysis of randomised controlled trials. Br J Nutr. 2014;112:457–66. https://pubmed.ncbi.nlm.nih.gov/24787712/

167. Shen XL, Zhao T, Zhou Y, Shi X, Zou Y, Zhao G. Effect of oat β-glucan intake on glycaemic control and insulin sensitivity of diabetic patients: a meta-analysis of randomized controlled trials. Nutrients. 2016;8. http://dx.doi.org/10.3390/nu8010039

168. Musa-Veloso K, Noori D, Venditti C, Poon T, Johnson J, Harkness LS, et al. A systematic review and meta-analysis of randomized controlled trials on the effects of oats and oat processing on postprandial blood glucose and insulin responses. J Nutr. 2021;151:341–51. https://europepmc.org/article/med/33296453

169. Chen C-YO, Milbury PE, Collins FW, Blumberg JB. Avenanthramides are bioavailable and have antioxidant activity in humans after acute consumption of an enriched mixture from oats. J Nutr. 2007;137:1375–82. https://pubmed.ncbi.nlm.nih.gov/17513394/

170. Zhang T, Zhao T, Zhang Y, Liu T, Gagnon G, Ebrahim J, et al. Avenanthramide supplementation reduces eccentric exercise-induced inflammation in young men and women. J Int Soc Sports Nutr. 2020;17:41. https://pubmed.ncbi.nlm.nih.gov/32711519/

171. Koenig RT, Dickman JR, Kang C-H, Zhang T, Chu Y-F, Ji LL. Avenanthramide supplementation attenuates eccentric exercise-inflicted blood inflammatory markers in women. Eur J Appl Physiol. 2016;116:67–76. https://www.ncbi .nlm.nih.gov/pmc/articles/PMC7382060/

172. Koenig R, Dickman JR, Kang C, Zhang T, Chu Y-F, Ji LL. Avenanthramide supplementation attenuates exercise-induced inflammation in postmenopausal women. Nutr J. 2014;13:21. https://pubmed.ncbi.nlm.nih .gov/24645793/

173. Reverri EJ, Randolph JM, Steinberg FM, Kappagoda CT, Edirisinghe I, Burton-Freeman BM. Black beans, fiber, and antioxidant capacity pilot study: examination of whole foods vs. functional components on postprandial metabolic, oxidative stress, and inflammation in adults with metabolic syndrome. Nutrients. 2015;7:6139–54. https://pubmed.ncbi.nlm.nih.gov/ 26225995/

174. Winham DM, Hutchins AM, Thompson SV. Glycemic response to black beans and chickpeas as part of a rice meal: a randomized cross-over trial. Nutrients. 2017;9. http://dx.doi.org/10.3390/nu9101095

175. Clark JL, Taylor CG, Zahradka P. Black beans and red kidney beans induce positive postprandial vascular responses in healthy adults: a pilot randomized cross-over study. Nutr Metab Cardiovasc Dis. 2021;31:216–26. https://pubmed.ncbi.nlm.nih.gov/32917495/

176. Li SS, Blanco Mejia S, Lytvyn L, Stewart SE, Viguiliouk E, Ha V, et al. Effect of plant protein on blood lipids: a systematic review and meta-analysis of randomized controlled trials. J Am Heart Assoc. 2017;6. http://dx.doi.org/ 10.1161/JAHA.117.006659

177. Liu XX, Li SH, Chen JZ, Sun K, Wang XJ, Wang XG, et al. Effect of soy isoflavones on blood pressure: a meta-analysis of randomized controlled trials. Nutr Metab Cardiovasc Dis. 2012;22:463–70. https://pubmed.ncbi .nlm.nih.gov/21310599/

178. Dong J-Y, Tong X, Wu Z-W, Xun P-C, He K, Qin L-Q. Effect of soya protein on blood pressure: a meta-analysis of randomised controlled trials. Br J Nutr. 2011;106:317–26. https://pubmed.ncbi.nlm.nih.gov/21342608/

179. Beavers DP, Beavers KM, Miller M, Stamey J, Messina MJ. Exposure to isoflavone-containing soy products and endothelial function: a Bayesian meta-analysis of randomized controlled trials. Nutr Metab Cardiovasc Dis. 2012;22:182–91. https://pubmed.ncbi.nlm.nih.gov/20709515/

180. Yan Z, Zhang X, Li C, Jiao S, Dong W. Association between consumption of soy and risk of cardiovascular disease: a meta-analysis of observational studies. Eur J Prev Cardiol. 2017;24:735–47. https://pubmed.ncbi.nlm.nih .gov/28067550/

Chapter 8

1. Misner B. Food alone may not provide sufficient micronutrients for preventing deficiency. J Int Soc Sports Nutr. 2006;3:51–55. https://www.ncbi.nlm.nih.gov/pmc/articles/PMC2129155/

2. Calton JB. Prevalence of micronutrient deficiency in popular diet plans. J Int Soc Sports Nutr. 2010;7:24. https://pubmed.ncbi.nlm.nih.gov/20537171/

3. Fulgoni VL 3rd, Keast DR, Bailey RL, Dwyer J. Foods, fortificants, and supplements: where do Americans get their nutrients? J Nutr. 2011;141:1847–54. https://pubmed.ncbi.nlm.nih.gov/21865568/

4. Bird JK, Murphy RA, Ciappio ED, McBurney MI. Risk of deficiency in multiple concurrent micronutrients in children and adults in the United States. Nutrients. 2017;9. http://dx.doi.org/10.3390/nu9070655

5. Tardy A-L, Pouteau E, Marquez D, Yilmaz C, Scholey A. Vitamins and minerals for energy, fatigue and cognition: a narrative review of the biochemical and clinical evidence. Nutrients. 2020;12. http://dx.doi.org/10.3390/nu12010228

6. Macpherson H, Pipingas A, Pase MP. Multivitamin-multimineral supplementation and mortality: a meta-analysis of randomized controlled trials. Am J Clin Nutr. 2013;97:437–44. https://www.ncbi.nlm.nih.gov/books/NBK126994/

7. Maric D, Brkic S, Tomic S, Novakov Mikic A, Cebovic T, Turkulov V. Multivitamin mineral supplementation in patients with chronic fatigue syndrome. Med Sci Monit. 2014;20:47–53. https://pubmed.ncbi.nlm.nih.gov/24419360/

8. Zingg J-M. Molecular and cellular activities of vitamin E analogues. Mini Rev Med Chem. 2007;7:543–58. https://pubmed.ncbi.nlm.nih.gov/17504191/

9. Russo P, Pala M, Parodi S, Ghiara C, Ferrari N, Vidali G. Effects of vitamin E on liver DNA. Cancer Lett. 1984;25:163–70. https://pubmed.ncbi.nlm.nih.gov/6509435/

10. Klein EA, Thompson IM Jr, Tangen CM, Crowley JJ, Lucia MS, Goodman PJ, et al. Vitamin E and the risk of prostate cancer: the selenium and vitamin E cancer prevention trial (SELECT). JAMA. 2011;306:1549–56. https://pubmed.ncbi.nlm.nih.gov/21990298/

11. Kuo H-K, Sorond FA, Chen J-H, Hashmi A, Milberg WP, Lipsitz LA. The role of homocysteine in multisystem age-related problems: a systematic review. J Gerontol A Biol Sci Med Sci. 2005;60:1190–201. https://academic.oup.com/biomedgerontology/article/60/9/1190/560525

12. Regland B, Andersson M, Abrahamsson L, Bagby J, Dyrehag LE, Gottfries CG. Increased concentrations of homocysteine in the cerebrospinal fluid in patients with fibromyalgia and chronic fatigue syndrome. Scand J Rheumatol. 1997;26:301–7. https://pubmed.ncbi.nlm.nih.gov/9310111/

13. Smith AD, Refsum H, Bottiglieri T, Fenech M, Hooshmand B, McCaddon A, et al. Homocysteine and dementia: an international consensus statement. J Alzheimers Dis. 2018;62:561–70. https://pubmed.ncbi.nlm.nih.gov/29480200/

14. Zhou F, Chen S. Hyperhomocysteinemia and risk of incident cognitive outcomes: an updated dose-response meta-analysis of prospective cohort studies. Ageing Res Rev. 2019;51:55–66. https://pubmed.ncbi.nlm.nih.gov/30826501/

15. Weisberg I, Tran P, Christensen B, Sibani S, Rozen R. A second genetic polymorphism in methylenetetrahydrofolate reductase (MTHFR) associated with decreased enzyme activity. Mol Genet Metab. 1998;64:169–72. https://pubmed.ncbi.nlm.nih.gov/9719624/

16. van der Put NM, Gabreëls F, Stevens EM, Smeitink JA, Trijbels FJ, Eskes TK, et al. A second common mutation in the methylenetetrahydrofolate reductase gene: an additional risk factor for neural-tube defects? Am J Hum Genet. 1998;62:1044–51. https://pubmed.ncbi.nlm.nih.gov/9545395/

17. Chango A, Boisson F, Barbé F, Quilliot D, Droesch S, Pfister M, et al. The effect of 677C-->T and 1298A-->C mutations on plasma homocysteine and 5,10-methylenetetrahydrofolate reductase activity in healthy subjects. Br J Nutr. 2000;83:593–96. https://pubmed.ncbi.nlm.nih.gov/10911766/

18. Gorelova V, Ambach L, Rébeillé F, Stove C, Van Der Straeten D. Folates in plants: research advances and progress in crop biofortification. Front Chem. 2017;5:21. https://pubmed.ncbi.nlm.nih.gov/28424769/

19. Paul C, Brady DM. Comparative bioavailability and utilization of particular forms of B_{12} supplements with potential to mitigate B12-related genetic polymorphisms. Integr Med. 2017;16:42–49. https://pubmed.ncbi.nlm.nih.gov/28223907/

20. Okuda K, Yashima K, Kitazaki T, Takara I. Intestinal absorption and concurrent chemical changes of methylcobalamin. J Lab Clin Med. 1973;81:557–67. https://pubmed.ncbi.nlm.nih.gov/4696188/

21. Chalmers JN, Shinton NK. Comparison of hydroxocobalamin and cyanocobalamin in the treatment of pernicious anaemia. Lancet. 1965;2:1305–8. https://pubmed.ncbi.nlm.nih.gov/4165301/

22. Nicolson GL, Ash ME. Lipid replacement therapy: a natural medicine approach to replacing damaged lipids in cellular membranes and organelles and restoring function. Biochim Biophys Acta. 2014;1838:1657–79. https://pubmed.ncbi.nlm.nih.gov/24269541/

23. Ibid.

24. Agadjanyan M, Vasilevko V, Ghochikyan A, Berns P, Kesslak P, Settineri RA, et al. Nutritional supplement (NT FactorTM) restores mitochondrial function and reduces moderately severe fatigue in aged subjects. J Chronic Fatigue Syndr. Taylor & Francis; 2003;11:23–36. https://www.tandfonline.com/doi/abs/10.1300/J092v11n03_03

25. Nicolson GL, Rosenblatt S, de Mattos GF, Settineri R, Breeding PC, Ellithorpe RR, et al. Clinical uses of membrane lipid replacement supplements in restoring membrane function and reducing fatigue in chronic diseases and cancer. Discoveries (Craiova). 2016;4:e54. https://pubmed.ncbi.nlm.nih.gov/32309576/

26. Dahash BA, Sankararaman S. *Carnitine Deficiency*. StatPearls. (Treasure Island, FL: StatPearls Publishing, 2020). https://www.ncbi.nlm.nih.gov/books/NBK559041/

27. Filler K, Lyon D, Bennett J, McCain N, Elswick R, Lukkahatai N, et al. Association of mitochondrial dysfunction and fatigue: a review of the literature. BBA Clin. 2014;1:12–23. https://pubmed.ncbi.nlm.nih.gov/25147756/

28. Malaguarnera M, Gargante MP, Cristaldi E, Colonna V, Messano M, Koverech A, et al. Acetyl L-carnitine (ALC) treatment in elderly patients with fatigue. Arch Gerontol Geriatr. 2008;46:181–90. https://pubmed.ncbi.nlm.nih.gov/17658628/

29. Aliev G, Liu J, Shenk JC, Fischbach K, Pacheco GJ, Chen SG, et al. Neuronal mitochondrial amelioration by feeding acetyl-L-carnitine and lipoic acid to aged rats. J Cell Mol Med. 2009;13:320–33. https://www.ncbi.nlm.nih.gov/pmc/articles/PMC2790425/

30. Nicassio L, Fracasso F, Sirago G, Musicco C, Picca A, Marzetti E, et al. Dietary supplementation with acetyl-l-carnitine counteracts age-related alterations of mitochondrial biogenesis, dynamics and antioxidant defenses in brain of old rats. Exp Gerontol. 2017;98:99–109. https://www.sciencedirect.com/science/article/abs/pii/S0531556517304849?via%3Dihub

31. Kobayashi S, Iwamoto M, Kon K, Waki H, Ando S, Tanaka Y. Acetyl-L-carnitine improves aged brain function. Geriatr Gerontol Int. 2010;10 Suppl 1:S99–106. https://pubmed.ncbi.nlm.nih.gov/20590847/

32. Imperato A, Ramacci MT, Angelucci L. Acetyl-L-carnitine enhances acetylcholine release in the striatum and hippocampus of awake freely moving rats. Neurosci Lett. 1989;107:251–55. https://pubmed.ncbi.nlm.nih.gov/2616037/

33. Smeland OB, Meisingset TW, Borges K, Sonnewald U. Chronic acetyl-L-carnitine alters brain energy metabolism and increases noradrenaline and serotonin content in healthy mice. Neurochem Int. 2012;61:100–7. https://pubmed.ncbi.nlm.nih.gov/22549035/

34. Dhitavat S, Ortiz D, Shea TB, Rivera ER. Acetyl-L-carnitine protects against amyloid-beta neurotoxicity: roles of oxidative buffering and ATP levels. Neurochem Res. 2002;27:501–5. https://pubmed.ncbi.nlm.nih.gov/12199155/

35. Liu J, Head E, Kuratsune H, Cotman CW, Ames BN. Comparison of the effects of L-carnitine and acetyl-L-carnitine on carnitine levels, ambulatory activity, and oxidative stress biomarkers in the brain of old rats. Ann N Y Acad Sci. 2004;1033:117–31. https://pubmed.ncbi.nlm.nih.gov/15591009/

36. Pennisi M, Lanza G, Cantone M, D'Amico E, Fisicaro F, Puglisi V, et al. Acetyl-L-carnitine in dementia and other cognitive disorders: a critical update. Nutrients. 2020;12. http://dx.doi.org/10.3390/nu12051389

37. Montgomery SA, Thal LJ, Amrein R. Meta-analysis of double blind randomized controlled clinical trials of acetyl-L-carnitine versus placebo in the treatment of mild cognitive impairment and mild Alzheimer's disease. Int Clin Psychopharmacol. 2003;18:61–71. https://pubmed.ncbi.nlm.nih.gov/12598816/

38. Veronese N, Stubbs B, Solmi M, Ajnakina O, Carvalho AF, Maggi S. Acetyl-L-carnitine supplementation and the treatment of depressive symptoms: a systematic review and meta-analysis. Psychosom Med. 2018;80:154–59. https://pubmed.ncbi.nlm.nih.gov/29076953/

39. Dempsey RL, Mazzone MF, Meurer LN. Does oral creatine supplementation improve strength? A meta-analysis. J Fam Pract. 2002;51:945–51. https://pubmed.ncbi.nlm.nih.gov/12485548/

40. Branch JD. Effect of creatine supplementation on body composition and performance: a meta-analysis. Int J Sport Nutr Exerc Metab. 2003;13:198–226. https://pubmed.ncbi.nlm.nih.gov/12945830/

41. Lanhers C, Pereira B, Naughton G, Trousselard M, Lesage F-X, Dutheil F. Creatine supplementation and upper limb strength performance: a systematic review and meta-analysis. Sports Med. 2017;47:163–73. https://pubmed.ncbi.nlm.nih.gov/27328852/

42. Lanhers C, Pereira B, Naughton G, Trousselard M, Lesage F-X, Dutheil F. Creatine Supplementation and Lower Limb Strength Performance: A Systematic Review and Meta-Analyses. Sports Med. 2015;45:1285–94. https://pubmed.ncbi.nlm.nih.gov/25946994/

43. Chilibeck PD, Kaviani M, Candow DG, Zello GA. Effect of creatine supplementation during resistance training on lean tissue mass and muscular strength in older adults: a meta-analysis. Open Access J Sports Med. 2017;8:213–26. https://pubmed.ncbi.nlm.nih.gov/29138605/

44. Sestili P, Barbieri E, Martinelli C, Battistelli M, Guescini M, Vallorani L, et al. Creatine supplementation prevents the inhibition of myogenic differentiation in oxidatively injured C2C12 murine myoblasts. Mol Nutr Food Res. 2009;53:1187–204. https://pubmed.ncbi.nlm.nih.gov/19653222/

45. Sestili P, Barbieri E, Stocchi V. Effects of creatine in skeletal muscle cells and in myoblasts differentiating under normal or oxidatively stressing conditions. Mini Rev Med Chem. 2016;16:4–11. https://pubmed.ncbi.nlm.nih.gov/26202198/

46. Barbieri E, Guescini M, Calcabrini C, Vallorani L, Diaz AR, Fimognari C, et al. Creatine prevents the structural and functional damage to mitochondria in myogenic, oxidatively stressed C2C12 cells and restores their differentiation capacity. Oxid Med Cell Longev. 2016;2016:5152029. https://www.hindawi.com/journals/omcl/2016/5152029/

47. Walsh B, Tonkonogi M, Söderlund K, Hultman E, Saks V, Sahlin K. The role of phosphorylcreatine and creatine in the regulation of mitochondrial respiration in human skeletal muscle. J Physiol. 2001;537:971–78. https://www.ncbi.nlm.nih.gov/pmc/articles/PMC2278998/

48. Andres RH, Ducray AD, Schlattner U, Wallimann T, Widmer HR. Functions and effects of creatine in the central nervous system. Brain Res Bull. 2008;76:329–43. https://pubmed.ncbi.nlm.nih.gov/18502307/

49. Dechent P, Pouwels PJ, Wilken B, Hanefeld F, Frahm J. Increase of total creatine in human brain after oral supplementation of creatine-monohydrate. Am J Physiol. 1999;277:R698–704. https://pubmed.ncbi.nlm.nih.gov/10484486/

50. Lyoo IK, Kong SW, Sung SM, Hirashima F, Parow A, Hennen J, et al. Multinuclear magnetic resonance spectroscopy of high-energy phosphate metabolites in human brain following oral supplementation of creatine-monohydrate. Psychiatry Res. 2003;123:87–100. https://pubmed.ncbi.nlm.nih.gov/12850248/

51. Pan JW, Takahashi K. Cerebral energetic effects of creatine supplementation in humans. Am J Physiol Regul Integr Comp Physiol. 2007;292:R1745–50. https://pubmed.ncbi.nlm.nih.gov/17185404/

52. Klein AM, Ferrante RJ. The neuroprotective role of creatine. Subcell Biochem. 2007;46:205–43. https://pubmed.ncbi.nlm.nih.gov/18652079/

53. Huxtable RJ. Physiological actions of taurine. Physiol Rev. 1992;72:101–63. https://pubmed.ncbi.nlm.nih.gov/1731369/

54. Schaffer S, Kim HW. Effects and mechanisms of taurine as a therapeutic agent. Biomol Ther. 2018;26:225–41. https://www.ncbi.nlm.nih.gov/pmc/articles/PMC5933890/

55. Ripps H, Shen W. Review: taurine: a "very essential" amino acid. Mol Vis. 2012;18:2673–86. https://pubmed.ncbi.nlm.nih.gov/23170060/

56. Hansen SH, Andersen ML, Birkedal H, Cornett C, Wibrand F. The important role of taurine in oxidative metabolism. Adv Exp Med Biol. 2006;583:129–35. https://pubmed.ncbi.nlm.nih.gov/17153596/

57. Jong CJ, Azuma J, Schaffer S. Mechanism underlying the antioxidant activity of taurine: prevention of mitochondrial oxidant production. Amino Acids. 2012;42:2223–32. https://pubmed.ncbi.nlm.nih.gov/21691752/

58. Maleki V, Mahdavi R, Hajizadeh-Sharafabad F, Alizadeh M. The effects of taurine supplementation on oxidative stress indices and inflammation biomarkers in patients with type 2 diabetes: a randomized, double-blind, placebo-controlled trial. Diabetol Metab Syndr. 2020;12:9. https://pubmed.ncbi.nlm.nih.gov/32015761/

59. Rosa FT, Freitas EC, Deminice R, Jordão AA, Marchini JS. Oxidative stress and inflammation in obesity after taurine supplementation: a double-blind, placebo-controlled study. Eur J Nutr. 2014;53:823–30. https://pubmed.ncbi.nlm.nih.gov/24065043/

60. Xiao C, Giacca A, Lewis GF. Oral taurine but not N-acetylcysteine ameliorates NEFA-induced impairment in insulin sensitivity and beta cell function in obese and overweight, non-diabetic men. Diabetologia. 2008;51:139–46. https://pubmed.ncbi.nlm.nih.gov/18026714/

61. Waldron M, Patterson SD, Tallent J, Jeffries O. The effects of an oral taurine dose and supplementation period on endurance exercise performance in humans: a meta-analysis. Sports Med. 2018;48:1247–53. https://pubmed.ncbi.nlm.nih.gov/29546641/

62. Guerin M, Huntley ME, Olaizola M. *Haematococcus* astaxanthin: applications for human health and nutrition. Trends Biotechnol. 2003;21:210–16. https://pubmed.ncbi.nlm.nih.gov/12727382/

63. Wolf AM, Asoh S, Hiranuma H, Ohsawa I, Iio K, Satou A, et al. Astaxanthin protects mitochondrial redox state and functional integrity against oxidative stress. J Nutr Biochem. 2010;21:381–89. https://pubmed.ncbi.nlm.nih.gov/19423317/

64. Yu T, Dohl J, Chen Y, Gasier HG, Deuster PA. Astaxanthin but not quercetin preserves mitochondrial integrity and function, ameliorates oxidative stress, and reduces heat-induced skeletal muscle injury. J Cell Physiol. 2019;234:13292–302. https://pubmed.ncbi.nlm.nih.gov/30609021/

65. Krestinina O, Baburina Y, Krestinin R, Odinokova I, Fadeeva I, Sotnikova L. Astaxanthin prevents mitochondrial impairment induced by isoproterenol in isolated rat heart mitochondria. Antioxidants (Basel). 2020;9. http://dx.doi .org/10.3390/antiox9030262

66. Kim SH, Kim H. Inhibitory effect of astaxanthin on oxidative stress-induced mitochondrial dysfunction—a mini-review. Nutrients. 2018;10. http:// dx.doi.org/10.3390/nu10091137

67. Park JS, Mathison BD, Hayek MG, Zhang J, Reinhart GA, Chew BP. Astaxanthin modulates age-associated mitochondrial dysfunction in healthy dogs. J Anim Sci. 2013;91:268–75. https://pubmed.ncbi.nlm.nih.gov/ 23100599/

68. Sztretye M, Dienes B, Gönczi M, Czirják T, Csernoch L, Dux L, et al. Astaxanthin: a potential mitochondrial-targeted antioxidant treatment in diseases and with aging. Oxid Med Cell Longev. 2019;2019:3849692. https:// pubmed.ncbi.nlm.nih.gov/31814873/

69. Choi HD, Kim JH, Chang MJ, Kyu-Youn Y, Shin WG. Effects of astaxanthin on oxidative stress in overweight and obese adults. Phytother Res. 2011;25:1813–8. https://pubmed.ncbi.nlm.nih.gov/21480416/

70. Liu SZ, Ali AS, Campbell MD, Kilroy K, Shankland EG, Roshanravan B, et al. Building strength, endurance, and mobility using an astaxanthin formulation with functional training in elderly. J Cachexia Sarcopenia Muscle. 2018;9:826–33. https://pubmed.ncbi.nlm.nih.gov/30259703/

71. Malmsten CL, Lignell A. Dietary supplementation with astaxanthin-rich algal meal improves strength endurance—a double blind placebo controlled study on male students. Carotenoid Sci. 2008;13:20–22. https://www .alifenutrition.cz/userfiles/dietary-supplementation-with-astaxanthin-rich -algal-meal-improves-strength-endurance.pdf

72. Fleischmann C, Horowitz M, Yanovich R, Raz H, Heled Y. Asthaxanthin improves aerobic exercise recovery without affecting heat tolerance in humans. Front Sports Act Living. 2019;1:17. https://pubmed.ncbi.nlm.nih .gov/33344941/

73. Djordjevic B, Baralic I, Kotur-Stevuljevic J, Stefanovic A, Ivanisevic J, Radivojevic N, et al. Effect of astaxanthin supplementation on muscle damage and oxidative stress markers in elite young soccer players. J Sports Med Phys Fitness. 2012;52:382–92. https://pubmed.ncbi.nlm.nih .gov/22828460/

74. Shay KP, Moreau RF, Smith EJ, Smith AR, Hagen TM. Alpha-lipoic acid as a dietary supplement: molecular mechanisms and therapeutic potential. Biochim Biophys Acta. 2009;1790:1149–60. https://pubmed.ncbi.nlm.nih .gov/19664690/

75. Savitha S, Sivarajan K, Haripriya D, Kokilavani V, Panneerselvam C. Efficacy of levo carnitine and alpha lipoic acid in ameliorating the decline in mitochondrial enzymes during aging. Clin Nutr. 2005;24:794–800. https://pubmed.ncbi.nlm.nih.gov/15919137/

76. Long J, Gao F, Tong L, Cotman CW, Ames BN, Liu J. Mitochondrial decay in the brains of old rats: ameliorating effect of alpha-lipoic acid and acetyl-L-carnitine. Neurochem Res. 2009;34:755–63. https://europepmc.org/article/PMC/2790461

77. Liu J, Killilea DW, Ames BN. Age-associated mitochondrial oxidative decay: improvement of carnitine acetyltransferase substrate-binding affinity and activity in brain by feeding old rats acetyl-L-carnitine and/or R-α-lipoic acid. Proc Natl Acad Sci U S A. 2002;99:1876–81. https://www.ncbi.nlm.nih.gov/pmc/articles/PMC122287/

78. Liu J. The effects and mechanisms of mitochondrial nutrient alpha-lipoic acid on improving age-associated mitochondrial and cognitive dysfunction: an overview. Neurochem Res. 2008;33:194–203. https://pubmed.ncbi.nlm.nih.gov/17605107/

79. Dos Santos SM, Romeiro CFR, Rodrigues CA, Cerqueira ARL, Monteiro MC. Mitochondrial dysfunction and alpha-lipoic acid: beneficial or harmful in Alzheimer's disease? Oxid Med Cell Longev. 2019;2019:8409329. https://pubmed.ncbi.nlm.nih.gov/31885820/

80. Panigrahi M, Sadguna Y, Shivakumar BR, Kolluri SV, Roy S, Packer L, et al. Alpha-lipoic acid protects against reperfusion injury following cerebral ischemia in rats. Brain Res. 1996;717:184–88. https://pubmed.ncbi.nlm.nih.gov/8738270/

81. Arivazhagan P, Shila S, Kumaran S, Panneerselvam C. Effect of DL-alpha-lipoic acid on the status of lipid peroxidation and antioxidant enzymes in various brain regions of aged rats. Exp Gerontol. 2002;37:803–11. https://pubmed.ncbi.nlm.nih.gov/12175480/

82. Zhang L, Xing GQ, Barker JL, Chang Y, Maric D, Ma W, et al. Alpha-lipoic acid protects rat cortical neurons against cell death induced by amyloid and hydrogen peroxide through the Akt signalling pathway. Neurosci Lett. 2001;312:125–28. https://pubmed.ncbi.nlm.nih.gov/11602326/

83. Shinto L, Quinn J, Montine T, Dodge HH, Woodward W, Baldauf-Wagner S, et al. A randomized placebo-controlled pilot trial of omega-3 fatty acids and alpha lipoic acid in Alzheimer's disease. J Alzheimers Dis. 2014;38:111–20. https://pubmed.ncbi.nlm.nih.gov/24077434/

84. Pershadsingh HA. Alpha-lipoic acid: physiologic mechanisms and indications for the treatment of metabolic syndrome. Expert Opin Investig Drugs. 2007;16:291–302. https://pubmed.ncbi.nlm.nih.gov/17302524/

85. Chen W-L, Kang C-H, Wang S-G, Lee H-M. α-lipoic acid regulates lipid metabolism through induction of sirtuin 1 (SIRT1) and activation of AMP-activated protein kinase. Diabetologia. 2012;55:1824–35. https://pubmed.ncbi.nlm.nih.gov/22456698/

86. Carbonelli MG, Di Renzo L, Bigioni M, Di Daniele N, De Lorenzo A, Fusco MA. Alpha-lipoic acid supplementation: a tool for obesity therapy? Curr Pharm Des. 2010;16:840–46. https://pubmed.ncbi.nlm.nih.gov/20388095/

87. Koh EH, Lee WJ, Lee SA, Kim EH, Cho EH, Jeong E, et al. Effects of alpha-lipoic acid on body weight in obese subjects. Am J Med. 2011;124:85.e1–8. https://pubmed.ncbi.nlm.nih.gov/21187189/

88. Li N, Yan W, Hu X, Huang Y, Wang F, Zhang W, et al. Effects of oral α-lipoic acid administration on body weight in overweight or obese subjects: a crossover randomized, double-blind, placebo-controlled trial. Clin Endocrinol. 2017;86:680–87. https://pubmed.ncbi.nlm.nih.gov/28239907/

89. Conley BA, Egorin MJ, Tait N, Rosen DM, Sausville EA, Dover G, et al. Phase I study of the orally administered butyrate prodrug, tributyrin, in patients with solid tumors. Clin Cancer Res. 1998;4:629–34. https://pubmed.ncbi .nlm.nih.gov/9533530/

90. Edelman MJ, Bauer K, Khanwani S, Tait N, Trepel J, Karp J, et al. Clinical and pharmacologic study of tributyrin: an oral butyrate prodrug. Cancer Chemother Pharmacol. 2003;51:439–44. https://pubmed.ncbi.nlm.nih .gov/12736763/

91. Miyoshi M, Sakaki H, Usami M, Iizuka N, Shuno K, Aoyama M, et al. Oral administration of tributyrin increases concentration of butyrate in the portal vein and prevents lipopolysaccharide-induced liver injury in rats. Clin Nutr. 2011;30:252–8. https://pubmed.ncbi.nlm.nih.gov/21051124/

92. Cresci GA, Glueck B, McMullen MR, Xin W, Allende D, Nagy LE. Prophylactic tributyrin treatment mitigates chronic-binge ethanol-induced intestinal barrier and liver injury. J Gastroenterol Hepatol. 2017;32:1587–97. https://pubmed.ncbi.nlm.nih.gov/28087985/

93. Vinolo MAR, Rodrigues HG, Festuccia WT, Crisma AR, Alves VS, Martins AR, et al. Tributyrin attenuates obesity-associated inflammation and insulin resistance in high-fat-fed mice. Am J Physiol Endocrinol Metab. 2012;303:E272–82. https://pubmed.ncbi.nlm.nih.gov/22621868/

94. Wang C, Cao S, Shen Z, Hong Q, Feng J, Peng Y, et al. Effects of dietary tributyrin on intestinal mucosa development, mitochondrial function and AMPK-mTOR pathway in weaned pigs. J Anim Sci Biotechnol. 2019;10:93. https://jasbsci.biomedcentral.com/articles/10.1186/s40104-019-0394-x

95. Murray RL, Zhang W, Iwaniuk M, Grilli E, Stahl CH. Dietary tributyrin, an HDAC inhibitor, promotes muscle growth through enhanced terminal differentiation of satellite cells. Physiol Rep. 2018;6:e13706. https://www .ncbi.nlm.nih.gov/pmc/articles/PMC5974723/

96. Szentirmai É, Millican NS, Massie AR, Kapás L. Butyrate, a metabolite of intestinal bacteria, enhances sleep. Sci Rep. 2019;9:7035. https://www .nature.com/articles/s41598-019-43502-1

97. Bourassa MW, Alim I, Bultman SJ, Ratan RR. Butyrate, neuroepigenetics and the gut microbiome: can a high fiber diet improve brain health? Neurosci Lett. 2016;625:56–63. https://pubmed.ncbi.nlm.nih.gov/26868600/

98. Filler K, Lyon D, Bennett J, McCain N, Elswick R, Lukkahatai N, et al. Association of mitochondrial dysfunction and fatigue: a review of the literature. BBA Clin. 2014;1:12–23. https://pubmed.ncbi.nlm.nih.gov/25147756/

99. Cordero MD, Moreno-Fernández AM, deMiguel M, Bonal P, Campa F, Jiménez-Jiménez LM, et al. Coenzyme Q10 distribution in blood is altered in patients with fibromyalgia. Clin Biochem. 2009;42:732–35. https://pubmed.ncbi.nlm.nih.gov/19133251/

100. Di Pierro F, Rossi A, Consensi A, Giacomelli C, Bazzichi L. Role for a water-soluble form of CoQ10 in female subjects affected by fibromyalgia. A preliminary study. Clin Exp Rheumatol. 2017;35 Suppl 105:20–27. https://pubmed.ncbi.nlm.nih.gov/27974102/

101. Cordero MD, Alcocer-Gómez E, de Miguel M, Culic O, Carrión AM, Alvarez-Suarez JM, et al. Can coenzyme q10 improve clinical and molecular parameters in fibromyalgia? Antioxid Redox Signal. 2013;19:1356–61. https://pubmed.ncbi.nlm.nih.gov/23458405/

102. Jafari M, Mousavi SM, Asgharzadeh A, Yazdani N. Coenzyme Q10 in the treatment of heart failure: A systematic review of systematic reviews. Indian Heart J. 2018;70 Suppl 1:S111–17. https://pubmed.ncbi.nlm.nih.gov/30122240/

103. DiNicolantonio JJ, Bhutani J, McCarty MF, O'Keefe JH. Coenzyme Q10 for the treatment of heart failure: a review of the literature. Open Heart. 2015;2:e000326. https://www.ncbi.nlm.nih.gov/pmc/articles/PMC4620231/

104. Sanoobar M, Dehghan P, Khalili M, Azimi A, Seifar F. Coenzyme Q10 as a treatment for fatigue and depression in multiple sclerosis patients: a double blind randomized clinical trial. Nutr Neurosci. 2016;19:138–43. https://pubmed.ncbi.nlm.nih.gov/25603363/

105. Sanoobar M, Eghtesadi S, Azimi A, Khalili M, Khodadadi B, Jazayeri S, et al. Coenzyme Q10 supplementation ameliorates inflammatory markers in patients with multiple sclerosis: a double blind, placebo, controlled randomized clinical trial. Nutr Neurosci. 2015;18:169–76. https://pubmed.ncbi.nlm.nih.gov/24621064/

106. Castro-Marrero J, Cordero MD, Segundo MJ, Sáez-Francàs N, Calvo N, Román-Malo L, et al. Does oral coenzyme Q10 plus NADH supplementation improve fatigue and biochemical parameters in chronic fatigue syndrome? Antioxid Redox Signal. 2015;22:679–85. https://pubmed.ncbi.nlm.nih.gov/25386668/

107. Fukuda S, Nojima J, Kajimoto O, Yamaguti K, Nakatomi Y, Kuratsune H, et al. Ubiquinol-10 supplementation improves autonomic nervous function and cognitive function in chronic fatigue syndrome. Biofactors. 2016;42:431–40. https://pubmed.ncbi.nlm.nih.gov/27125909/

108. Mizuno K, Tanaka M, Nozaki S, Mizuma H, Ataka S, Tahara T, et al. Antifatigue effects of coenzyme Q10 during physical fatigue. Nutrition. 2008;24:293–99. https://pubmed.ncbi.nlm.nih.gov/18272335/

109. Castro-Marrero J, Sáez-Francàs N, Segundo MJ, Calvo N, Faro M, Aliste L, et al. Effect of coenzyme Q10 plus nicotinamide adenine dinucleotide supplementation on maximum heart rate after exercise testing in chronic fatigue syndrome—a randomized, controlled, double-blind trial. Clin Nutr. 2016;35:826–34. https://pubmed.ncbi.nlm.nih.gov/26212172/

110. Mizuno K, Sasaki AT, Watanabe K, Watanabe Y. Ubiquinol-10 intake is effective in relieving mild fatigue in healthy individuals. Nutrients. 2020;12. http://dx.doi.org/10.3390/nu12061640

111. Sarmiento A, Diaz-Castro J, Pulido-Moran M, Moreno-Fernandez J, Kajarabille N, Chirosa I, et al. Short-term ubiquinol supplementation reduces oxidative stress associated with strenuous exercise in healthy adults: a randomized trial. Biofactors. 2016;42:612–22. https://pubmed.ncbi.nlm.nih.gov/27193497/

112. Soto-Urquieta MG, López-Briones S, Pérez-Vázquez V, Saavedra-Molina A, González-Hernández GA, Ramírez-Emiliano J. Curcumin restores mitochondrial functions and decreases lipid peroxidation in liver and kidneys of diabetic db/db mice. Biol Res. 2014;47:74. https://pubmed.ncbi.nlm.nih.gov/25723052/

113. de Oliveira MR, Jardim FR, Setzer WN, Nabavi SM, Nabavi SF. Curcumin, mitochondrial biogenesis, and mitophagy: exploring recent data and indicating future needs. Biotechnol Adv. 2016;34:813–26. https://pubmed.ncbi.nlm.nih.gov/27143655/

114. Hewlings SJ, Kalman DS. Curcumin: a review of its effects on human health. Foods. 2017;6. http://dx.doi.org/10.3390/foods6100092

115. van Campen C (Linda) MC van C. The effect of curcumin in patients with chronic fatigue syndrome (or) myalgic encephalomyelitis disparate responses in different disease severities. Pharmacovigilance and Pharmacoepidemiology. Edelweiss Publications Inc; 2019;22–27. https://www.researchgate.net/publication/337628848_The_Effect_of_Curcumin_in_Patients_with_Chronic_Fatigue_Syndrome_or_Myalgic_Encephalomyelitis_Disparate_Responses_in_Different_Disease_Severities

116. van Campen C (linda) MC, Riepma K, Visser FC. The effect of curcumin on patients with chronic fatigue syndrome/myalgic encephalomyelitis: an open label study. IJCM. 2018;09:356–66. https://www.scirp.org/journal/paperinformation.aspx?paperid=84389

117. Suhett LG, de Miranda Monteiro Santos R, Silveira BKS, Leal ACG, de Brito ADM, de Novaes JF, et al. Effects of curcumin supplementation on sport and physical exercise: a systematic review. Crit Rev Food Sci Nutr. 2021;61:946–58. https://pubmed.ncbi.nlm.nih.gov/32282223/

118. Jamwal R. Bioavailable curcumin formulations: a review of pharmacokinetic studies in healthy volunteers. J Integr Med. 2018;16:367–74. https://pubmed.ncbi.nlm.nih.gov/30006023/

119. Pauly DF, Pepine CJ. D-Ribose as a supplement for cardiac energy metabolism. J Cardiovasc Pharmacol Ther. 2000;5:249–58. https://pubmed.ncbi.nlm.nih.gov/11150394/

120. Omran H, Illien S, MacCarter D, St Cyr J, Lüderitz B. D-Ribose improves diastolic function and quality of life in congestive heart failure patients: a prospective feasibility study. Eur J Heart Fail. 2003;5:615–19. https://pubmed .ncbi.nlm.nih.gov/14607200/

121. MacCarter D, Vijay N, Washam M, Shecterle L, Sierminski H, St Cyr JA. D-ribose aids advanced ischemic heart failure patients. Int J Cardiol. 2009;137:79–80. https://pubmed.ncbi.nlm.nih.gov/18674831/

122. Pliml W, von Arnim T, Stäblein A, Hofmann H, Zimmer HG, Erdmann E. Effects of ribose on exercise-induced ischaemia in stable coronary artery disease. Lancet. 1992;340:507–10. https://pubmed.ncbi.nlm.nih.gov/ 1354276/

123. Hellsten Y, Skadhauge L, Bangsbo J. Effect of ribose supplementation on resynthesis of adenine nucleotides after intense intermittent training in humans. Am J Physiol Regul Integr Comp Physiol. 2004;286:R182–88. https://pubmed.ncbi.nlm.nih.gov/14660478/

124. Seifert JG, Brumet A, St Cyr JA. The influence of D-ribose ingestion and fitness level on performance and recovery. J Int Soc Sports Nutr. 2017;14:47. https://pubmed.ncbi.nlm.nih.gov/29296106/

125. Teitelbaum JE, Johnson C, St Cyr J. The use of D-ribose in chronic fatigue syndrome and fibromyalgia: a pilot study. J Altern Complement Med. 2006;12:857–62. https://pubmed.ncbi.nlm.nih.gov/17109576/

126. Gebhart B, Jorgenson JA. Benefit of ribose in a patient with fibromyalgia. Pharmacotherapy. 2004;24:1646–48. https://pubmed.ncbi.nlm.nih.gov/ 15537568/

127. Alasbahi RH, Melzig MF. Forskolin and derivatives as tools for studying the role of cAMP. Pharmazie. 2012;67:5–13. https://pubmed.ncbi.nlm.nih.gov/ 22393824/

128. Zhang F, Zhang L, Qi Y, Xu H. Mitochondrial cAMP signaling. Cell Mol Life Sci. 2016;73:4577–90. https://www.ncbi.nlm.nih.gov/pmc/articles/ PMC5097110/

129. Henderson S, Magu B, Rasmussen C, Lancaster S, Kerksick C, Smith P, et al. Effects of coleus forskohlii supplementation on body composition and hematological profiles in mildly overweight women. J Int Soc Sports Nutr. 2005;2:54–62. https://pubmed.ncbi.nlm.nih.gov/18500958/

130. Godard MP, Johnson BA, Richmond SR. Body composition and hormonal adaptations associated with forskolin consumption in overweight and obese men. Obes Res. 2005;13:1335–43. https://pubmed.ncbi.nlm.nih.gov/ 16129715/

131. Loftus HL, Astell KJ, Mathai ML, Su XQ. Coleus forskohlii extract supplementation in conjunction with a hypocaloric diet reduces the risk factors of metabolic syndrome in overweight and obese subjects: a randomized controlled trial. Nutrients. 2015;7:9508–22. https://pubmed .ncbi.nlm.nih.gov/26593941/

132. Singhal K, Raj N, Gupta K, Singh S. Probable benefits of green tea with genetic implications. J Oral Maxillofac Pathol. 2017;21:107–14. https://www .ncbi.nlm.nih.gov/pmc/articles/PMC5406788/

133. Suzuki Y, Miyoshi N, Isemura M. Health-promoting effects of green tea. Proc Jpn Acad Ser B Phys Biol Sci. 2012;88:88–101. https://pubmed.ncbi.nlm.nih.gov/22450537/

134. Chacko SM, Thambi PT, Kuttan R, Nishigaki I. Beneficial effects of green tea: a literature review. Chin Med. 2010;5:13. https://www.ncbi.nlm.nih.gov/pmc/articles/PMC2855614/

135. Ortiz-López L, Márquez-Valadez B, Gómez-Sánchez A, Silva-Lucero MDC, Torres-Pérez M, Téllez-Ballesteros RI, et al. Green tea compound epigallo-catechin-3-gallate (EGCG) increases neuronal survival in adult hippocampal neurogenesis in vivo and in vitro. Neuroscience. 2016;322:208–20. https://pubmed.ncbi.nlm.nih.gov/26917271/

136. Pervin M, Unno K, Ohishi T, Tanabe H, Miyoshi N, Nakamura Y. Beneficial effects of green tea catechins on neurodegenerative diseases. Molecules. 2018;23. http://dx.doi.org/10.3390/molecules23061297

137. Babu PVA, Liu D. Green tea catechins and cardiovascular health: an update. Curr Med Chem. 2008;15:1840–50. https://pubmed.ncbi.nlm.nih.gov/18691042/

138. Bhardwaj P, Khanna D. Green tea catechins: defensive role in cardiovascular disorders. Chin J Nat Med. 2013;11:345–53. https://pubmed.ncbi.nlm.nih.gov/23845542/

139. Rains TM, Agarwal S, Maki KC. Antiobesity effects of green tea catechins: a mechanistic review. J Nutr Biochem. 2011;22:1–7. https://pubmed.ncbi.nlm.nih.gov/21115335/

140. Hursel R, Westerterp-Plantenga MS. Catechin- and caffeine-rich teas for control of body weight in humans. Am J Clin Nutr. 2013;98:1682S–93S. https://pubmed.ncbi.nlm.nih.gov/24172301/

141. Hursel R, Viechtbauer W, Westerterp-Plantenga MS. The effects of green tea on weight loss and weight maintenance: a meta-analysis. Int J Obes. 2009;33:956–61. https://pubmed.ncbi.nlm.nih.gov/19597519/

142. Cooper R, Morré DJ, Morré DM. Medicinal benefits of green tea: part II. Review of anticancer properties. J Altern Complement Med. 2005;11:639–52. https://pubmed.ncbi.nlm.nih.gov/16131288/

143. Lambert JD. Does tea prevent cancer? Evidence from laboratory and human intervention studies. Am J Clin Nutr. 2013;98:1667S–1675S. https://pubmed.ncbi.nlm.nih.gov/24172300/

144. Park J-H, Bae J-H, Im S-S, Song D-K. Green tea and type 2 diabetes. Integr Med Res. 2014;3:4–10. https://www.ncbi.nlm.nih.gov/pmc/articles/PMC5481694/

145. Oliveira MR de, Nabavi SF, Daglia M, Rastrelli L, Nabavi SM. Epigallocatechin gallate and mitochondria—a story of life and death. Pharmacol Res. 2016;104:70–85. https://pubmed.ncbi.nlm.nih.gov/26731017/

146. Schroeder EK, Kelsey NA, Doyle J, Breed E, Bouchard RJ, Loucks FA, et al. Green tea epigallocatechin 3-gallate accumulates in mitochondria and displays a selective antiapoptotic effect against inducers of mitochondrial oxidative stress in neurons. Antioxid Redox Signal. 2009;11:469–80. https://pubmed.ncbi.nlm.nih.gov/18754708/

147. Most J, Timmers S, Warnke I, Jocken JW, van Boekschoten M, de Groot P, et al. Combined epigallocatechin-3-gallate and resveratrol supplementation for 12 wk increases mitochondrial capacity and fat oxidation, but not insulin sensitivity, in obese humans: a randomized controlled trial. Am J Clin Nutr. 2016;104:215–27. https://pubmed.ncbi.nlm.nih.gov/27194304/

148. Jurgens TM, Whelan AM, Killian L, Doucette S, Kirk S, Foy E. Green tea for weight loss and weight maintenance in overweight or obese adults. Cochrane Database Syst Rev. 2012;12:CD008650. https://pubmed.ncbi.nlm .nih.gov/23235664/

149. Baladia E, Basulto J, Manera M, Martínez R, Calbet D. [Effect of green tea or green tea extract consumption on body weight and body composition; systematic review and meta-analysis]. Nutr Hosp. 2014;29:479–90. https:// pubmed.ncbi.nlm.nih.gov/24558988/

150. Zhong X, Zhang T, Liu Y, Wei X, Zhang X, Qin Y, et al. Short-term weight-centric effects of tea or tea extract in patients with metabolic syndrome: a meta-analysis of randomized controlled trials. Nutr Diabetes. 2015;5:e160. https://pubmed.ncbi.nlm.nih.gov/26075637/

151. Vázquez Cisneros LC, López-Uriarte P, López-Espinoza A, Navarro Meza M, Espinoza-Gallardo AC, Guzmán Aburto MB. [Effects of green tea and its epigallocatechin (EGCG) content on body weight and fat mass in humans: a systematic review.] Nutr Hosp. 2017;34:731–37. https://pubmed.ncbi.nlm .nih.gov/28627214/

152. Hibi M, Takase H, Iwasaki M, Osaki N, Katsuragi Y. Efficacy of tea catechin-rich beverages to reduce abdominal adiposity and metabolic syndrome risks in obese and overweight subjects: a pooled analysis of 6 human trials. Nutr Res. 2018;55:1–10. https://europepmc.org/article/med/29914623

153. Nguyen PH, Gauhar R, Hwang SL, Dao TT, Park DC, Kim JE, et al. New dammarane-type glucosides as potential activators of AMP-activated protein kinase (AMPK) from *Gynostemma pentaphyllum*. Bioorg Med Chem. 2011;19:6254–60. https://pubmed.ncbi.nlm.nih.gov/21978948/

154. Lee HS, Lim S-M, Jung JI, Kim SM, Lee JK, Kim YH, et al. *Gynostemma pentaphyllum* extract ameliorates high-fat diet-induced obesity in C57BL/6N mice by upregulating SIRT1. Nutrients. 2019;11. http://dx.doi.org/10.3390/ nu11102475

155. Choi E-K, Won YH, Kim S-Y, Noh S-O, Park S-H, Jung S-J, et al. Supplementation with extract of *Gynostemma pentaphyllum* leaves reduces anxiety in healthy subjects with chronic psychological stress: a randomized, double-blind, placebo-controlled clinical trial. Phytomedicine. 2019;52:198–205. https://www.sciencedirect.com/science/article/pii/S094471131830165X

156. Park S-H, Huh T-L, Kim S-Y, Oh M-R, Tirupathi Pichiah PB, Chae S-W, et al. Antiobesity effect of *Gynostemma pentaphyllum* extract (actiponin): a randomized, double-blind, placebo-controlled trial. Obesity. 2014;22:63–71. https://pubmed.ncbi.nlm.nih.gov/23804546/

157. Huyen VTT, Phan DV, Thang P, Hoa NK, Ostenson CG. Antidiabetic effect of *Gynostemma pentaphyllum* tea in randomly assigned type 2 diabetic patients. Horm Metab Res. 2010;42:353–7. https://pubmed.ncbi.nlm.nih .gov/20213586/

158. Atkuri KR, Mantovani JJ, Herzenberg LA, Herzenberg LA. N-Acetylcysteine—a safe antidote for cysteine/glutathione deficiency. Curr Opin Pharmacol. 2007;7:355–59. https://pubmed.ncbi.nlm.nih.gov/17602868/

159. Pendyala L, Creaven PJ. Pharmacokinetic and pharmacodynamic studies of N-acetylcysteine, a potential chemopreventive agent during a phase I trial. Cancer Epidemiol Biomarkers Prev. 1995;4:245–51. https://pubmed.ncbi .nlm.nih.gov/7606199/

160. Lauterburg BH, Corcoran GB, Mitchell JR. Mechanism of action of N-acetylcysteine in the protection against the hepatotoxicity of acetaminophen in rats in vivo. J Clin Invest. 1983;71:980–91. https:// pubmed.ncbi.nlm.nih.gov/6833497/

161. Pizzorno J. Glutathione! Integr Med. 2014;13:8–12. https://www.ncbi.nlm .nih.gov/pmc/articles/PMC4684116/

162. Polyak E, Ostrovsky J, Peng M, Dingley SD, Tsukikawa M, Kwon YJ, et al. N-acetylcysteine and vitamin E rescue animal longevity and cellular oxidative stress in pre-clinical models of mitochondrial complex I disease. Mol Genet Metab. 2018;123:449–62. https://www.ncbi.nlm.nih.gov/pmc/ articles/PMC5891356/

163. Aparicio-Trejo OE, Reyes-Fermín LM, Briones-Herrera A, Tapia E, León-Contreras JC, Hernández-Pando R, et al. Protective effects of N-acetyl-cysteine in mitochondria bioenergetics, oxidative stress, dynamics and S-glutathionylation alterations in acute kidney damage induced by folic acid. Free Radic Biol Med. 2019;130:379–96. https://pubmed.ncbi.nlm.nih.gov/ 30439416/

164. Sandhir R, Sood A, Mehrotra A, Kamboj SS. N-Acetylcysteine reverses mitochondrial dysfunctions and behavioral abnormalities in 3-nitropropionic acid-induced Huntington's disease. Neurodegener Dis. 2012;9:145–57. https://pubmed.ncbi.nlm.nih.gov/22327485/

165. Wright DJ, Renoir T, Smith ZM, Frazier AE, Francis PS, Thorburn DR, et al. N-Acetylcysteine improves mitochondrial function and ameliorates behavioral deficits in the R6/1 mouse model of Huntington's disease. Transl Psychiatry. 2015;5:e492. https://pubmed.ncbi.nlm.nih.gov/25562842/

166. Devrim-Lanpir A, Hill L, Knechtle B. How N-acetylcysteine supplementation affects redox regulation, especially at mitohormesis and sarcohormesis level: current perspective. Antioxidants (Basel). 2021;10. http://dx.doi.org/ 10.3390/antiox10020153

167. Faghfouri AH, Zarezadeh M, Tavakoli-Rouzbehani OM, Radkhah N, Faghfuri E, Kord-Varkaneh H, et al. The effects of N-acetylcysteine on inflammatory and oxidative stress biomarkers: a systematic review and meta-analysis of controlled clinical trials. Eur J Pharmacol. 2020;884:173368. https://pubmed .ncbi.nlm.nih.gov/32726657/

168. Ghezzi P. Role of glutathione in immunity and inflammation in the lung. Int J Gen Med. 2011;4:105–13. https://www.ncbi.nlm.nih.gov/pmc/articles/ PMC3048347/

169. Dröge W, Breitkreutz R. Glutathione and immune function. Proc Nutr Soc. 2000;59:595–600. https://pubmed.ncbi.nlm.nih.gov/11115795/

170. Bounous G, Molson J. Competition for glutathione precursors between the immune system and the skeletal muscle: pathogenesis of chronic fatigue syndrome. Med Hypotheses. 1999;53:347–49. https://pubmed.ncbi.nlm.nih.gov/10608272/

171. Mikirova N, Casciari J, Hunninghake R. The assessment of the energy metabolism in patients with chronic fatigue syndrome by serum fluorescence emission. Altern Ther Health Med. 2012;18:36–40. https://pubmed.ncbi.nlm.nih.gov/22516851/

172. Airhart SE, Shireman LM, Risler LJ, Anderson GD, Nagana Gowda GA, Raftery D, et al. An open-label, non-randomized study of the pharmacokinetics of the nutritional supplement nicotinamide riboside (NR) and its effects on blood NAD+ levels in healthy volunteers. PLoS One. 2017;12:e0186459. https://pubmed.ncbi.nlm.nih.gov/29211728/

173. Martens CR, Denman BA, Mazzo MR, Armstrong ML, Reisdorph N, McQueen MB, et al. Chronic nicotinamide riboside supplementation is well-tolerated and elevates NAD+ in healthy middle-aged and older adults. Nat Commun. 2018;9:1286. https://pubmed.ncbi.nlm.nih.gov/29599478/

174. Elhassan YS, Kluckova K, Fletcher RS, Schmidt MS, Garten A, Doig CL, et al. Nicotinamide riboside augments the aged human skeletal muscle NAD+ metabolome and induces transcriptomic and anti-inflammatory signatures. Cell Rep. 2019;28:1717–28.e6. https://pubmed.ncbi.nlm.nih.gov/31412242/

175. Dollerup OL, Christensen B, Svart M, Schmidt MS, Sulek K, Ringgaard S, et al. A randomized placebo-controlled clinical trial of nicotinamide riboside in obese men: safety, insulin-sensitivity, and lipid-mobilizing effects. Am J Clin Nutr. 2018;108:343–53. https://pubmed.ncbi.nlm.nih.gov/29992272/

176. Dollerup OL, Chubanava S, Agerholm M, Søndergård SD, Altıntaş A, Møller AB, et al. Nicotinamide riboside does not alter mitochondrial respiration, content or morphology in skeletal muscle from obese and insulin-resistant men. J Physiol. 2020;598:731–54. https://pubmed.ncbi.nlm.nih.gov/31710095/

177. Conze D, Brenner C, Kruger CL. Safety and metabolism of long-term administration of NIAGEN (nicotinamide riboside chloride) in a randomized, double-blind, placebo-controlled clinical trial of healthy overweight adults. Sci Rep. 2019;9:9772. https://pubmed.ncbi.nlm.nih.gov/31278280/

178. Remie CME, Roumans KHM, Moonen MPB, Connell NJ, Havekes B, Mevenkamp J, et al. Nicotinamide riboside supplementation alters body composition and skeletal muscle acetylcarnitine concentrations in healthy obese humans. Am J Clin Nutr. 2020;112:413–26. https://pubmed.ncbi.nlm.nih.gov/32320006/

179. Li X-T, Chen R, Jin L-M, Chen H-Y. Regulation on energy metabolism and protection on mitochondria of Panax ginseng polysaccharide. Am J Chin Med. 2009;37:1139–52. https://pubmed.ncbi.nlm.nih.gov/19938222/

180. Huang Y, Kwan KKL, Leung KW, Yao P, Wang H, Dong TT, et al. Ginseng extracts modulate mitochondrial bioenergetics of live cardiomyoblasts: a functional comparison of different extraction solvents. J Ginseng Res. 2019;43:517–26. https://pubmed.ncbi.nlm.nih.gov/31695560/

181. Jin T-Y, Rong P-Q, Liang H-Y, Zhang P-P, Zheng G-Q, Lin Y. Clinical and preclinical systematic review of *Panax ginseng* C. A. Mey and its compounds for fatigue. Front Pharmacol. 2020;11:1031. https://pubmed.ncbi.nlm.nih.gov/32765262/

182. Lee N, Lee S-H, Yoo H-R, Yoo HS. Anti-fatigue effects of enzyme-modified ginseng extract: a randomized, double-blind, placebo-controlled trial. J Altern Complement Med. 2016;22:859–64. https://pubmed.ncbi.nlm.nih.gov/27754709/

183. Kim H-G, Cho J-H, Yoo S-R, Lee J-S, Han J-M, Lee N-H, et al. Antifatigue effects of *Panax ginseng* C.A. Meyer: a randomised, double-blind, placebo-controlled trial. PLoS One. Public Library of Science; 2013;8. https://www.ncbi.nlm.nih.gov/pmc/articles/PMC3629193/

184. Chowanadisai W, Bauerly KA, Tchaparian E, Wong A, Cortopassi GA, Rucker RB. Pyrroloquinoline quinone stimulates mitochondrial biogenesis through cAMP response element-binding protein phosphorylation and increased PGC-1alpha expression. J Biol Chem. 2010;285:142–52. https://pubmed.ncbi.nlm.nih.gov/19861415/

185. Saihara K, Kamikubo R, Ikemoto K, Uchida K, Akagawa M. Pyrroloquinoline quinone, a redox-active o-quinone, stimulates mitochondrial biogenesis by activating the SIRT1/PGC-1α signaling pathway. Biochemistry. 2017;56:6615–25. https://pubmed.ncbi.nlm.nih.gov/29185343/

186. Hwang P, Willoughby DS. Mechanisms behind pyrroloquinoline quinone supplementation on skeletal muscle mitochondrial biogenesis: possible synergistic effects with exercise. J Am Coll Nutr. 2018;37:738–48. https://pubmed.ncbi.nlm.nih.gov/29714638/

187. Nakano M, Yamamoto T, Okamura H, Tsuda A, Kowatari Y. Effects of oral supplementation with pyrroloquinoline quinone on stress, fatigue, and sleep. Functional Foods in Health and Disease. 2012;2:307–24. https://www.ffhdj.com/index.php/ffhd/article/view/81

188. Harris CB, Chowanadisai W, Mishchuk DO, Satre MA, Slupsky CM, Rucker RB. Dietary pyrroloquinoline quinone (PQQ) alters indicators of inflammation and mitochondrial-related metabolism in human subjects. J Nutr Biochem. 2013;24:2076–84. https://pubmed.ncbi.nlm.nih.gov/24231099/

189. de Oliveira MR, Nabavi SM, Braidy N, Setzer WN, Ahmed T, Nabavi SF. Quercetin and the mitochondria: a mechanistic view. Biotechnol Adv. 2016;34:532–49. https://pubmed.ncbi.nlm.nih.gov/26740171/

190. Davis JM, Murphy EA, Carmichael MD, Davis B. Quercetin increases brain and muscle mitochondrial biogenesis and exercise tolerance. Am J Physiol Regul Integr Comp Physiol. 2009;296:R1071–77. https://pubmed.ncbi.nlm.nih.gov/19211721/

191. Pelletier DM, Lacerte G, Goulet EDB. Effects of quercetin supplementation on endurance performance and maximal oxygen consumption: a meta-analysis. Int J Sport Nutr Exerc Metab. 2013;23:73–82. https://pubmed.ncbi.nlm.nih.gov/22805526/

192. Kressler J, Millard-Stafford M, Warren GL. Quercetin and endurance exercise capacity: a systematic review and meta-analysis. Med Sci Sports Exerc. 2011;43:2396–404. https://pubmed.ncbi.nlm.nih.gov/21606866/

193. Ou Q, Zheng Z, Zhao Y, Lin W. Impact of quercetin on systemic levels of inflammation: a meta-analysis of randomised controlled human trials. Int J Food Sci Nutr. 2020;71:152–63. https://pubmed.ncbi.nlm.nih.gov/31213101/

194. Mohammadi-Sartang M, Mazloom Z, Sherafatmanesh S, Ghorbani M, Firoozi D. Effects of supplementation with quercetin on plasma C-reactive protein concentrations: a systematic review and meta-analysis of randomized controlled trials. Eur J Clin Nutr. 2017;71:1033–99. https://pubmed.ncbi .nlm.nih.gov/28537580/

195. Tabrizi R, Tamtaji OR, Mirhosseini N, Lankarani KB, Akbari M, Heydari ST, et al. The effects of quercetin supplementation on lipid profiles and inflammatory markers among patients with metabolic syndrome and related disorders: a systematic review and meta-analysis of randomized controlled trials. Crit Rev Food Sci Nutr. 2020;60:1855–68. https://pubmed.ncbi.nlm .nih.gov/31017459/

196. Guo W, Gong X, Li M. Quercetin actions on lipid profiles in overweight and obese individuals: a systematic review and meta-analysis. Curr Pharm Des. 2019;25:3087–95. https://pubmed.ncbi.nlm.nih.gov/31465275/

197. Sahebkar A. Effects of quercetin supplementation on lipid profile: a systematic review and meta-analysis of randomized controlled trials. Crit Rev Food Sci Nutr. 2017;57:666–76. https://pubmed.ncbi.nlm.nih.gov/25897620/

198. Tamtaji OR, Milajerdi A, Dadgostar E, Kolahdooz F, Chamani M, Amirani E, et al. The effects of quercetin supplementation on blood pressures and endothelial function among patients with metabolic syndrome and related disorders: a systematic review and meta-analysis of randomized controlled trials. Curr Pharm Des. 2019;25:1372–84. https://pubmed.ncbi.nlm.nih.gov/ 31092175/

199. Serban M-C, Sahebkar A, Zanchetti A, Mikhailidis DP, Howard G, Antal D, et al. Effects of quercetin on blood pressure: a systematic review and meta-analysis of randomized controlled trials. J Am Heart Assoc. 2016;5. http:// dx.doi.org/10.1161/JAHA.115.002713

200. Riva A, Ronchi M, Petrangolini G, Bosisio S, Allegrini P. Improved oral absorption of quercetin from Quercetin Phytosome®, a new delivery system based on food grade lecithin. Eur J Drug Metab Pharmacokinet. 2019;44:169–77. https://pubmed.ncbi.nlm.nih.gov/30328058/

201. Singh N, Bhalla M, de Jager P, Gilca M. An overview on Ashwagandha: a Rasayana (rejuvenator) of Ayurveda. Afr J Tradit Complement Altern Med. 2011;8:208–13. https://www.ncbi.nlm.nih.gov/pmc/articles/PMC3252722/

202. Pratte MA, Nanavati KB, Young V, Morley CP. An alternative treatment for anxiety: a systematic review of human trial results reported for the Ayurvedic herb ashwagandha (*Withania somnifera*). J Altern Complement Med. 2014;20:901–8. https://pubmed.ncbi.nlm.nih.gov/25405876/

203. Andrade C. Ashwagandha for anxiety disorders. World J. Biol. Psychiatry. 2009;10(4 Pt2):686–87. https://pubmed.ncbi.nlm.nih.gov/19363747/

204. Zahiruddin S, Basist P, Parveen A, Parveen R, Khan W, Gaurav, et al. Ashwagandha in brain disorders: A review of recent developments. J Ethnopharmacol. 2020;257:112876. https://pubmed.ncbi.nlm.nih.gov/ 32305638/

205. Candelario M, Cuellar E, Reyes-Ruiz JM, Darabedian N, Feimeng Z, Miledi R, et al. Direct evidence for GABAergic activity of *Withania somnifera* on mammalian ionotropic GABAA and GABAρ receptors. J Ethnopharmacol. 2015;171:264–72. https://pubmed.ncbi.nlm.nih.gov/26068424/

206. Salve J, Pate S, Debnath K, Langade D. Adaptogenic and anxiolytic effects of Ashwagandha root extract in healthy adults: a double-blind, randomized, placebo-controlled clinical study. Cureus. 2019;11:e6466. https://pubmed .ncbi.nlm.nih.gov/32021735/

207. Langade D, Kanchi S, Salve J, Debnath K, Ambegaokar D. Efficacy and safety of Ashwagandha (Withania somnifera) root extract in insomnia and anxiety: a double-blind, randomized, placebo-controlled study. Cureus. 2019;11:e5797. https://pubmed.ncbi.nlm.nih.gov/31728244/

208. Chandrasekhar K, Kapoor J, Anishetty S. A prospective, randomized double-blind, placebo-controlled study of safety and efficacy of a high-concentration full-spectrum extract of ashwagandha root in reducing stress and anxiety in adults. Indian J Psychol Med. 2012;34:255–62. https://pubmed.ncbi.nlm.nih .gov/23439798/

209. Fuladi S, Emami SA, Mohammadpour AH, Karimani A, Manteghi AA, Sahebkar A. Assessment of *Withania somnifera* root extract efficacy in patients with generalized anxiety disorder: a randomized double-blind placebo-controlled trial. Curr Clin Pharmacol. 2021;16(2):191–96. https:// pubmed.ncbi.nlm.nih.gov/32282308/

210. Salve, Pate, Debnath, Langade. Adaptogenic and anxiolytic effects of Ashwagandha root extract.

211. Kelgane SB, Salve J, Sampara P, Debnath K. Efficacy and tolerability of Ashwagandha root extract in the elderly for improvement of general well-being and sleep: a prospective, randomized, double-blind, placebo-controlled study. Cureus. 2020;12:e7083. https://pubmed.ncbi.nlm.nih.gov/32226684/

212. Langade. Efficacy and safety of Ashwagandha (Withania somnifera) root extract in insomnia and anxiety.

213. Lopresti AL, Smith SJ, Malvi H, Kodgule R. An investigation into the stress-relieving and pharmacological actions of an ashwagandha (*Withania somnifera*) extract: a randomized, double-blind, placebo-controlled study. Medicine. 2019;98:e17186. https://www.ncbi.nlm.nih.gov/pmc/articles/ PMC6750292/

214. Larsen C, Shahinas J. Dosage, efficacy and safety of cannabidiol administration in adults: a systematic review of human trials. J Clin Med Res. 2020;12:129–41. https://pubmed.ncbi.nlm.nih.gov/32231748/

215. VanDolah HJ, Bauer BA, Mauck KF. Clinicians' guide to cannabidiol and hemp oils. Mayo Clin Proc. 2019;94:1840–51. https://pubmed.ncbi.nlm.nih .gov/31447137/

216. Babson KA, Sottile J, Morabito D. Cannabis, cannabinoids, and sleep: a review of the literature. Curr Psychiatry Rep. 2017;19:23. https://pubmed.ncbi.nlm.nih.gov/28349316/

217. Murillo-Rodriguez E, Blanco-Centurion C, Sanchez C, Piomelli D, Shiromani PJ. Anandamide enhances extracellular levels of adenosine and induces sleep: an in vivo microdialysis study. Sleep. 2003;26:943–47. https://pubmed.ncbi.nlm.nih.gov/14746372/

218. Monti JM. Hypnoticlike effects of cannabidiol in the rat. Psychopharmacology. 1977;55:263–65. https://pubmed.ncbi.nlm.nih.gov/414288/

219. Chagas MHN, Eckeli AL, Zuardi AW, Pena-Pereira MA, Sobreira-Neto MA, Sobreira ET, et al. Cannabidiol can improve complex sleep-related behaviours associated with rapid eye movement sleep behaviour disorder in Parkinson's disease patients: a case series. J Clin Pharm Ther. 2014;39:564–66. https://pubmed.ncbi.nlm.nih.gov/24845114/

220. Shannon S, Opila-Lehman J. Effectiveness of cannabidiol oil for pediatric anxiety and insomnia as part of posttraumatic stress disorder: a case report. Perm J. 2016;20:16–005. https://pubmed.ncbi.nlm.nih.gov/27768570/

221. Shannon S, Lewis N, Lee H, Hughes S. Cannabidiol in anxiety and sleep: a large case series. Perm J. 2019;23:18–041. https://pubmed.ncbi.nlm.nih.gov/30624194/

222. Srivastava JK, Shankar E, Gupta S. Chamomile: a herbal medicine of the past with bright future. Mol Med Rep. 2010;3:895–901. https://www.ncbi.nlm.nih.gov/pmc/articles/PMC2995283/

223. Hieu TH, Dibas M, Surya Dila KA, Sherif NA, Hashmi MU, Mahmoud M, et al. Therapeutic efficacy and safety of chamomile for state anxiety, generalized anxiety disorder, insomnia, and sleep quality: a systematic review and meta-analysis of randomized trials and quasi-randomized trials. Phytother Res. 2019;33:1604–15. https://pubmed.ncbi.nlm.nih.gov/31006899/

224. Amsterdam JD, Li Y, Soeller I, Rockwell K, Mao JJ, Shults J. A randomized, double-blind, placebo-controlled trial of oral *Matricaria recutita* (chamomile) extract therapy for generalized anxiety disorder. J Clin Psychopharmacol. 2009;29:378–82. https://pubmed.ncbi.nlm.nih.gov/19593179/

225. Keefe JR, Mao JJ, Soeller I, Li QS, Amsterdam JD. Short-term open-label chamomile (*Matricaria chamomilla* L.) therapy of moderate to severe generalized anxiety disorder. Phytomedicine. 2016;23:1699–1705. https://pubmed.ncbi.nlm.nih.gov/27912871/

226. Mao JJ, Xie SX, Keefe JR, Soeller I, Li QS, Amsterdam JD. Long-term chamomile (*Matricaria chamomilla* L.) treatment for generalized anxiety disorder: a randomized clinical trial. Phytomedicine. 2016;23:1735–42. https://pubmed.ncbi.nlm.nih.gov/27912875/

227. Shakeri A, Sahebkar A, Javadi B. *Melissa officinalis* L. —a review of its traditional uses, phytochemistry and pharmacology. J Ethnopharmacol. 2016;188:204–28. https://pubmed.ncbi.nlm.nih.gov/27167460/

228. Kennedy DO, Scholey AB, Tildesley NTJ, Perry EK, Wesnes KA. Modulation of mood and cognitive performance following acute administration of *Melissa officinalis* (lemon balm). Pharmacol Biochem Behav. 2002;72:953–64. https://pubmed.ncbi.nlm.nih.gov/12062586/

229. Kennedy DO, Wake G, Savelev S, Tildesley NTJ, Perry EK, Wesnes KA, et al. Modulation of mood and cognitive performance following acute administration of single doses of *Melissa officinalis* (lemon balm) with human CNS nicotinic and muscarinic receptor-binding properties. Neuropsychopharmacology. 2003;28:1871–81. https://pubmed.ncbi.nlm.nih.gov/12888775/

230. Kennedy DO, Little W, Scholey AB. Attenuation of laboratory-induced stress in humans after acute administration of *Melissa officinalis* (lemon balm). Psychosom Med. 2004;66:607–13. https://pubmed.ncbi.nlm.nih.gov/15272110/

231. Scholey A, Gibbs A, Neale C, Perry N, Ossoukhova A, Bilog V, et al. Anti-stress effects of lemon balm-containing foods. Nutrients. 2014;6:4805–21. https://pubmed.ncbi.nlm.nih.gov/25360512/

232. Cases J, Ibarra A, Feuillère N, Roller M, Sukkar SG. Pilot trial of Melissa officinalis L. leaf extract in the treatment of volunteers suffering from mild-to-moderate anxiety disorders and sleep disturbances. Med J Nutrition Metab. 2011;4:211–18. https://pubmed.ncbi.nlm.nih.gov/22207903/

233. Müller SF, Klement S. A combination of valerian and lemon balm is effective in the treatment of restlessness and dyssomnia in children. Phytomedicine. 2006;13:383–87. https://pubmed.ncbi.nlm.nih.gov/16487692/

234. Taavoni S, Nazem Ekbatani N, Haghani H. Valerian/lemon balm use for sleep disorders during menopause. Complement Ther Clin Pract. 2013;19:193–96. https://pubmed.ncbi.nlm.nih.gov/24199972/

235. Auld F, Maschauer EL, Morrison I, Skene DJ, Riha RL. Evidence for the efficacy of melatonin in the treatment of primary adult sleep disorders. Sleep Med Rev. 2017;34:10–22. https://pubmed.ncbi.nlm.nih.gov/28648359/

236. Ferracioli-Oda E, Qawasmi A, Bloch MH. Meta-analysis: melatonin for the treatment of primary sleep disorders. PLoS One. 2013;8:e63773. https://pubmed.ncbi.nlm.nih.gov/23691095/

237. Li T, Jiang S, Han M, Yang Z, Lv J, Deng C, et al. Exogenous melatonin as a treatment for secondary sleep disorders: a systematic review and meta-analysis. Front Neuroendocrinol. 2019;52:22–8. https://pubmed.ncbi.nlm.nih.gov/29908879/

238. Wang Y-Y, Zheng W, Ng CH, Ungvari GS, Wei W, Xiang Y-T. Meta-analysis of randomized, double-blind, placebo-controlled trials of melatonin in Alzheimer's disease. Int J Geriatr Psychiatry. 2017;32:50–57. https://pubmed.ncbi.nlm.nih.gov/27645169/

239. Zhang W, Chen X-Y, Su S-W, Jia Q-Z, Ding T, Zhu Z-N, et al. Exogenous melatonin for sleep disorders in neurodegenerative diseases: a meta-analysis of randomized clinical trials. Neurol Sci. 2016;37:57–65. https://pubmed.ncbi.nlm.nih.gov/26255301/

240. Abdelgadir IS, Gordon MA, Akobeng AK. Melatonin for the management of sleep problems in children with neurodevelopmental disorders: a systematic review and meta-analysis. Arch Dis Child. 2018;103:1155–62. https://pubmed.ncbi.nlm.nih.gov/29720494/

241. Rossignol DA, Frye RE. Melatonin in autism spectrum disorders: a systematic review and meta-analysis. Dev Med Child Neurol. 2011;53:783–92. https://pubmed.ncbi.nlm.nih.gov/21518346/

242. Doosti-Irani A, Ostadmohammadi V, Mirhosseini N, Mansournia MA, Reiter RJ, Kashanian M, et al. The effects of melatonin supplementation on glycemic control: a systematic review and meta-analysis of randomized controlled trials. Horm Metab Res. 2018;50:783–90. https://pubmed.ncbi.nlm.nih.gov/30396207/

243. Akbari M, Ostadmohammadi V, Mirhosseini N, Lankarani KB, Tabrizi R, Keshtkaran Z, et al. The effects of melatonin supplementation on blood pressure in patients with metabolic disorders: a systematic review and meta-analysis of randomized controlled trials. J Hum Hypertens. 2019;33:202–9. https://pubmed.ncbi.nlm.nih.gov/30647466/

244. Akbari M, Ostadmohammadi V, Tabrizi R, Lankarani KB, Heydari ST, Amirani E, et al. The effects of melatonin supplementation on inflammatory markers among patients with metabolic syndrome or related disorders: a systematic review and meta-analysis of randomized controlled trials. Inflammopharmacology. 2018;26:899–907. https://pubmed.ncbi.nlm.nih.gov/29907916/

245. Morvaridzadeh M, Sadeghi E, Agah S, Nachvak SM, Fazelian S, Moradi F, et al. Effect of melatonin supplementation on oxidative stress parameters: a systematic review and meta-analysis. Pharmacol Res. 2020;161:105210. https://pubmed.ncbi.nlm.nih.gov/33007423/

246. Ghorbaninejad P, Sheikhhossein F, Djafari F, Tijani AJ, Mohammadpour S, Shab-Bidar S. Effects of melatonin supplementation on oxidative stress: a systematic review and meta-analysis of randomized controlled trials. Horm Mol Biol Clin Investig. 2020;41. http://dx.doi.org/10.1515/hmbci-2020-0030

247. van Heukelom RO, Prins JB, Smits MG, Bleijenberg G. Influence of melatonin on fatigue severity in patients with chronic fatigue syndrome and late melatonin secretion. Eur J Neurol. 2006;13:55–60. https://pubmed.ncbi.nlm.nih.gov/16420393/

248. Ekmekcioglu C. Melatonin receptors in humans: biological role and clinical relevance. Biomed Pharmacother. 2006;60:97–108. https://pubmed.ncbi.nlm.nih.gov/16527442/

249. Morgan PJ, Barrett P, Howell HE, Helliwell R. Melatonin receptors: localization, molecular pharmacology and physiological significance. Neurochem Int. 1994;24:101–46. https://pubmed.ncbi.nlm.nih.gov/8161940/

250. Harpsøe NG, Andersen LPH, Gögenur I, Rosenberg J. Clinical pharmacokinetics of melatonin: a systematic review. Eur J Clin Pharmacol. 2015;71:901–9. https://pubmed.ncbi.nlm.nih.gov/26008214/

251. Matsumoto M, Sack RL, Blood ML, Lewy AJ. The amplitude of endogenous melatonin production is not affected by melatonin treatment in humans. J Pineal Res. 1997;22:42–44. https://pubmed.ncbi.nlm.nih.gov/9062869/

252. Wright J, Aldhous M, Franey C, English J, Arendt J. The effects of exogenous melatonin on endocrine function in man. Clin Endocrinol. 1986;24:375–82. https://pubmed.ncbi.nlm.nih.gov/3742833/

253. Arendt J, Bojkowski C, Folkard S, Franey C, Marks V, Minors D, et al. Some effects of melatonin and the control of its secretion in humans. Ciba Found Symp. 1985;117:266–83. https://pubmed.ncbi.nlm.nih.gov/3836818/

254. Matsumoto, Sack, Blood, Lewy. The amplitude of endogenous melatonin production is not affected by melatonin treatment in humans. J Pineal Res. 1997;22(1):42–44. https://onlinelibrary.wiley.com/doi/10.1111/j.1600-079X.1997.tb00301.x

255. Dhawan K, Kumar R, Kumar S, Sharma A. Correct identification of Passiflora incarnata Linn., a promising herbal anxiolytic and sedative. J Med Food. 2001;4:137–44. https://pubmed.ncbi.nlm.nih.gov/12639407/

256. da Fonseca LR, Rodrigues R de A, Ramos A de S, da Cruz JD, Ferreira JLP, Silva JR de A, et al. Herbal medicinal products from Passiflora for anxiety: an unexploited potential. ScientificWorldJournal. 2020;2020:6598434. https://www.hindawi.com/journals/tswj/2020/6598434/

257. Lee J, Jung H-Y, Lee SI, Choi JH, Kim S-G. Effects of Passiflora incarnata Linnaeus on polysomnographic sleep parameters in subjects with insomnia disorder: a double-blind randomized placebo-controlled study. Int Clin Psychopharmacol. 2020;35:29–35. https://pubmed.ncbi.nlm.nih.gov/31714321/

258. Ngan A, Conduit R. A double-blind, placebo-controlled investigation of the effects of Passiflora incarnata (passionflower) herbal tea on subjective sleep quality. Phytother Res. 2011;25:1153–59. https://pubmed.ncbi.nlm.nih.gov/21294203/

259. Guerrero FA, Medina GM. Effect of a medicinal plant (Passiflora incarnata L) on sleep. Sleep Sci. 2017;10:96–100. https://pubmed.ncbi.nlm.nih.gov/29410738/

260. Kim G-H, Yi SS. Chronic oral administration of Passiflora incarnata extract has no abnormal effects on metabolic and behavioral parameters in mice, except to induce sleep. Lab Anim Res. 2019;35:31. https://labanimres.biomedcentral.com/articles/10.1186/s42826-019-0034-9

261. Movafegh A, Alizadeh R, Hajimohamadi F, Esfehani F, Nejatfar M. Preoperative oral Passiflora incarnata reduces anxiety in ambulatory surgery patients: a double-blind, placebo-controlled study. Anesth Analg. 2008;106:1728–32. https://pubmed.ncbi.nlm.nih.gov/18499602/

262. Aslanargun P, Cuvas O, Dikmen B, Aslan E, Yuksel MU. Passiflora incarnata Linneaus as an anxiolytic before spinal anesthesia. J Anesth. 2012;26:39–44. https://pubmed.ncbi.nlm.nih.gov/22048283/

263. Dantas L-P, de Oliveira-Ribeiro A, de Almeida-Souza L-M, Groppo F-C. Effects of passiflora incarnata and midazolam for control of anxiety in patients

undergoing dental extraction. Med Oral Patol Oral Cir Bucal. 2017;22:e95–101. https://pubmed.ncbi.nlm.nih.gov/27918731/

264. Akhondzadeh S, Naghavi HR, Vazirian M, Shayeganpour A, Rashidi H, Khani M. Passionflower in the treatment of generalized anxiety: a pilot double-blind randomized controlled trial with oxazepam. J Clin Pharm Ther. 2001;26:363–67. https://pubmed.ncbi.nlm.nih.gov/11679026/

265. Kakuda T. Neuroprotective effects of theanine and its preventive effects on cognitive dysfunction. Pharmacol Res. 2011;64:162–68. https://europepmc.org/article/med/21477654

266. Yamada T, Terashima T, Okubo T, Juneja LR, Yokogoshi H. Effects of theanine, r-glutamylethylamide, on neurotransmitter release and its relationship with glutamic acid neurotransmission. Nutr Neurosci. 2005;8:219–26. https://pubmed.ncbi.nlm.nih.gov/16493792/

267. Kobayashi K, Nagato Y, Aoi N, Juneja LR, Kim M, Yamamoto T, et al. Effects of L-theanine on the release of alpha-brain waves in human volunteers. Journal of the Agricultural Chemical Society of Japan. 1998. http://agris.fao.org/agris-search/search.do?recordID=JP1998003883

268. Juneja LR, Chu D-C, Okubo T, Nagato Y, Yokogoshi H. L-theanine—a unique amino acid of green tea and its relaxation effect in humans. Trends Food Sci Technol. 1999;10:199–204. https://www.sciencedirect.com/science/article/abs/pii/S0924224499000448

269. Nobre AC, Rao A, Owen GN. L-theanine, a natural constituent in tea, and its effect on mental state. Asia Pac J Clin Nutr. 2008;17 Suppl 1:167–68. https://pubmed.ncbi.nlm.nih.gov/18296328/

270. Gomez-Ramirez M, Kelly SP, Montesi JL, Foxe JJ. The effects of L-theanine on alpha-band oscillatory brain activity during a visuo-spatial attention task. Brain Topogr. 2009;22:44–51. https://pubmed.ncbi.nlm.nih.gov/18841456/

271. Higashiyama A, Htay HH, Ozeki M, Juneja LR, Kapoor MP. Effects of l-theanine on attention and reaction time response. J Funct Foods. 2011;3:171–78. https://www.sciencedirect.com/science/article/pii/S1756464611000351

272. Dietz C, Dekker M. Effect of green tea phytochemicals on mood and cognition. Curr Pharm Des. 2017;23:2876–905. https://pubmed.ncbi.nlm.nih.gov/28056735/

273. Williams JL, Everett JM, D'Cunha NM, Sergi D, Georgousopoulou EN, Keegan RJ, et al. The effects of green tea amino acid L-theanine consumption on the ability to manage stress and anxiety levels: a systematic review. Plant Foods Hum Nutr. 2020;75:12–23. https://pubmed.ncbi.nlm.nih.gov/31758301/

274. Lyon MR, Kapoor MP, Juneja LR. The effects of L-theanine (Suntheanine®) on objective sleep quality in boys with attention deficit hyperactivity disorder (ADHD): a randomized, double-blind, placebo-controlled clinical trial. Altern Med Rev. 2011;16:348–54. https://pubmed.ncbi.nlm.nih.gov/22214254/

275. Kim S, Jo K, Hong K-B, Han SH, Suh HJ. GABA and l-theanine mixture decreases sleep latency and improves NREM sleep. Pharm Biol. 2019;57:65–73. https://pubmed.ncbi.nlm.nih.gov/30707852/

276. Jang H-S, Jung JY, Jang I-S, Jang K-H, Kim S-H, Ha J-H, et al. L-theanine partially counteracts caffeine-induced sleep disturbances in rats. Pharmacol Biochem Behav. 2012;101:217–21. https://pubmed.ncbi.nlm.nih.gov/22285321/

277. Kakuda T, Nozawa A, Unno T, Okamura N, Okai O. Inhibiting effects of theanine on caffeine stimulation evaluated by EEG in the rat. Biosci Biotechnol Biochem. 2000;64:287–93. https://pubmed.ncbi.nlm.nih.gov/10737183/

278. Shinjyo N, Waddell G, Green J. Valerian root in treating sleep problems and associated disorders—a systematic review and meta-analysis. J Evid Based Integr Med. 2020;25:2515690X20967323. https://pubmed.ncbi.nlm.nih.gov/33086877/

279. Thapa BR. Health factors in colostrum. Indian J Pediatr. 2005;72:579–81. https://pubmed.ncbi.nlm.nih.gov/16077241/

280. Sienkiewicz M, Szymańska P, Fichna J. Supplementation of bovine colostrum in inflammatory bowel disease: benefits and contraindications. Adv Nutr. 2020;12:533–45. http://dx.doi.org/10.1093/advances/nmaa120

281. Li J, Xu Y-W, Jiang J-J, Song Q-K. Bovine colostrum and product intervention associated with relief of childhood infectious diarrhea. Sci Rep. 2019;9:3093. https://www.nature.com/articles/s41598-019-39644-x

282. Marchbank T, Davison G, Oakes JR, Ghatei MA, Patterson M, Moyer MP, et al. The nutriceutical bovine colostrum truncates the increase in gut permeability caused by heavy exercise in athletes. Am J Physiol Gastrointest Liver Physiol. 2011;300:G477–84. https://pubmed.ncbi.nlm.nih.gov/21148400/

283. Davison G, Marchbank T, March DS, Thatcher R, Playford RJ. Zinc carnosine works with bovine colostrum in truncating heavy exercise-induced increase in gut permeability in healthy volunteers. Am J Clin Nutr. 2016;104:526–36. https://pubmed.ncbi.nlm.nih.gov/27357095/

284. March DS, Jones AW, Thatcher R, Davison G. The effect of bovine colostrum supplementation on intestinal injury and circulating intestinal bacterial DNA following exercise in the heat. Eur J Nutr. 2019;58:1441–51. https://www.ncbi.nlm.nih.gov/pmc/articles/PMC6561991/

285. Hałasa M, Maciejewska D, Baśkiewicz-Hałasa M, Machaliński B, Safranow K, Stachowska E. Oral supplementation with bovine colostrum decreases intestinal permeability and stool concentrations of zonulin in athletes. Nutrients. 2017;9. http://dx.doi.org/10.3390/nu9040370

286. Achamrah N, Déchelotte P, Coëffier M. Glutamine and the regulation of intestinal permeability: from bench to bedside. Curr Opin Clin Nutr Metab Care. 2017;20:86–91. https://pubmed.ncbi.nlm.nih.gov/27749689/

287. Rao R, Samak G. Role of glutamine in protection of intestinal epithelial tight junctions. J Epithel Biol Pharmacol. 2012;5:47–54. https://pubmed.ncbi.nlm.nih.gov/25810794/

288. Potsic B, Holliday N, Lewis P, Samuelson D, DeMarco V, Neu J. Glutamine supplementation and deprivation: effect on artificially reared rat small intestinal morphology. Pediatr Res. 2002;52:430–36. https://www.nature.com/articles/pr2002202

289. Lima AAM, Brito LFB, Ribeiro HB, Martins MCV, Lustosa AP, Rocha EM, et al. Intestinal barrier function and weight gain in malnourished children taking glutamine supplemented enteral formula. J Pediatr Gastroenterol Nutr. 2005;40:28–35. https://pubmed.ncbi.nlm.nih.gov/15625423/

290. Hulsewé KWE, van Acker BAC, Hameeteman W, van der Hulst RRWJ, Vainas T, Arends J-W, et al. Does glutamine-enriched parenteral nutrition really affect intestinal morphology and gut permeability? Clin Nutr. 2004;23:1217–25. https://www.academia.edu/23494101/Does_glutamine-enriched _parenteral_nutrition_really_affect_intestinal_morphology_and_gut _permeability

291. Zuhl M, Dokladny K, Mermier C, Schneider S, Salgado R, Moseley P. The effects of acute oral glutamine supplementation on exercise-induced gastrointestinal permeability and heat shock protein expression in peripheral blood mononuclear cells. Cell Stress Chaperones. 2015;20:85–93. https:// pubmed.ncbi.nlm.nih.gov/25062931/

292. Pugh JN, Sage S, Hutson M, Doran DA, Fleming SC, Highton J, et al. Glutamine supplementation reduces markers of intestinal permeability during running in the heat in a dose-dependent manner. Eur J Appl Physiol. 2017;117:2569–77. https://pubmed.ncbi.nlm.nih.gov/29058112/

293. L'Huillier C, Jarbeau M, Achamrah N, Belmonte L, Amamou A, Nobis S, et al. Glutamine, but not branched-chain amino acids, restores intestinal barrier function during activity-based anorexia. Nutrients. 2019;11. http://dx.doi .org/10.3390/nu11061348

294. Slavin JL, Greenberg NA. Partially hydrolyzed guar gum: clinical nutrition uses. Nutrition. 2003;19:549–52. https://pubmed.ncbi.nlm.nih.gov/ 12781858/

295. Quartarone G. Role of PHGG as a dietary fiber: a review article. Minerva Gastroenterol Dietol. 2013;59:329–40. https://pubmed.ncbi.nlm.nih.gov/ 24212352/

296. Giannini EG, Mansi C, Dulbecco P, Savarino V. Role of partially hydrolyzed guar gum in the treatment of irritable bowel syndrome. Nutrition. 2006;22:334–42. https://pubmed.ncbi.nlm.nih.gov/16413751/

297. Polymeros D, Beintaris I, Gaglia A, Karamanolis G, Papanikolaou IS, Dimitriadis G, et al. Partially hydrolyzed guar gum accelerates colonic transit time and improves symptoms in adults with chronic constipation. Dig Dis Sci. 2014;59:2207–14. https://pubmed.ncbi.nlm.nih.gov/24711073/

298. Parisi G, Bottona E, Carrara M, Cardin F, Faedo A, Goldin D, et al. Treatment effects of partially hydrolyzed guar gum on symptoms and quality of life of patients with irritable bowel syndrome. A multicenter randomized open trial. Dig Dis Sci. 2005;50:1107–12. https://pubmed.ncbi.nlm.nih.gov/15986863/

299. Niv E, Halak A, Tiommny E, Yanai H, Strul H, Naftali T, et al. Randomized clinical study: partially hydrolyzed guar gum (PHGG) versus placebo in the treatment of patients with irritable bowel syndrome. Nutr Metab. 2016;13:10. https://pubmed.ncbi.nlm.nih.gov/26855665/

300. Yasukawa Z, Inoue R, Ozeki M, Okubo T, Takagi T, Honda A, et al. Effect of repeated consumption of partially hydrolyzed guar gum on fecal characteristics and gut microbiota: a randomized, double-blind, placebo-controlled, and parallel-group clinical trial. Nutrients. 2019;11. http://dx.doi.org/10.3390/nu11092170.

301. Reider SJ, Moosmang S, Tragust J, Trgovec-Greif L, Tragust S, Perschy L, et al. Prebiotic effects of partially hydrolyzed guar gum on the composition and function of the human microbiota—results from the PAGODA Trial. Nutrients. 2020;12. https://www.ncbi.nlm.nih.gov/pmc/articles/PMC7281958/

302. Skrovanek S, DiGuilio K, Bailey R, Huntington W, Urbas R, Mayilvaganan B, et al. Zinc and gastrointestinal disease. World J Gastrointest Pathophysiol. 2014;5:496–513. https://pubmed.ncbi.nlm.nih.gov/25400994/

303. Siva S, Rubin DT, Gulotta G, Wroblewski K, Pekow J. Zinc deficiency is associated with poor clinical outcomes in patients with inflammatory bowel disease. Inflamm Bowel Dis. 2017;23:152–57. https://pubmed.ncbi.nlm.nih.gov/27930412/

304. Sturniolo GC, Di Leo V, Ferronato A, D'Odorico A, D'Incà R. Zinc supplementation tightens "leaky gut" in Crohn's disease. Inflamm Bowel Dis. 2001;7:94–98. https://pubmed.ncbi.nlm.nih.gov/11383597/

305. Sturniolo GC, Fries W, Mazzon E, Di Leo V, Barollo M, D'inca R. Effect of zinc supplementation on intestinal permeability in experimental colitis. J Lab Clin Med. 2002;139:311–15. https://pubmed.ncbi.nlm.nih.gov/12032492/

306. Mahmood A, FitzGerald AJ, Marchbank T, Ntatsaki E, Murray D, Ghosh S, et al. Zinc carnosine, a health food supplement that stabilises small bowel integrity and stimulates gut repair processes. Gut. 2007;56:168–75. https://www.ncbi.nlm.nih.gov/pmc/articles/PMC1856764/

307. Davison. Zinc carnosine works with bovine colostrum in truncating heavy exercise-induced increase.

308. Suliman NA, Mat Taib CN, Mohd Moklas MA, Adenan MI, Hidayat Baharuldin MT, Basir R. Establishing natural nootropics: recent molecular enhancement influenced by natural nootropic. Evid Based Complement Alternat Med. 2016;2016:4391375. https://pubmed.ncbi.nlm.nih.gov/27656235/

309. Lanni C, Lenzken SC, Pascale A, Del Vecchio I, Racchi M, Pistoia F, et al. Cognition enhancers between treating and doping the mind. Pharmacol Res. 2008;57:196–213. https://pubmed.ncbi.nlm.nih.gov/18353672/

310. Malik R, Sangwan A, Saihgal R, Jindal DP, Piplani P. Towards better brain management: nootropics. Curr Med Chem. 2007;14:123–31. https://pubmed.ncbi.nlm.nih.gov/17266573/

311. Abdul Manap AS, Vijayabalan S, Madhavan P, Chia YY, Arya A, Wong EH, et al. *Bacopa monnieri*, a neuroprotective lead in Alzheimer disease: a review on its properties, mechanisms of action, and preclinical and clinical studies. Drug Target Insights. 2019;13:1177392819866412. https://pubmed.ncbi.nlm.nih.gov/31391778/

312. Dubey T, Chinnathambi S. Brahmi (*Bacopa monnieri*): an ayurvedic herb against the Alzheimer's disease. Arch Biochem Biophys. 2019;676:108153. https://pubmed.ncbi.nlm.nih.gov/31622587/

313. Kwon HJ, Jung HY, Hahn KR, Kim W, Kim JW, Yoo DY, et al. *Bacopa monnieri* extract improves novel object recognition, cell proliferation, neuroblast differentiation, brain-derived neurotrophic factor, and phosphorylation of cAMP response element-binding protein in the dentate gyrus. Lab Anim Res. 2018;34:239–47. https://pubmed.ncbi.nlm.nih.gov/30671111/

314. Chaudhari KS, Tiwari NR, Tiwari RR, Sharma RS. Neurocognitive effect of nootropic drug *Brahmi* (*Bacopa monnieri*) in Alzheimer's disease. Ann Neurosci. 2017;24:111–22. https://www.karger.com/Article/Fulltext/475900

315. Aguiar S, Borowski T. Neuropharmacological review of the nootropic herb *Bacopa monnieri*. Rejuvenation Res. 2013;16:313–26. https://pubmed.ncbi.nlm.nih.gov/23772955/

316. Kumar N, Abichandani LG, Thawani V, Gharpure KJ, Naidu MUR, Venkat Ramana G. Efficacy of standardized extract of *Bacopa monnieri* (Bacognize®) on cognitive functions of medical students: a six-week, randomized placebo-controlled trial. Evid Based Complement Alternat Med. 2016;2016:4103423. https://pubmed.ncbi.nlm.nih.gov/27803728/

317. Stough C, Lloyd J, Clarke J, Downey LA, Hutchison CW, Rodgers T, et al. The chronic effects of an extract of Bacopa monniera (Brahmi) on cognitive function in healthy human subjects. Psychopharmacology. 2001;156:481–84. https://pubmed.ncbi.nlm.nih.gov/11498727/

318. Stough C, Downey LA, Lloyd J, Silber B, Redman S, Hutchison C, et al. Examining the nootropic effects of a special extract of Bacopa monniera on human cognitive functioning: 90 day double-blind placebo-controlled randomized trial. Phytother Res. 2008;22:1629–34. https://pubmed.ncbi.nlm.nih.gov/18683852/

319. Morgan A, Stevens J. Does Bacopa monnieri improve memory performance in older persons? Results of a randomized, placebo-controlled, double-blind trial. J Altern Complement Med. 2010;16:753–59. https://pubmed.ncbi.nlm.nih.gov/20590480/

320. Calabrese C, Gregory WL, Leo M, Kraemer D, Bone K, Oken B. Effects of a standardized Bacopa monnieri extract on cognitive performance, anxiety, and depression in the elderly: a randomized, double-blind, placebo-controlled trial. J Altern Complement Med. 2008;14:707–13. https://pubmed.ncbi.nlm.nih.gov/18611150/

321. Peth-Nui T, Wattanathorn J, Muchimapura S, Tong-Un T, Piyavhatkul N, Rangseekajee P, et al. Effects of 12-week Bacopa monnieri consumption on attention, cognitive processing, working memory, and functions of both cholinergic and monoaminergic systems in healthy elderly volunteers. Evid Based Complement Alternat Med. 2012;2012:606424. https://pubmed.ncbi.nlm.nih.gov/23320031/

322. Singh SK, Srivastav S, Castellani RJ, Plascencia-Villa G, Perry G. Neuroprotective and Antioxidant Effect of Ginkgo biloba Extract Against AD and Other Neurological Disorders. Neurotherapeutics. 2019;16:666–74. https://pubmed.ncbi.nlm.nih.gov/31376068/

323. Yuan Q, Wang C-W, Shi J, Lin Z-X. Effects of Ginkgo biloba on dementia: an overview of systematic reviews. J Ethnopharmacol. 2017;195:1–9. https://europepmc.org/article/med/27940086

324. Liu H, Ye M, Guo H. An updated review of randomized clinical trials testing the improvement of cognitive function of *Ginkgo biloba* extract in healthy people and Alzheimer's patients. Front Pharmacol. 2019;10:1688. https://www.ncbi.nlm.nih.gov/pmc/articles/PMC7047126/

325. Sabaratnam V, Kah-Hui W, Naidu M, Rosie David PR. Neuronal health—can culinary and medicinal mushrooms help? Afr J Tradit Complement Altern Med. 2013;3:62–68. https://www.ncbi.nlm.nih.gov/pmc/articles/PMC3924982/

326. Lai P-L, Naidu M, Sabaratnam V, Wong K-H, David RP, Kuppusamy UR, et al. Neurotrophic properties of the Lion's mane medicinal mushroom, *Hericium erinaceus* (Higher Basidiomycetes) from Malaysia. Int J Med Mushrooms. 2013;15:539–54. https://pubmed.ncbi.nlm.nih.gov/24266378/

327. Kawagishi H, Shimada A, Shirai R, Okamoto K, Ojima F, Sakamoto H, et al. Erinacines A, B and C, strong stimulators of nerve growth factor (NGF)-synthesis, from the mycelia of Hericium erinaceum. *Tetrahedron* Lett. 1994;35:1569–72. https://www.sciencedirect.com/science/article/abs/pii/S0040403900767608

328. Kawagishi H, Simada A, Shizuki K, Ojima F, Mori H, Okamoto K, et al. Erinacine D, a stimulator of NGF-synthesis, from the mycelia of *Hericum erinaceum*. Heterocycl Commun. 1996;2:4561. https://doi.org/10.1515/HC.1996.2.1.51

329. Mori K, Obara Y, Hirota M, Azumi Y, Kinugasa S, Inatomi S, et al. Nerve growth factor-inducing activity of *Hericium erinaceus* in 1321N1 human astrocytoma cells. Biol Pharm Bull. 2008;31:1727–32. https://pubmed.ncbi.nlm.nih.gov/18758067/

330. Aloe L, Rocco ML, Balzamino BO, Micera A. Nerve growth factor: a focus on neuroscience and therapy. Curr Neuropharmacol. 2015;13:294–303. https://pubmed.ncbi.nlm.nih.gov/26411962/

331. Chiu C-H, Chyau C-C, Chen C-C, Lee L-Y, Chen W-P, Liu J-L, et al. Erinacine A-enriched *Hericium erinaceus* mycelium produces antidepressant-like effects through modulating BDNF/PI3K/Akt/GSK-3β signaling in mice. Int J Mol Sci. 2018;19. http://dx.doi.org/10.3390/ijms19020341

332. Ibid.

333. Yao W, Zhang J-C, Dong C, Zhuang C, Hirota S, Inanaga K, et al. Effects of amycenone on serum levels of tumor necrosis factor-α, interleukin-10, and depression-like behavior in mice after lipopolysaccharide administration. Pharmacol Biochem Behav. 2015;136:7–12. https://pubmed.ncbi.nlm.nih.gov/26150007/

334. Chiu. Erinacine A-enriched *Hericium erinaceus* mycelium produces antidepressant-like effects.

335. Kowiański P, Lietzau G, Czuba E, Waśkow M, Steliga A, Moryś J. BDNF: a key factor with multipotent impact on brain signaling and synaptic plasticity.

Cell Mol Neurobiol. 2018;38:579–93. https://pubmed.ncbi.nlm.nih.gov/ 28623429/

336. Ratto D, Corana F, Mannucci B, Priori EC, Cobelli F, Roda E, et al. *Hericium erinaceus* improves recognition memory and induces hippocampal and cerebellar neurogenesis in frail mice during aging. Nutrients. 2019;11. http:// dx.doi.org/10.3390/nu11040715

337. Jang H-J, Kim J-E, Jeong KH, Lim SC, Kim SY, Cho K-O. The neuroprotective effect of *Hericium erinaceus* extracts in mouse hippocampus after pilocarpine-induced status epilepticus. Int J Mol Sci. 2019;20. http://dx.doi.org/10.3390/ ijms20040859

338. Chiu. Erinacine A-enriched *Hericium erinaceus* mycelium produces antidepressant-like effects.

339. Mori K, Inatomi S, Ouchi K, Azumi Y, Tuchida T. Improving effects of the mushroom Yamabushitake (*Hericium erinaceus*) on mild cognitive impairment: a double-blind placebo-controlled clinical trial. Phytother Res. 2009;23:367–72. https://pubmed.ncbi.nlm.nih.gov/18844328/

340. Vigna L, Morelli F, Agnelli GM, Napolitano F, Ratto D, Occhinegro A, et al. *Hericium erinaceus* improves mood and sleep disorders in patients affected by overweight or obesity: could circulating pro-BDNF and BDNF be potential biomarkers? Evid Based Complement Alternat Med. 2019;2019:7861297. https://pubmed.ncbi.nlm.nih.gov/31118969/

341. Swaminathan R. Magnesium metabolism and its disorders. Clin Biochem Rev. 2003;24:47–66. https://pubmed.ncbi.nlm.nih.gov/18568054/

342. Igamberdiev AU, Kleczkowski LA. Optimization of ATP synthase function in mitochondria and chloroplasts via the adenylate kinase equilibrium. Front Plant Sci. 2015;6:10. https://www.ncbi.nlm.nih.gov/pmc/articles/ PMC4309032/

343. Pilchova I, Klacanova K, Tatarkova Z, Kaplan P, Racay P. The Involvement of Mg^{2+} in regulation of cellular and mitochondrial functions. Oxid Med Cell Longev. 2017;2017:6797460. https://www.ncbi.nlm.nih.gov/pmc/articles/ PMC5516748/

344. Clerc P, Young CA, Bordt EA, Grigore AM, Fiskum G, Polster BM. Magnesium sulfate protects against the bioenergetic consequences of chronic glutamate receptor stimulation. PLoS One. 2013;8:e79982. https://www.ncbi.nlm.nih .gov/pmc/articles/PMC3827425/

345. Lambuk L, Jafri AJA, Arfuzir NNN, Iezhitsa I, Agarwal R, Rozali KNB, et al. Neuroprotective effect of magnesium acetyltaurate against NMDA-induced excitotoxicity in rat retina. Neurotox Res. 2017;31:31–45. https:// onlinelibrary.wiley.com/doi/10.1111/ejn.14662

346. Yasui M, Kihira T, Ota K. Calcium, magnesium and aluminum concentrations in Parkinson's disease. Neurotoxicology. 1992;13:593–600. https://pubmed .ncbi.nlm.nih.gov/1475063/

347. Uitti RJ, Rajput AH, Rozdilsky B, Bickis M, Wollin T, Yuen WK. Regional metal concentrations in Parkinson's disease, other chronic neurological diseases, and control brains. Can J Neurol Sci. 1989;16:310–14. https:// pubmed.ncbi.nlm.nih.gov/2766123/

348. Veronese N, Zurlo A, Solmi M, Luchini C, Trevisan C, Bano G, et al. Magnesium status in Alzheimer's disease: a systematic review. Am J Alzheimers Dis Other Demen. 2016;31:208–13. https://pubmed.ncbi.nlm .nih.gov/26351088/

349. Andrási E, Igaz S, Molnár Z, Makó S. Disturbances of magnesium concentrations in various brain areas in Alzheimer's disease. Magnes Res. 2000;13:189–96. https://pubmed.ncbi.nlm.nih.gov/11008926/

350. Glick JL. Dementias: the role of magnesium deficiency and an hypothesis concerning the pathogenesis of Alzheimer's disease. Med Hypotheses. 1990;31:211–25. https://pubmed.ncbi.nlm.nih.gov/2092675/

351. Li W, Yu J, Liu Y, Huang X, Abumaria N, Zhu Y, et al. Elevation of brain magnesium prevents synaptic loss and reverses cognitive deficits in Alzheimer's disease mouse model. Mol Brain. 2014;7:65. https://pubmed .ncbi.nlm.nih.gov/25213836/

352. Slutsky I, Abumaria N, Wu L-J, Huang C, Zhang L, Li B, et al. Enhancement of learning and memory by elevating brain magnesium. Neuron. 2010;65:165–77. https://pubmed.ncbi.nlm.nih.gov/20152124/

353. Uysal N, Kizildag S, Yuce Z, Guvendi G, Kandis S, Koc B, et al. Timeline (bioavailability) of magnesium compounds in hours: which magnesium compound works best? Biol Trace Elem Res. 2019;187:128–36. https:// pubmed.ncbi.nlm.nih.gov/29679349/

354. Ates M, Kizildag S, Yuksel O, Hosgorler F, Yuce Z, Guvendi G, et al. Dose-dependent absorption profile of different magnesium compounds. Biol Trace Elem Res. 2019;192:244–51. https://pubmed.ncbi.nlm.nih.gov/30761462/

355. Panossian A, Wikman G, Sarris J. Rosenroot (*Rhodiola rosea*): traditional use, chemical composition, pharmacology and clinical efficacy. Phytomedicine. 2010;17:481–93. https://pubmed.ncbi.nlm.nih.gov/20378318/

356. Panossian A, Hamm R, Wikman G, Efferth T. Mechanism of action of *Rhodiola*, salidroside, tyrosol and triandrin in isolated neuroglial cells: an interactive pathway analysis of the downstream effects using RNA microarray data. Phytomedicine. 2014;21:1325–48. https://pubmed.ncbi .nlm.nih.gov/25172797/

357. Edwards D, Heufelder A, Zimmermann A. Therapeutic effects and safety of *Rhodiola rosea* extract WS® 1375 in subjects with life-stress symptoms— results of an open-label study. Phytother Res. 2012;26:1220–25. https:// pubmed.ncbi.nlm.nih.gov/22228617/

358. Lekomtseva Y, Zhukova I, Wacker A. *Rhodiola rosea* in subjects with prolonged or chronic fatigue symptoms: results of an open-label clinical trial. Complement Med Res. 2017;24:46–52. https://pubmed.ncbi.nlm.nih .gov/28219059/

359. Kasper S, Dienel A. Multicenter, open-label, exploratory clinical trial with *Rhodiola rosea* extract in patients suffering from burnout symptoms. Neuropsychiatr Dis Treat. 2017;13:889–98. https://pubmed.ncbi.nlm.nih .gov/28367055/

360. Spasov AA, Wikman GK, Mandrikov VB, Mironova IA, Neumoin VV. A double-blind, placebo-controlled pilot study of the stimulating and adaptogenic effect of *Rhodiola rosea* SHR-5 extract on the fatigue of students caused by stress during an examination period with a repeated low-dose regimen. Phytomedicine. 2000;7:85–89. https://pubmed.ncbi.nlm.nih.gov/10839209/

361. Shevtsov VA, Zholus BI, Shervarly VI, Vol'skij VB, Korovin YP, Khristich MP, et al. A randomized trial of two different doses of a SHR-5 *Rhodiola rosea* extract versus placebo and control of capacity for mental work. Phytomedicine. 2003;10:95–105. https://pubmed.ncbi.nlm.nih.gov/12725561/

362. Olsson EM, von Schéele B, Panossian AG. A randomised, double-blind, placebo-controlled, parallel-group study of the standardised extract shr-5 of the roots of *Rhodiola rosea* in the treatment of subjects with stress-related fatigue. Planta Med. 2009;75:105–12. https://pubmed.ncbi.nlm.nih.gov/19016404/

363. Serbinova E, Kagan V, Han D, Packer L. Free radical recycling and intramembrane mobility in the antioxidant properties of alpha-tocopherol and alpha-tocotrienol. Free Radic Biol Med. 1991;10:263–75. https://pubmed.ncbi.nlm.nih.gov/1649783/

364. Serbinova EA, Packer L. Antioxidant properties of alpha-tocopherol and alpha-tocotrienol. Methods Enzymol. 1994;234:354–66. https://pubmed.ncbi.nlm.nih.gov/7808307/

365. Suzuki YJ, Tsuchiya M, Wassall SR, Choo YM, Govil G, Kagan VE, et al. Structural and dynamic membrane properties of alpha-tocopherol and alpha-tocotrienol: implication to the molecular mechanism of their antioxidant potency. Biochemistry. 1993;32:10692–99. https://pubmed.ncbi.nlm.nih.gov/8399214/

366. Chan AC. Partners in defense, vitamin E and vitamin C. Can J Physiol Pharmacol. 1993;71:725–31. https://pubmed.ncbi.nlm.nih.gov/8313238/

367. Patel V, Rink C, Gordillo GM, Khanna S, Gnyawali U, Roy S, et al. Oral tocotrienols are transported to human tissues and delay the progression of the model for end-stage liver disease score in patients. J Nutr. 2012;142:513–19. https://pubmed.ncbi.nlm.nih.gov/22298568/

368. Sen CK, Khanna S, Roy S. Tocotrienol: the natural vitamin E to defend the nervous system? Ann N Y Acad Sci. 2004;1031:127–42. https://pubmed.ncbi.nlm.nih.gov/15753140/

369. Chin K-Y, Tay SS. A review on the relationship between Tocotrienol and Alzheimer disease. Nutrients. 2018;10:881. http://dx.doi.org/10.3390/nu10070881

370. Gopalan Y, Shuaib IL, Magosso E, Ansari MA, Abu Bakar MR, Wong JW, et al. Clinical investigation of the protective effects of palm vitamin E tocotrienols on brain white matter. Stroke. 2014;45:1422–28. https://pubmed.ncbi.nlm.nih.gov/24699052/

371. Modi KP, Patel NM, Goyal RK. Estimation of L-dopa from *Mucuna pruriens* LINN and formulations containing M. pruriens by HPTLC method. Chem Pharm Bull. 2008;56:357–59. https://pubmed.ncbi.nlm.nih.gov/18310948/

372. Hardebo JE, Owman C. Barrier mechanisms for neurotransmitter monoamines and their precursors at the blood-brain interface. Ann Neurol. 1980;8:1–31. https://pubmed.ncbi.nlm.nih.gov/6105837/

373. Daubner SC, Le T, Wang S. Tyrosine hydroxylase and regulation of dopamine synthesis. Arch Biochem Biophys. 2011;508:1–12. https://www.ncbi.nlm.nih.gov/pmc/articles/PMC3065393/

374. Lieu CA, Kunselman AR, Manyam BV, Venkiteswaran K, Subramanian T. A water extract of *Mucuna pruriens* provides long-term amelioration of parkinsonism with reduced risk for dyskinesias. Parkinsonism Relat Disord. 2010;16:458–65. https://pubmed.ncbi.nlm.nih.gov/20570206/

375. Katzenschlager R, Evans A, Manson A, Patsalos PN, Ratnaraj N, Watt H, et al. *Mucuna pruriens* in Parkinson's disease: a double blind clinical and pharmacological study. J Neurol Neurosurg Psychiatry. 2004;75:1672–77. https://pubmed.ncbi.nlm.nih.gov/15548480/

376. Cilia R, Laguna J, Cassani E, Cereda E, Pozzi NG, Isaias IU, et al. *Mucuna pruriens* in Parkinson disease: a double-blind, randomized, controlled, crossover study. Neurology. 2017;89:432–38. https://pubmed.ncbi.nlm.nih.gov/28679598/

377. Cilia R, Laguna J, Cassani E, Cereda E, Raspini B, Barichella M, et al. Daily intake of *Mucuna pruriens* in advanced Parkinson's disease: a 16-week, noninferiority, randomized, crossover, pilot study. Parkinsonism Relat Disord. 2018;49:60–66. https://pubmed.ncbi.nlm.nih.gov/29352722/

378. Fernstrom JD, Fernstrom MH. Tyrosine, phenylalanine, and catecholamine synthesis and function in the brain. J Nutr. 2007;137:1539S–1547S; discussion 1548S. https://pubmed.ncbi.nlm.nih.gov/17513421/

379. Goldstein DS. Catecholamines 101. Clin Auton Res. 2010;20:331–52. https://www.ncbi.nlm.nih.gov/pmc/articles/PMC3046107/

380. Lehnert H, Reinstein DK, Strowbridge BW, Wurtman RJ. Neurochemical and behavioral consequences of acute, uncontrollable stress: effects of dietary tyrosine. Brain Res. 1984;303:215–23. https://www.sciencedirect.com/science/article/abs/pii/0006899384912071

381. Hase A, Jung SE, aan het Rot M. Behavioral and cognitive effects of tyrosine intake in healthy human adults. Pharmacol Biochem Behav. 2015;133:1–6. https://pubmed.ncbi.nlm.nih.gov/25797188/

382. Jongkees BJ, Hommel B, Kühn S, Colzato LS. Effect of tyrosine supplementation on clinical and healthy populations under stress or cognitive demands—a review. J Psychiatr Res. 2015;70:50–57. https://pubmed.ncbi.nlm.nih.gov/26424423/

383. Abbiati G, Fossati T, Lachmann G, Bergamaschi M, Castiglioni C. Absorption, tissue distribution and excretion of radiolabelled compounds in rats after administration of [14C]-L-alpha-glycerylphosphorylcholine. Eur J Drug Metab Pharmacokinet. 1993;18:173–80. https://link.springer.com/article/10.1007/BF03188793

384. Parnetti L, Mignini F, Tomassoni D, Traini E, Amenta F. Cholinergic precursors in the treatment of cognitive impairment of vascular origin: ineffective approaches or need for re-evaluation? J Neurol Sci. 2007;257:264–69. https://pubmed.ncbi.nlm.nih.gov/17331541/

385. Ibid.

386. Ziegenfuss T, Landis J, Hofheins J. Acute supplementation with alpha-glycerylphosphorylcholine augments growth hormone response to, and peak force production during, resistance exercise. J Int Soc Sports Nutr. 2008;5 (suppl 1):P15. https://jissn.biomedcentral.com/articles/10.1186/1550-2783-5-S1-P15

387. Bellar D, LeBlanc NR, Campbell B. The effect of 6 days of alpha glycerylphosphorylcholine on isometric strength. J Int Soc Sports Nutr. 2015;12:42. https://pubmed.ncbi.nlm.nih.gov/26582972/

388. Marcus L, Soileau J, Judge LW, Bellar D. Evaluation of the effects of two doses of alpha glycerylphosphorylcholine on physical and psychomotor performance. J Int Soc Sports Nutr. 2017;14:39. https://jissn.biomedcentral.com/articles/10.1186/s12970-017-0196-5

389. Cruse JL. The acute effects of alpha-GPC on hand grip strength, jump height, power output, mood, and reaction-time in recreationally trained, college-aged individuals [Master of Science]. Eastern Kentucky University; 2018. https://encompass.eku.edu//etd/518

390. Parker AG, Byars A, Purpura M, Jäger R. The effects of alpha-glycerylphosphorylcholine, caffeine or placebo on markers of mood, cognitive function, power, speed, and agility. J Int Soc Sports Nutr. BioMed Central; 2015;12 (Suppl 1):P41. https://www.ncbi.nlm.nih.gov/pmc/articles/PMC4595381/

391. Fioravanti M, Yanagi M. Cytidinediphosphocholine (CDP-choline) for cognitive and behavioural disturbances associated with chronic cerebral disorders in the elderly. Cochrane Database Syst Rev. 2005;CD000269. https://pubmed.ncbi.nlm.nih.gov/15846601/

392. Castagna A, Cotroneo AM, Ruotolo G, Gareri P. The CITIRIVAD Study: CITIcoline plus RIVAstigmine in elderly patients affected with dementia study. Clin Drug Investig. 2016;36:1059–65. https://pubmed.ncbi.nlm.nih.gov/27587069/

393. Gareri P, Castagna A, Cotroneo AM, Putignano D, Conforti R, Santamaria F, et al. The Citicholinage Study: citicoline plus cholinesterase inhibitors in aged patients affected with Alzheimer's disease study. J Alzheimers Dis. 2017;56:557–65. https://pubmed.ncbi.nlm.nih.gov/28035929/

394. Cotroneo AM, Castagna A, Putignano S, Lacava R, Fantò F, Monteleone F, et al. Effectiveness and safety of citicoline in mild vascular cognitive impairment: the IDEALE study. Clin Interv Aging. 2013;8:131–37. https://pubmed.ncbi.nlm.nih.gov/23403474/

395. McGlade E, Agoston AM, DiMuzio J, Kizaki M, Nakazaki E, Kamiya T, et al. The effect of citicoline supplementation on motor speed and attention in adolescent males. J Atten Disord. 2019;23:121–34. https://pubmed.ncbi.nlm.nih.gov/26179181/

396. McGlade E, Locatelli A, Hardy J, Kamiya T, Morita M, Morishita K, et al. Improved attentional performance following citicoline administration in healthy adult women. FNS. 2012;03:769–73. https://www.scirp.org/journal/paperinformation.aspx?paperid=19921

397. Patocka J. Huperzine A—an interesting anticholinesterase compound from the Chinese herbal medicine. Acta Medica. 1998;41:155–57. https://pubmed.ncbi.nlm.nih.gov/9951045/

398. Dos Santos TC, Gomes TM, Pinto BAS, Camara AL, Paes AM de A. Naturally occurring acetylcholinesterase inhibitors and their potential use for Alzheimer's disease therapy. Front Pharmacol. 2018;9:1192. https://pubmed.ncbi.nlm.nih.gov/30405413/

399. Yang G, Wang Y, Tian J, Liu J-P. Huperzine A for Alzheimer's disease: a systematic review and meta-analysis of randomized clinical trials. PLoS One. 2013;8:e74916. https://pubmed.ncbi.nlm.nih.gov/24086396/

400. Xing S-H, Zhu C-X, Zhang R, An L. Huperzine A in the treatment of Alzheimer's disease and vascular dementia: a meta-analysis. Evid Based Complement Alternat Med. 2014;2014:363985. https://www.hindawi.com/journals/ecam/2014/363985/

401. Zheng W, Xiang Y-Q, Ungvari GS, Chiu FKH, H Ng C, Wang Y, et al. Huperzine A for treatment of cognitive impairment in major depressive disorder: a systematic review of randomized controlled trials. Shanghai Arch Psychiatry. 2016;28:64–71. https://minerva-access.unimelb.edu.au/handle/11343/256395

402. Hepsomali P, Groeger JA, Nishihira J, Scholey A. Effects of oral gamma-aminobutyric acid (GABA) administration on stress and sleep in humans: a systematic review. Front Neurosci. 2020;14:923. https://www.ncbi.nlm.nih.gov/pmc/articles/PMC7527439/

403. Birdsall TC. 5-Hydroxytryptophan: a clinically-effective serotonin precursor. Altern Med Rev. 1998;3:271–80. https://pubmed.ncbi.nlm.nih.gov/9727088/

404. Shaw K, Turner J, Del Mar C. Tryptophan and 5-hydroxytryptophan for depression. Cochrane Database Syst Rev. 2002;CD003198. https://pubmed.ncbi.nlm.nih.gov/11869656/

405. Javelle F, Lampit A, Bloch W, Häussermann P, Johnson SL, Zimmer P. Effects of 5-hydroxytryptophan on distinct types of depression: a systematic review and meta-analysis. Nutr Rev. 2020;78:77–88. https://pubmed.ncbi.nlm.nih.gov/31504850/

406. Jacobsen JPR, Krystal AD, Krishnan KRR, Caron MG. Adjunctive 5-hydroxytryptophan slow-release for treatment-resistant depression: clinical and preclinical rationale. Trends Pharmacol Sci. 2016;37:933–44. https://pubmed.ncbi.nlm.nih.gov/27692695/

407. Lopresti AL, Drummond PD. Saffron (*Crocus sativus*) for depression: a systematic review of clinical studies and examination of underlying antidepressant mechanisms of action. Hum Psychopharmacol. 2014;29:517–27. https://pubmed.ncbi.nlm.nih.gov/25384672/

408. Bukhari SI, Manzoor M, Dhar MK. A comprehensive review of the pharmacological potential of *Crocus sativus* and its bioactive apocarotenoids. Biomed Pharmacother. 2018;98:733–45. https://pubmed.ncbi.nlm.nih.gov/29306211/

409. Khaksarian M, Behzadifar M, Behzadifar M, Alipour M, Jahanpanah F, Re TS, et al. The efficacy of *Crocus sativus* (Saffron) versus placebo and Fluoxetine in treating depression: a systematic review and meta-analysis. Psychol Res Behav Manag. 2019;12:297–305. https://pubmed.ncbi.nlm.nih.gov/31118846/

410. Tóth B, Hegyi P, Lantos T, Szakács Z, Kerémi B, Varga G, et al. The efficacy of saffron in the treatment of mild to moderate depression: a meta-analysis. Planta Med. 2019;85:24–31. https://pubmed.ncbi.nlm.nih.gov/30036891/

411. Yang X, Chen X, Fu Y, Luo Q, Du L, Qiu H, et al. Comparative efficacy and safety of *Crocus sativus* L. for treating mild to moderate major depressive disorder in adults: a meta-analysis of randomized controlled trials. Neuropsychiatr Dis Treat. 2018;14:1297–305. https://pubmed.ncbi.nlm.nih.gov/29849461/

412. Hausenblas HA, Saha D, Dubyak PJ, Anton SD. Saffron (*Crocus sativus* L.) and major depressive disorder: a meta-analysis of randomized clinical trials. J Integr Med. 2013;11:377–83. https://pubmed.ncbi.nlm.nih.gov/24299602/

413. Khaksarian M, The efficacy of *Crocus sativus* (Saffron) versus placebo and Fluoxetine.

Conclusion

1.   Ito TA, Larsen JT, Smith NK, Cacioppo JT. Negative information weighs more heavily on the brain: the negativity bias in evaluative categorizations. J Pers Soc Psychol. 1998;75:887–900. https://pubmed.ncbi.nlm.nih.gov/9825526/

2.   Smith NK, Cacioppo JT, Larsen JT, Chartrand TL. May I have your attention, please: electrocortical responses to positive and negative stimuli. Neuropsychologia. 2003;41:171–83. https://psycnet.apa.org/record/2003-04041-010

INDEX

ACKNOWLEDGMENTS

This book was only possible because I had a phenomenal team behind me. Many thanks to our team at *The Energy Blueprint*, whose expertise, passion, and deep commitment to helping people reclaim their lives from fatigue inspires me to keep doing this work. Thanks to Amanda Ibey, whose writing prowess and ability to quickly understand complex topics and explain them in ways anyone can access is unparalleled. I'm deeply grateful for the brilliance in the way Amanda seamlessly blended our scientific concepts with our client stories. Thanks to Alex Leaf, for being a lifelong science geek like me, for having such a brilliant scientific mind, for the thoroughness in digging into every body of research to ensure complete accuracy and integrity of each section, and for having spent so many years building a world-class level of knowledge on nutrition science, which allowed me to have a true partner in writing this book. To Lucinda Halpern, our phenomenal agent who helped us to connect with the world-class team at Hay House. We are grateful that she has been our shepherd through the publishing process and world. To the entire Hay House publishing team, especially our brilliant editor, Lisa Cheng, whose suggestions elevated our thinking and shaped this book. Finally, many thanks to my wife, Marcela, for her relentless love and support, and for always being up for a new adventure. And to my kids, Mateo and Kaia, who bring me greater happiness than I ever thought possible, and whose smiles and laughter continually inspire me to create an incredible life for our little tribe.

ABOUT THE AUTHORS

Ari Whitten is the founder of *The Energy Blueprint* system, a comprehensive lifestyle and supplement program which has helped more than two million people (and counting) experience optimal health, better performance, and more energy. He is also the best-selling author of *The Ultimate Guide to Red Light Therapy* and the host of the popular *The Energy Blueprint Podcast*, which features the world's leading natural health experts. In 2020, Ari was voted #1 Health Influencer by Mindshare, the largest natural and functional medicine community. For more than 25 years, Ari has been dedicated to the study of human health science. He holds a M.S. in Human Nutrition and Functional Medicine, a B.S. in Kinesiology, and certifications as a Corrective Exercise Specialist and Performance Enhancement Specialist from the National Academy of Sports Medicine, and he has completed the coursework for a Ph.D. in Clinical Psychology. You can find his podcast, programs, and supplement formulas at www.theenergyblueprint.com.

Alex Leaf, M.S., holds a master's degree in Nutrition from Bastyr University and has been writing about the science of nutrition, health, and fitness for over a decade. Currently, Alex is a content creator and research writer alongside Ari Whitten at *The Energy Blueprint*. You can visit him online at alexleaf.com.

OUR PRODUCTS AND PROGRAMS

SUPPLEMENTS

At *The Energy Blueprint*, we strive to make leading-edge, best-in-category formulas designed to provide results that you can actually feel. Whereas most companies put in 1/5th to 1/20th the actual clinical dosage of the various ingredients in their formulas, we put in real clinical dosages for all our ingredients (making our costs to manufacture these formulas 5 to 10 times higher than most manufacturers). We do this because our goal is to provide the absolute best product on the market in each category and, most importantly, to get you noticeable and hopefully life-changing results.

Here's the quick rundown of what we offer.

Energenesis

This is our flagship mitochondrial formula. Instead of stimulant- and caffeine-based products, which give you a quick boost but actually worsen your energy when used regularly, this formula is designed to build up your own body's capacity to produce energy by supporting your mitochondria with cutting-edge ingredients with proven fatigue-fighting and energy-boosting effects like NTFactor®, PQQ, acetyl-L-carnitine, R-alpha lipoic acid, and shoden Ashwagandha. It's also our best-selling product that has changed thousands of lives.

Energy Essentials & Superfoods

More than 9 out of 10 people in the U.S. have at least one nutrient deficiency, and more than 7 out of 10 people have at least three nutrient deficiencies! This is a major cause of fatigue for many people. These nutrients—various vitamins and minerals—play key roles in your hormone balance, brain function, risk of dozens of diseases, and the ability of your cells to produce energy! With full doses of whole-food sources vitamins, the most bioavailable methylated B vitamins, disease-fighting tocotrienols, and real clinical doses of powerful superfoods like spirulina, chlorella, pomegranate, and fulvic/humic acid to enhance bioavailability and absorption, Energy Essentials & Superfoods is the most powerful and comprehensive multivitamin/multimineral and superfoods supplement on the market—designed to plug the holes in your diet and provide your body with the nutrients and cofactors it needs for optimal health, disease prevention, and energy production.

Immune Genesis

Immune Genesis is our comprehensive immune support formula that we designed explicitly for increasing your resistance to viral respiratory infections. It has science-backed compounds like BerryShield, Seleno-Excell, reishi mushroom, vitamin D, zinc, astragalus, andrographis, and Wellmune—ingredients that are proven in clinical trials to reduce the incidence, severity, and duration of respiratory infections.

UltraBrain

UltraBrain is a premium, next-generation brain health–optimizing, anxiety- and depression-fighting nootropic that's designed to combat brain fog, boost your mood, and get your brain functioning at its peak potential. All while supporting long-term brain health! (Again, completely free of stimulants and sugar.) Packed with the most powerful, evidence-based brain-boosting compounds available like *Rhodiola rosea*, lion's mane mushroom (dual extract), cognatiQ, L-theanine, choline CDP, alpha-GPC, huperzine A, saffron extract, and more—all in real clinically effective dosages—this formula is for anyone looking to step into their brain's full potential.

PROGRAMS

The Energy Blueprint

This is our flagship course that's the culmination of over seven years of work. This program covers all the different factors that play into our energy levels and the practical lifestyle habits to optimize everything from circadian rhythm and sleep, to gut health, to detoxification, to light therapies, to hormesis. It's an ultra-comprehensive 60-day program that takes you deep into the science of virtually every aspect of human energy optimization.

Breathing for Energy

We partnered with world-leading breathing expert Patrick McKeown to create a cutting-edge program specifically for the purpose of enhancing energy levels. This program centers around using breathing practice to retrain optimal autonomic nervous system function (to de-stress the brain and body) and particularly the hormetic practice of breath holding (intermittent hypoxic training) to systematically upregulate one of the biggest needle movers for energy optimization—the pulmonary and cardiovascular systems. We've created a systematized program to take people from 10- to 15-second breath hold capacities up to multi-minute breath holds. This creates profound adaptations in lung capacity and mitochondrial adaptations that result in massive improvements in oxygen utilization and ultimately, cellular energy production. If you're looking for one specific practice you can do each day to dramatically improve your energy levels, this breathwork training system is the single most powerful and fastest way I've ever found to increase energy levels in my over 25 years of studying and teaching health science.

To access two bonus chapters on optimizing detoxification pathways and energy flux, and for more energy-enhancing strategies, visit theenergyblueprint.com/efebook.

Hay House Titles of Related Interest

YOU CAN HEAL YOUR LIFE, the movie,
starring Louise Hay & Friends
(available as an online streaming video)
www.hayhouse.com/louise-movie

THE SHIFT, the movie,
starring Dr. Wayne W. Dyer
(available as an online streaming video)
www.hayhouse.com/the-shift-movie

***

ALCHEMY OF HERBS: Transform Everyday Ingredients into Foods and Remedies That Heal, by Rosalee de la Forêt

BEAT CANCER KITCHEN: Deliciously Simple Plant-Based Anticancer Recipes, by Chris & Micah Wark

OUTSIDE THE BOX CANCER THERAPIES: Alternative Therapies That Treat and Prevent Cancer, by Dr. Mark Stengler & Dr. Paul Anderson

All of the above are available at www.hayhouse.co.uk.

***

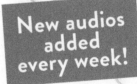

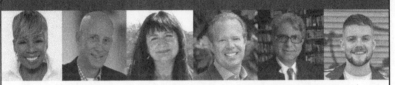

CONNECT WITH
HAY HOUSE
ONLINE

🌐 hayhouse.co.uk   **f** @hayhouse

📷 @hayhouseuk   🐦 @hayhouseuk

▶️ @hayhouseuk   🎵 @hayhouseuk

*Find out all about our latest books & card decks • Be the first
to know about exclusive discounts • Interact with our authors
in live broadcasts • Celebrate the cycle of the seasons with us
• Watch free videos from your favourite authors •
Connect with like-minded souls*

'*The gateways to wisdom and knowledge
are always open.*'

Louise Hay